*Vivian Kaufman*

P9-EEA-663

# HOMEOPATHIC PSYCHOLOGY

# HOMEOPATHIC PSYCHOLOGY

*Personality Profiles of the
Major Constitutional Remedies*

## Philip M. Bailey, M.D.

M.B.,B.S.  MFHom.

North Atlantic Books
Berkeley, California

Homeopathic Educational Services
Berkeley, California

**Homeopathic Psychology**

Copyright © 1995 Philip M. Bailey. All Rights Reserved.
 No portion of this book, except for brief review, may be reproduced, stored in a retrieval system, or transmitted, in any form or by any means, electronic, mechanical, photocopying, recording or otherwise without the written permission of the publisher. For information contact North Atlantic Books.

Published by

North Atlantic Books
P.O. Box 12327
Berkeley, California 94712

Homeopathic Educational Services
2124 Kittredge Street
Berkeley, California 94704

Cover and book design by Legacy Media, Inc.
Cover drawings by Angie Lyndon and Patricia House
"Biting the Hand that Feeds Them," first published in *Fremantle Stories,* Cliff Street Publishing, 1994.
Printed in the United States of America

*Homeopathic Psychology* is sponsored by the Society for the Study of Native Arts and Sciences, a nonprofit educational organization whose goals are to develop an ecological and crosscultural perspective linking various scientific, social, and artistic fields; to nurture a holistic view of arts, sciences humanities, and healing; and to publish and distribute literature on the relationship of mind, body, and nature.

**Library of Congress Cataloging-in-Publication Data**
Bailey, Philip M.
    Homeopathic psychology : personality profiles of the major constitutional remedies / Philip M. Bailey
        p.   cm.
    Includes bibliographical references and index.
    ISBN 1-55643-099-X
    1. Mental illness—Homeopathic treatment.   I. Title.
    [DNLM:   1. Personality Disorders—drug therapy.   2. Homeopathy—methods.   WM 190 B155h 1995]
RX301,M45B35   1995
615.5'32—dc20
DNLM/DLC
for Library of Congress                                                    95-9242
                                                                              CIP

                    7   8   9   10   11   12   /   09   08   07   06   05

To Sharon Leanne Bailey

# Acknowledgments

I am endebted to L.D. for his generosity in supporting the project with such faith, to my wife Sharon for endless hours of help typing and editing, and to Professor Bob White for his thorough and willing proof-reading. I also wish to thank Angie and Patricia for their cover drawings.

# Contents

Vivian Kaufman
415 - 215 - 8480

# Contents

# *Introduction*

It is my hope that this book will help satisfy a need that, to a large extent, has remained inadequately served to this date; the need of homeopaths for an accurate and realistic description of the personalities of the constitutional remedies. The old materia medicas that we rely upon so heavily describe only the crudest and most extreme elements of the mental picture of each remedy, missing the subtleties that we actually find in the minds of our patients. I hope that this book will help to bridge that gap, and hence enable both the student and practising homeopath to relate more easily to real personalities, rather than caricatures.

In my experience, the mentals are still the least understood, and the most underdeveloped aspect of homeopathic prescribing. Yet the personality of the patient is at least as important as the physical characteristics in individualising the case and finding the similimum. So often remedies are prescribed on the basis of a few physical symptoms, along with gross simplifications of the patient's personality, and fail to act. This gives the unfortunate impression that homeopathy is a vague and unreliable practice. It also gives rise to the relatively common attitude amongst homeopaths that the patient belongs to several constitutional types simultaneously, any of which will help at any given time. This is nothing more than an excuse for inaccuracy, and it results in the homeopath failing to persist with case taking and analysis to the point where the mentals are truly understood.

It is true that some patients have more than one layer of pathology, and that each layer corresponds to a different remedy, but the layers must be dealt with in the right sequence if progress is to be made, and the personality of the patient at any given time will correspond primarily to the most superficial layer, which represents the present frequency of the patient's vital force.

By familiarising himself or herself thoroughly with the personalities of the major constitutional remedies, the homeopath can avoid endless hours of confusion and uncertainty in case taking, and can rapidly become an effective prescriber.

The profiles that are contained in this book are the result entirely of my own clinical experience. They are not derived from previous materia medicas, and they sometimes differ considerably from the classical profiles that have been handed down through the years. I believe that this is due to the tendency for the original remedy pictures to be copied over the years from teacher to teacher, and from materia medica to materia medica, with the result that the most obvious characteristics remain, and tend to be magnified, whilst the more subtle tendencies are left out, since they are not regarded as reliable. Furthermore, the subtle understanding of personality is a relatively recent phenomenon, growing out of Freud's discoveries of the unconscious, and the subsequent developments of depth psychology. This is another reason for the crudeness that we find in the mental profiles of the old materia medicas. Thus Natrum Muriaticum is generally portrayed as an introvert, yet I have come across many highly extrovert cases of this type. Similarly, Thuja tends to be portrayed as a nasty character who is bordering on the psychotic, whereas the truth is far more normal and varied. (I have never come across a Thuja patient who felt that his legs were made of glass!)

In portraying the mentals, I have tried to get across the 'essence' of each type, which is often perceivable in the absence of more localised specifics, and indeed may even seem to contradict them. Thus the essence of Lycopodium is a lack of self-confidence, and this must be recognised by the homeopath through the confident exterior that many Lycopodiums adopt. An understanding of the essence of the mentals is just as important as an understanding of the specific symptoms of a remedy. Sometimes the former is more apparent, sometimes the latter.

Wherever possible I have indicated the approximate ratio of males to females within each constitutional type. I have done this because in many cases there is a clear preponderance of one gender, sometimes amounting to almost one hundred percent. The homeopath should be very careful, for example, before assuming that he has found a Sepia man or a Sulphur woman. The former does exist, but the homeopath should be aware of its rarity. Furthermore, I have tried to portray the ways in which a single constitutional type may be expressed differently in men and women. For instance, male Lycopodiums often hide their lack of confidence with bravado, whereas female Lycopodiums tend to express their anxiety quite undisguised.

Many readers will be struck by the emphasis on negative characteristics in my descriptions of each type. I have done my best to list the positive traits of each remedy, but it is true that it is easier to spot most constitutional types on the basis of their weaknesses and excesses, than on their merits. As people become more aware, and overcome their personality 'flaws', they tend to develop the same positive characteristics, (such as openness, flexibility and confidence), regardless of their constitutional type. The negative characteristics that remain tend to be the best guide to the remedy, (along with the generals and physicals). As for those portraits in the book that seem relatively positive when compared to the rest, I can only describe what I have seen, and in some types I have indeed seen more positive traits than in others. It may be that the less developed members of these types do not frequent homeo-pathic surgeries!

At the end of each profile I give a short description of the characteristic appearances of the type. I have included these because physical appearance is so closely connected to personality, and also because I feel it is an aspect of prescribing that has been inadequately covered previously. These descriptions are meant only as a guide. They are not exhaustive, and there are many cases of patients who do not have the typical physical appearance of their type.

I do not pretend that this book covers all the possible constitutional remedies, but it covers those that are most commonly seen, and will provide an understanding of the mentals of the vast majority of patients that seek help for chronic complaints. (I have seen Psorinum constitutionally, but the mentals were so indistinct to me that they merged with the personality of the underlying layer, hence it is not included.)

## *A note about Constitution, Layers and Acute Mentals.*

The term 'constitutional' is used in more than one way by homeopaths. There are three main uses for the term, as follows:

1. 'Constitutional prescribing' refers to selecting the one remedy which covers the totality of the patient's symptoms, (both mental and physical) at a given time. It contrasts with 'local prescribing', based on only a few localised symptoms, ignoring other 'unrelated' features of the case. Thus an acute remedy may be prescribed in a constitutional manner for an acute illness, and a polychrest may be prescribed unconstitutionally for the local symptoms of either acute or chronic disease.

2. A 'constitutional remedy' is one which covers the totality of a patient's mental and physical characteristics over a long period of time, excluding temporary changes during acute illnesses. This is the context in which I use the term 'constitutional' in this book.

3. Some homeopaths use the term 'constitutional remedy' to refer to the deepest layers of a person's constitution, which may be partially obscured by more superficial layers. This is an unfortunate and misleading use of the term, since one cannot know for sure what remedy types, if any, lie beneath the surface layer, until that layer has been adequately treated. Furthermore, the most superficial layer is the most apparent one.

## *Layers*

The human organism appears to retain a memory of all preceding chronic states of the body and mind. This memory includes certain inherited traits. Each stable state of body and mind can be considered a layer of the person's constitution. When it has been superseded by a different stable state, it remains as a cellular memory, which can be reactivated in the future. This takes place when the more recent layers have been 'peeled off' by correct homeopathic prescribing.

In my experience the majority of people remain in the same constitutional state for the whole of their lives. In other words, their vital force will resonate to the same remedy from birth till death, excluding periods of acute illness. Traumatic experiences, both physical and psychic, can shift a person's vital force to a different frequency, forming a new layer, but more often they cause a deterioration of functioning within the same layer. Thus a relatively healthy, symptom-free Natrum Muriaticum person will develop chronic sinusitis and claustrophobia following a long divorce settlement, which remain until homeopathic help or other deep healing methods are used. These new symptoms are still within the scope of Natrum Muriaticum, and the remedy will simply return the patient's vital force to a healthier 'octave' of the Natrum Muriaticum wavelength. Without treatment the new symptoms may remain until further trauma causes another deterioration in health, this time to (say) chronic bronchitis and recurrent depression, still within the Natrum Muriaticum layer.

Given the stability of the chronic layers, a patient's past medical and psychological history can provide useful information which can help to confirm the constitutional remedy.

Some people are born with several layers of pathology, which they inherited from their parents. They will usually continue to express the uppermost layer until the correct homeopathic remedy dissolves it, revealing the one underneath. However, some characteristics of the deeper layers can show through from time to time, both physically and psychologically. Thus a Natrum Muriaticum person with an underlying Phosphorus layer may exhibit some of the spontaneity, naivety and openness of Phosphorus but the most dominant characteristics will fit Natrum Muriaticum, especially those that constitute a problem for the patient.

In my experience, inherited layers of pathology frequently correspond to the miasmatic remedies—Psorinum, Syphilinum, Medorrhinum and Tuberculinum. When these layers have been removed one often finds 'non-miasmatic' remedy layers underneath. However, it often happens that a person is born with only one constitutional layer, whether it be miasmatic or not, and treatment will simply rebalance the vital force within the same layer. Thus a person may benefit from occasional doses of the same constitutional remedy throughout his or her life.

Additional layers of pathology may be acquired after birth by exposure to traumatic influences, be it psychological trauma, direct physical injury, or infective disease. For example, a person may develop a Medorrhinum state after acquiring gonorrhoea, or a Natrum Sulphuricum state after a head injury. A relatively common example is the acquisition of a Natrum Muriaticum state after a shock. It must be remembered, however, that the majority of patients who present in a Natrum Muriaticum state after a bereavement or shock were already Natrum before the event. Similarly, many patients who present with venereal disease in a Thuja state were already Thuja before acquiring the disease.

Apart from acute diseases which produce a temporary change in level, change from one layer to another is uncommon except as a result of homeopathic treatment. It does sometimes happen that a person spontaneously 'grows out' of one constitutional state and into another. This occurs particularly during childhood, when some Calcareas and Pulsatillas change into other types. Calcarea is especially common in infancy, which means that many Calcarea infants will change into different types as they get older. This is not a pathological change, and is not reversed by correct prescribing, unless the previous state involved pathology that was not cured, but was suppressed. Most toddlers go through a Pulsatilla stage between the ages of one or two and four. Again, the majority of these Pulsatilla children grow into a different adult type by the age of five. Very few remain constitutionally Pulsatilla after this age.

### *Potencies and Aggravations*

In my experience, the 10M potency is the most effective in bringing about lasting psychological improvement, and I give it in most cases of psychological pathology unless the body is too frail to take it, or there is a danger of serious physical aggravation. In these cases the potency can be raised stepwise over several months, strengthening the body to the point where it can take higher potencies safely. I have found that LM potencies are more likely to help the patient psychologically than low to middle centesimal potencies, hence I tend to use a daily dose of an LM potency when there is psychological pathology and the body is too sick to take a 1M or 10M potency. It is not necessary to begin with the first LM potency. Indeed this is often too weak to effect much change. As a rough guide, if it is safe to give a 30c potency, it is safe to start with LM3, and if it is safe to give a 200c potency, it is safe to start with LM6. Once the physical pathology has lessened to the point where a 1M or 10M can be given, these potencies will bring about further psychological improvement.

I have not found that 10M produces psychological aggravations that are dangerous, or that lasted longer than four weeks. However, considerable aggravations do occur when the potency has not been raised stepwise, and the patient should be warned of these, assured that they are part of the process of healing, and will be followed by great psychological improvement.

## *Hints on Taking the Mentals History and Analysing it*

Every homeopath has his or her own style when it comes to case taking, and no style is inherently right or wrong. However, the following hints may help the student homeopath to avoid common mistakes in taking and analysing the mentals history, mistakes which often lead to the wrong remedy being prescribed. I will also describe some techniques which I have found useful for eliciting information from the patient which is not immediately obvious or forthcoming; information which is sometimes vital in identifying the similimum.

Let us begin by examining what information can be gained from the first impression of the patient as they walk in and sit down. As always, first impressions can be misleading, but with experience the discerning homeopath can gather much useful information from the first few moments of the interview, which can then be analysed in the context of the subsequent history. Obviously the appearance of the patient can say a great deal. A thin delicate woman with black hair is not likely to need Calcarea Carbonica, (although the homeopath must be flexible enough to realise that exceptions always exist). The degree of caution or enthusiasm with which the patient greets you should be noted. The following remedy-types are likely to greet the homeopath with some degree of caution, fear or reserve; Arsenicum, Aurum, Baryta, China, the Kalis, the Natrums, Nux, Silica, and Thuja. Nux is not usually reserved, but is often suspicious of unorthodox practices such as homeopathy.

The types likely to greet the homeopath with enthusiasm, even on the first consultation, are: Argentum, Causticum, Ignatia, Lachesis, Medorrhinum, Mercurius, Phosphorus, Sulphur, (Natrum Muriaticum). The more extrovert Natrums can put the homeopath on the wrong track with their enthusiasm, which may hide misgivings about putting themselves in a vulnerable position.

Those patients who come in visibly irritated by being kept waiting for ten minutes are likely to be Arsenicum, Natrum Muriaticum, Mercurius or Nux.

Observe the position that the patient adopts on sitting down. A patient who sits as far back as they can, or who chooses a chair more distant than the one meant for them is likely to be one of the cautious types listed above. Similarly, someone who leans forward in the chair, or even moves it forwards, probably belongs to one of the enthusiastic types, especially Phosphorus.

The clothes that the patient is wearing may provide much relevant information. A flamboyantly dressed patient is likely to need Argentum, Medorrhinum, Phosphorus or Sulphur. Certain types are more likely to wear black, particularly Ignatia, Natrum Muriaticum and Sepia. The emotional types Phosphorus, Pulsatilla, and Graphites often wear pink, (at least the females!). Slovenly, dirty or untidy dress sense favours Baryta, Mercurius and

Sulphur. The woman who wears a rather manly suit is probably Ignatia, Natrum Muriaticum, or Nux.

Look for the formal, bolt upright posture of Aurum, the Kalis, and some Natrums. It will probably make you feel a bit tense yourself.

During the taking of the physical case history observe the degree of detail with which the patient describes his or her symptoms. The following types are likely to be objective and precise in their descriptions; Arsenicum, Aurum, Causticum, the Kalis, Lachesis, Lycopodium, Medorrhinum, Mercurius, the Natrums, Nux, Silica, Sulphur, and Tuberculinum.

Look for the clearly hypochondriacal concern with which some members of the following types describe their symptoms; Arsenicum, Calcarea, the Kalis, Phosphorus and Natrum Muriaticum. Ignatia tends to dramatise whatever she says, and hence is likely to exaggerate, as are Sulphur and Phosphorus. If the physical history touches upon sexuality, look out for the reluctance of Thuja and some Natrums to discuss the subject, and if reluctance is found, consider exploring it further during the mental history.

By the time one reaches the mentals history, one should already have some feeling for the personality of the patient, even if it is just a vague sense that one cannot identify clearly. Often there is a sense of liking or disliking the patient, and this can be useful, since each homeopath will learn with time which types tend to attract or repel him or her.

When taking the mentals history, I recommend asking patients to talk about themselves first, before asking them specific questions. Their initial few words often go straight to the point, reducing the possibilities to just a few remedies. For example, the patient may begin with, "Well, I'm really quite a reserved person," or, "I'm a very nervous person." Negative traits are usually more reliable than positive ones. Common positive remarks like, "I like people," or "I'm sociable" are virtually worthless, since they apply to so many types, even the more reserved ones, who have often learned to compensate. Having said that, patients who initially reply, "I'm creative" are usually Natrum Muriaticum, Sulphur or Nux constitutionally.

If the patient's first remarks are a denial of a negative trait (which has not been brought up by the homeopath) one should suspect the opposite of what the patient says. When asked about relationships in general, one rather proud Lachesis man said, "I'm not a jealous type," telling me immediately that jealousy was an issue for him. (This was confirmed on further questioning.) If you suspect that the patient is not being entirely accurate, further detailed questioning often helps to clarify whether or not your suspicion is correct. Never take the patient's words at face value. This is the surest way to the wrong prescription.

Once the patient has exhausted his or her self-description, it is time for specific questioning. This should continue until the similimum is clear. After this, further questions tend to obscure the issue (at least for myself), since you may not be able to see the wood for the trees.

I find that a useful initial question is, "What would you like to change about your personality?" This often gets to the heart of the weaknesses that are so useful in identifying the remedy. If the patient cannot think of a single thing that they would like to change, they are either perfect or they belong to one of the proud types, which include Arsenicum, Lachesis, Lycopodium, Nux, Platina, Sulphur, and sometimes Natrum and Tuberculinum.

If the patient's main concern is lack of self-confidence, one should think of Alumina, Argentum, Baryta, China, Graphites, Lycopodium, Pulsatilla, Sepia, Silica and the Natrums. Ask the patient in which situations they feel this lack of confidence. If they reply, "In groups of people," the Natrums are particularly likely. If the answer is "All the time," think of Baryta, Lycopodium Argentum and Alumina. Shyness on first meeting people, which soon disappears is typical of Pulsatilla and Silica, whereas shyness which remains is more characteristic of Baryta and China. Anticipatory anxiety, the dread of failure before an important event that demands something of the patient is most often seen in Argentum, Lycopodium, and Silica. (These three are very different personalities and should be relatively easy to distinguish.)

If worrying is the patient's main complaint, ask what the worries are about. If the reply is, "everything," think of Alumina, Calcarea, Lycopodium, the Kalis, Natrum Carbonicum, Phosphorus and Sepia. The patient whose worries centre around work is especially likely to be Lycopodium. Worries about health that are not realistic are found in the hypochondriacal types listed previously, and less commonly in Lachesis, Lycopodium and the Natrums. The patient who worries excessively about the health and welfare of relatives is often Calcarea, Natrum or Phosphorus. Financial worries are common, but if they are clearly unrealistic think of Arsenicum.

I always ask about the patient's fears and phobias. Many Lycopodium patients report a fear that their lives will amount to nothing. Natrum Muriaticum fears situations in which they do not feel in control, such as flying in an aeroplane, or a blind date. Claustrophobia is most commonly seen in Natrums, but also in Argentum and Stramonium. Lachesis has a kind of claustrophobia which occurs when the air supply is poor, or when the mouth and nostrils are partially obstructed, such as in the operating theatre when a mask is put over the face. Medorrhinum often has a fear of going insane, as does Stramonium. Paranoid fears can be subtle, but are very useful when spotted. An example is a tendency by the patient to assume that people are talking about them or laughing at them on frequent occasions. Another common paranoid symptom is the fear on seeing a policeman that they will be arrested. Paranoid fears are most often seen in Anacardium, Argentum, Arsenicum, China, Hyocyamus, Lachesis, Mercurius, Natrum, Stramonium,

Veratrum and Thuja. Most people are afraid of snakes, but if the sight of a snake on the television makes a patient's heart pound, this suggests that the patient is most probably needing Lachesis or Natrum Muriaticum. Fear of the dark is commonly seen in Baryta, Graphites, Medorrhinum, Phosphorus, Pulsatilla, Stramonium and sometimes in Natrum Muriaticum and Arsenicum. Fear of death is most often seen in Arsenicum, and manifests as a reluctance to even think about the subject, or else as an intruding fearful thought. It is also common amongst Natrums. An excessive fear of catching a contagious disease is seen in Arsenicum, Calcarea, and Syphilinum. Fear that a loved one will die is especially common in Ignatia and Natrum Muriaticum, and these remedies also have a strong fear of abandonment.

Some patients admit to experiencing very little or no fear in their lives. They are usually either fiery types (Causticum, Lachesis, Nux and Sulphur), or two of the more intellectual types, Medorrhinum and Tuberculinum. Lycopodium may claim to be free from fear, but this usually an example of bravado and wishful thinking on his part.

Patients often complain of a difficulty in relating to other people, which is more then just shyness or lack of confidence. It is a barrier that they put up automatically to protect themselves, which prevents them from experiencing intimacy with other people. This is typical of Natrums, but is also seen in Alumina, Arsenicum, Aurum, Ignatia, the Kalis, Lycopodium, Mercurius, Sepia, Staphysagria, and Thuja.

Guilt feelings are common, but become particularly persistent and damaging in Natrum Muriaticum, Lachesis and Thuja. The patient who feels responsible for everyone else is more often than not Natrum Muriaticum. The latter is so common that I routinely ask certain questions to identify Natrum Muriaticum when the remedy is not easy to spot. These include;

"Have you had any bereavements in your life?' and if the answer is yes, "and how did you react to them?"

"Do you find it easier to give than to receive?" (Most Natrums emphatically answer, "to give." Others that may give the same answer, though usually less emphatically, are Lycopodium, Sepia and Staphysagria.)

"Do you suffer from depression, and if so, do you prefer company or solitude when depressed?"

"Are you a perfectionist, and if so, in what way?" (Other perfectionist types include Arsenicum, Silica, and Nux.)

"Are you able to cry when sad?"

Anger is an important aspect of life which I usually enquire into if the patient does not mention it. Many patients are prone to feelings of anger and irritation, yet say they are not, since they do not express their feelings. If a patient says, "I don't get angry very often," it is worth asking, "But do you feel angry inside?" This gets an affirmative answer far more often. Since expressing anger is generally not socially acceptable, even the more volatile types like Nux and Sepia tend to keep much of it inside. Because of this I find that the degree of anger felt is a better guide to the remedy type. Types that tend to feel anger and irritation relatively easily include Alumina, Arsenicum, Ignatia, Lachesis, Mercurius, Natrum Muriaticum, Nux, Sepia, Sulphur, Syphilinum, Stramonium, Thuja, Tuberculinum and Veratrum. The kind of situations which bring forth anger help to differentiate between these types. Thus Arsenicum is irritated by untidiness, but also by people who are unreliable, whilst Ignatia is particularly sensitive to any form of rejection or criticism, and will react angrily as a defence. Nux and Sulphur, the natural leaders, are angered by anyone who gets in the way of their plans, and Sepia is often resentful towards men who try to give her orders, or who neglect her. Tuberculinum and Lachesis both love freedom, and will not take kindly to being restricted in any way.

Those patients who do flare up in a temper fairly regularly are likely to be one of the following volatile types; Alumina, Anacardium, Ignatia, Lachesis, Nux, Mercurius, Sepia, Sulphur, Stramonium, and Veratrum. Some Staphysagria people are also very prone to anger, though only the "wild" type (see chapter on Staphysagria) is likely to express it.

In general, the more sophisticated a patient is, the less they will admit to weaknesses. Patients who have changed consciously through their own efforts, or with the help of therapists, tend to deny negative traits that they possessed until quite recently. If you suspect that a person is a particular type, but they deny having the weaknesses of that type, ask if they used to possess them. Very often the patient will willingly confirm this. Personal growth does not change the constitutional type, hence previous characteristics can be used in the homeopath's assessment. In this regard, I find that an enquiry into the personality of the patient during childhood is often very helpful. As people get older, they learn to compensate for their weaknesses, to control their excesses, and to hide traits which are not socially acceptable. The personality of the child is relatively unmodified by such adaptations, and often reveals the constitutional type very clearly. Only Pulsatilla and Calcarea children are likely to change types as they grow older.

Just as patients often possess the trait which they go to great lengths to deny, so patients who are determined not to be like their father or mother often share the same constitutional type with this parent. Thus I sometimes make enquiries about the personality of such parents. The person who showers her child with love and attention, determined not to be like her cold mother, is likely to be Natrum Muriaticum, whilst the man who drops out from society, and professes to be indifferent to what others think of him, probably belongs to the same type as his Lycopodium father, who tried hard to make it in the world, and always courted popularity.

A patient's profession can reveal a good deal of useful information, and should not be ignored. Arsenicum and Natrum Muriaticum have good organisational skills, and are often to be found in administrative positions. Counsellors and therapists are often Natrums, being very good at listening to others, but not so keen to talk about themselves. Calcarea is often to be found in jobs that are either practically oriented, such as a mechanic, or else in clerical and secretarial roles. Calcarea tends to avoid taking on too much responsibility, and often accepts work well below his intellectual capabilities. Lycopodiums are often to be found in scientific and computing positions, in salesman jobs and also in businesses of their own. They are also common in the teaching professions.

Artistic skills are seen most commonly in Lachesis, Natrum Muriaticum, Phosphorus, Sepia, Ignatia, Silica and Medorrhinum.

Sulphur and Nux Vomica are natural leaders, and are unlikely to remain in subordinate positions for long. If they are not at the top of an institution, they are likely to be self-employed.

Sepia is often attracted to the healing professions, particularly to nursing, physiotherapy, and other 'hands-on' therapies.

Pulsatilla, if she works at all outside the home, often chooses one of the caring professions, whilst Tuberculinum seeks either mental stimulation from his work, or adventure.

There is a saying amongst homeopaths that one should never believe what the patient says. Whilst this is deliberately provocative, and overstates the case, there is some truth behind it. Not only do many patients try to hide their weaknesses from the homeopath, many more succeed in hiding them from themselves. Hence one should not expect patients to give accurate accounts of themselves. Often the way a patient says something is more important than what they say. I remember an interview with a young campus religious minister who was seeking treatment for post-viral malaise. He appeared open and friendly, and professed to being relatively liberal and progressive as ministers go. There were few helpful mental features, and the physicals were also rather non-specific. It eventually became clear that the most noticeable aspect of his personality was a certain formality and politeness that was more commonly seen in his grandparents' generation than in his own. Furthermore, his very position as a religious minister on a university campus, surrounded by predominantly boisterous and hedonistic students (who were of the same age as he, or only slightly younger) served to emphasise his formality and 'squareness'. It was this stiffness of character that led to the prescription of Kali Carbonicum, rather than the words he chose to describe himself. Very often the impression that patient gives is more useful than the content of his speech. Thus the patient who is very matter of fact, and is visibly impatient at having to discuss his emotions, when all he wants is treatment for his backache, may well be Nux Vomica. Similarly, the patient who denies being fastidious or prone to anxiety, but who observes the homeopath throughout the interview with an air of wariness or suspicion, and wants to know exactly what side-effects to expect, is likely to be Arsenicum. With experience, the homeopath learns to give as much importance to the non-verbal cues as to the verbal ones.

Sex is a subject that many patients and homeopaths avoid, yet it can reveal a lot of helpful information, and is worth inquiring into when the remedy is not clear. Again, the attitude with which the patient responds is as important as the words they use, or more so. An obvious reluctance to talk about sex is common with Natrum Muriaticum and Thuja, both of whom are prone to guilt feelings. On the other hand, an easy and even enthusiastic approach to the subject is often seen in Causticum, some Ignatias, Lachesis, Medorrhinum, Mercurius, Phosphorus, Sulphur and Argentum. The rest tend to be in-between. Lycopodium men often have issues about virility, which can lead to one of several approaches to talking about sex. If they are aware that they doubt their virility, they may brush over the subject, saying simply, "There's no problem there." Alternately, they may boast of their sexual prowess, either directly, or using their tone of voice in the manner of a men's locker-room exchange, "Well, there's CERTAINLY no problem on THAT account." An honest and direct third approach is also seen quite often.

Some types are rather shy but still relatively straightforward when talking about sex. These include Alumina, Baryta, Calcarea, China, the Kalis, Phosphorus, Silica and Staphysagria. They will probably exhibit some embarrassment when asked about their sex life, but this will not usually stop them from speaking about it.

I like to get some idea of the strength of the patient's libido. One way of doing this is to simply ask, "Would you say your sex-drive is high, low or average?" Most people reply average, but those with a particularly high sex-drive usually say so, especially Argentum, Hyoscyamus, Lachesis, Lycopodium, Medorrhinum, Nux, Platina and Sulphur. A low sex-drive is reported by worn-out Sepias, and also by China, and by those Natrums who are having difficulties in relating emotionally to their partner. If, for some reason, I doubt the accuracy of a patient's reply, I may enquire further, asking, "In a good relationship, how often would you ideally like to have intercourse?"

Often during a difficult case I find it helpful to narrow the personality of the patient down to one that is primarily mental, emotional, intuitive or practical. Once the case has been narrowed down to a few remedies, selective questioning can be used to rule out all but the correct remedy. Thus, if the choice is between Causticum, Medorrhinum, Lachesis, and Phosphorus, an enquiry into the patient's sense of social justice may help to support or eliminate Causticum, whilst a specific question about "spacing out" may help to identify Medorrhinum.

Sometimes it happens that the physicals seem to favour one remedy whilst the mentals favour another. In my experience, in chronic conditions the mentals tend to be more reliable in helping to find the correct remedy when the two don't agree. This is partly due to the enormous overlap in physical characteristics between the remedy types, and also to the fact that the list of possible physicals for each polychrest is so vast that it cannot be comprehensively learned, or even covered thoroughly by the repertory. There will always be physical symptoms of any given remedy that are not familiar to the homeopath. Obviously, if the physicals of the case are keynotes of one remedy, and the mentals only vaguely fit a different remedy, the physicals should be given more weight.

There are atypical cases of just about every type from the mental point of view, which can mislead the homeopath. In such cases, the essence of the personality, if it can be divined, may be more useful than the particulars. The essence is a theme that runs through every aspect of the personality, such as the physical insecurity of Arsenicum. In other cases, a single strange, rare or peculiar mental trait can reveal the correct remedy. The hand-washing compulsion of Syphilinum is a good example.

Every homeopath must realise that information that is volunteered by the patient is far more reliable than that which is given as a response to a specific question, especially if it is a leading question (one that can only be answered by "yes" or "no"). For example, I have found that patients who volunteer that they get the feeling that someone is behind them when out walking at night are almost always Medorrhinum, whereas those that say "yes" when asked if they get this experience may belong to any of the constitutional types. As a compromise, if the patient does not volunteer a particular keynote, an open question can be asked to try to flush it out. For example, one might ask the patient if she is prone to sixth-sense feelings when out alone at night, or whether her imagination tends to be very active when alone at night. If she says yes, asking her to elaborate will usually reveal Medorrhinum's characteristic symptom if it is present.

It is extremely important to begin the interview with as much of an open mind as possible. Although a remedy or two will usually occur to the homeopath early on in the interview, he must be flexible enough to abandon it at a moment's notice if new information changes the picture.

There is another saying that during a good homeopathic interview the patient will laugh and cry at least once. Although not literally true, it expresses an important point; that the interview should be of sufficient breadth and depth to reach the heart of the patient. All too often homeopaths obtain a superficial and misleading impression of the patient's personality by failing to delve beyond the immediate replies that are given. This may be due to laziness on the part of the homeopath, but it is just as often due to fear of embarrassing not the patient, but himself, and to feeling uncomfortable with the expression of painful emotions. The more a homeopath is in touch with, and comfortable with his own self, the more easily he will win the confidence of his patients, and discover the real person that lies beneath the appearance.

# *Alumina*

*Keynote:* Mental instability

Alumina is not a common constitutional type. It is one of that group of remedies that the homeopath thinks of when he has a patient who is mentally unstable, with a tendency towards hysteria. Such patients often have a history of unstable childhood circumstances, including a family history of mental illness and alcoholism, a reflection of the syphilitic miasm in the family. The few Alumina cases I have seen have all been women.

## *Mental Deterioration*

The first impression that the Alumina patient often gives is usually one of confusion. She complains of being unable to think straight, and she confirms this by hesitating as she speaks, and by struggling to find the right words (Kent: 'Inability to follow a train of thought', 'makes mistakes in writing and speaking'). One Alumina patient told me that her brain would 'scramble' all the time, making clear thinking impossible. She had to constantly make lists in order to remind herself what she was supposed to be doing, because her mind would often go blank, leaving her disorientated when she 'switched back on'. (It may help to imagine the Alumina brain like a faulty computer, which frequently shuts down momentarily, and when it starts up again the programme is lost and has to be searched for. This computer is also prone to scrambling, a fault which results in information being mixed up and appearing randomly on the screen as nonsense.)

In many cases Alumina's mental confusion is present from childhood. The Alumina child has difficulty learning, especially with regard to speech and writing, and Alumina patients will say that others have said that as a child they seemed vague and dreamy. This apparent dreaminess is really just confusion. It becomes more obvious when the Alumina individual leaves home and tries to cope as an adult in the world. She then begins to feel overwhelmed, and incapable of making decisions and looking after herself. This generates anxiety, which reduces her self-confidence, making her thinking even less clear.

One of the characteristic results of Alumina's confusion is indecision (Kent: 'Irresolution'). Most Alumina patients complain of this, and for many it is a major problem. One patient, a young woman in her twenties who came to see me for treatment of anxiety and confusion, said that she would lie awake for hours at night trying to decide between two courses of action, terrified that she might make the wrong decision. The decisions before her

1

at such times were not necessarily crucial ones. Often they were small matters in which either of the possible choices were appropriate, such as what to cook for dinner the next day. After a dose of Alumina 10M she was visibly more 'together', and she smiled gratefully as she reported that she no longer lay awake at night agonising over petty decisions.

The fear of making the wrong decision is a natural consequence of the confusion which Alumina experiences. It is really a fear that if she cannot think straight, her external life will collapse into chaos, a not unreasonable concern. Very often Alumina will rely heavily upon a parent or a partner to make decisions for her, and she will be aware that this is unhealthy, but she cannot help herself.

### Loss of Self

Another highly characteristic feature of Alumina's mental instability is a sense of unreality. This may be described in various ways. Some patients say, "It's like I'm not here." By this they do not mean that their mind has gone blank, but rather that their sense of self has gone. It is a state that is hard to imagine, in which the perception of the outside world continues, without a sense of the person herself. Others say, "It is as though it is not me but another person watching these things." Hahnemann in his Chronic Diseases uses the same description; 'When he says anything he feels as if another person has said it'. This is a state in which the mind is detached and witnessing events (including the subjects own thoughts and actions) from a distance. One patient of mine who subsequently responded well to the remedy said, "It's like I'm looking at the world from behind a glass case." (After taking the remedy this sensation gradually disappeared.) Naturally, this feeling of detachment can be very disturbing, confirming to the Alumina individual that there is something seriously wrong with her mind.

Alumina may sometimes be confused with Medorrhinum, and even Cannabis Indica, since both of these types experience a sense of unreality or duality. Medorrhinum often reports episodes of feeling 'spaced out' or far away from the world, but these are transient compared to the constant loss of ego of Alumina. I have never heard a Medorrhinum person say that they felt that they did not exist, or that someone else seemed to speak when they spoke. It seems that these two states are superficially similar, but really very different. Medorrhinum's detachment is similar to the detachment which anyone who practises a lot of meditation may experience, where the self is experienced as silent and expanded, and separate from the thinking mind. In contrast, Alumina experiences a complete loss of the sense of self, which is entirely pathological. (Other features of the mentals will usually be sufficiently distinct for the careful homeopath to distinguish between Alumina, Medorrhinum and Cannabis Indica.)

Some Alumina people describe a milder form of identity confusion. When asked about their personality in the interview, they say "I haven't got one", and they are not joking. When asked what they mean, they say that they have no sense of a personality, since all they do is try to make sense of their confusion, and cope with their anxiety.

One Alumina patient, an extremely thin, nervous woman who was having relationship problems, was quite analytical about this. She said that she had no personality because she had no role models as a child, since her father was seldom at home and her mother was aloof. Whilst the latter conditions will not help to give a child a sense of identity, they will not produce such a profound lack of sense of self in other constitutional types as that seen in Alumina.

### Depression and Self-Destructive Impulses

The confusion and lack of identity may bring to mind another remedy - Phosphoric Acid. Unlike the latter, however, Alumina is prone to powerful emotions, particularly despair, anger and anxiety. The mood often alternates between despair and a relatively contented state, changing several times within a day (Kent: 'Mood changeable'). During depressive moods Alumina will feel hopeless, and will often contemplate suicide. There may be a great deal of weeping, or the patient may not weep at all, but simply withdraws into silence like Natrum and Aurum. One Alumina patient would burst into floods of tears as soon as she sat down in the consulting room (Kent: 'Weeping, involuntary), and cried throughout the consultation, until, having tried Sepia with only slight effect, I gave her Alumina 10M, after which she did not cry at all during the consultation, and said that her moods had become a lot more stable.

Alumina is predominantly a female remedy, and there is often a marked increase in moodiness before the menses. Both despair and aggression may increase at this time, along with the fear that the patient will hurt herself. Alumina has a very characteristic impulse to kill herself when she sees a knife or other sharp object. One patient was constantly resisting the impulse to kill herself with a razor (Kent: 'Seeing blood or a knife, she has horrid thoughts of killing herself, though she abhors the idea'). As Kent suggests, Alumina is prone to these impulses even when she is not feeling depressed.

The same moods that possess the Alumina patient premenstrually may endure longer in the form of post-natal depression. At this time the impulse to kill the child may be more prominent than the suicidal tendency, and this may produce both horror and profound feelings of guilt in the poor Alumina mother.

Alumina is not listed in Kent's repertory for either desire or aversion to company, and I have not found either to be consistent. Some Alumina patients want company when depressed, whilst others avoid it. One depressed Alumina woman reported a strong feeling of self-loathing, and a feeling that she didn't want to see or talk to anyone, which lifted after taking the remedy.

### Violence

Alumina should come to mind whenever the homeopath comes across a case which combines mental confusion with violent thoughts and impulses. Alumina feels violent at times towards herself, and at other times towards those around her. She may be subject to sudden bouts of rage, although often she will not take out her rage on others, but rather slams doors and smashes things, or curses out loud. Alumina is usually a quiet, gentle person who hates her violent side (Kent: 'Quiet disposition'). Very often the homeopath must gain her confidence before she will admit to feeling violent impulses. She will often complain of anger, but will not reveal the murderous impulses to which she is prone until specifically asked. (The same can be said for the sexual and violent impulses of Hyoscyamus and Platina.) Once she realises that the homeopath will not be shocked by such things, she will usually be relieved to be able to talk about her strange impulses. One Alumina patient said that she felt when angry as if she had poison coming out of her. Another felt at times that she could kill, and imagined chopping off the head of her child or husband. These violent thoughts of Alumina nearly always involve cutting, be they suicidal or homicidal. The patient is usually sensitive, and has enough self-control to resist her impulses, but they cause her a great deal of distress, and there is presumably the potential for the violent impulses to be acted upon.

Alumina can easily be confused with Sepia, who is also prone to violent thoughts towards loved ones, particularly premenstrually, and may feel that her mind is falling apart. However, the mental and emotional pathology of Alumina is more serious than that seen in Sepia. Sepia is seldom on the verge of insanity, is not nearly so prone to suicidal impulses, and does not have a fixation upon cutting and stabbing. Neither does Sepia experience the unreality that Alumina does. Furthermore, the pre-morbid personality of Sepia is generally far more integrated and healthy than that of Alumina.

### Anxiety

Given the mental and emotional instability of Alumina, it is not surprising that Alumina individuals are prone to anxiety problems. Alumina is an extremely anxious type, prone to panic attacks and phobias. There is usually a fear of insanity, and related to this is a fear of succumbing to the suicidal or homicidal impulses. Almost any other fear may develop. Commonly there is a fear of meeting people, especially groups of people, a fear that is seen in most individuals prone to severe anxiety. Alumina's fear often leads to insomnia. She will lie awake at night obsessively worrying about how she will cope with the next day, or with some anticipated ordeal in the near future. Given Alumina's scattered mental processes, even little tasks like writing a thankyou note can generate anxiety, and Alumina can be thrown into a panic by any change in her surroundings or her daily routine. She is unlikely to risk venturing forth on holiday for example, unless she has a strong and reliable partner, and even then holidays are likely to be too stressful for her to cope with.

One of my Alumina patients had a tremendous fear of failure, and on account of this she became a perfectionist, and would seldom attempt anything beyond her essential daily tasks.

Like other types who are prone to mental disintegration, (Argentum, Mercurius, Nitricum, Phosphoric Acid), Alumina tends to become hurried when she is anxious (Kent: 'Propensity to hurry'). This is usually an aimless hurry in which very little is achieved, since the mind is so scattered. The more she hurries, the less she is able to cope, and so a vicious circle sets in. It may culminate in admission to a psychiatric ward with a 'nervous breakdown'. Alumina's hurriedness is often accompanied by a feeling of wanting to get away, to escape, although the patient has no idea where she wants to go to.

### Physical Appearance

I have seen only a few Alumina patients, hence comments on their physical appearance are only tentative. Most were very thin, with bony facial features, and wrinkled brows. The hair was sometimes light and sometimes dark, and was nearly always very long. (The appearance was thus often reminiscent of Sepia, further increasing the possibility of confusion between these two types. Unlike Sepia, however, the skin is usually pale.)

# *Anacardium*

*Keynote:* Good versus evil

This is a rare constitutional type, and my observations must be tentative, since they are based on only a few patients. However, the central characteristic of the Anacardium personality is quite dramatic, and hard to miss, providing that the patient feels sufficiently at ease with the homeopath to be open with him. The old materia medicas stress the divided nature of Anacardium's will (Kent: 'Will-contradiction of', 'feels as if he had two wills') In my experience this division is between a normal, sensitive personality, and a sharply contrasting perverse or 'demonic' subpersonality, which attempts to possess the individual and prompt him to commit obscene acts. (Kent: 'He is persuaded by his evil will to do acts of violence and injustice, but is restrained by a good will'.) The Repertory lists many of the characteristics of Anacardium's 'evil' side (malicious, paranoia, cruelty, propensity to curse, unfeeling, rage). The Anacardium patients that I have seen, however, were sufficiently in control of themselves to resist the promptings of their demonic side, although at times this involved a great struggle between the two wills (the resemblance to classic descriptions of demon possession was striking).

The most consistent compulsion that I have seen in Anacardium patients is a compulsion to curse at others in violent sexual language. One such patient was a highly sophisticated young man, whose main interests in life were spiritual. He practised meditation regularly, and had a fine understanding of mystical philosophy. This spiritual side contrasted starkly with his other side, which had been with him since birth. Even as a small child it was clear to his family that he was strange, since he used a potty to urinate until he was ten years old, and still sat on the toilet to urinate after that age. Furthermore, he had a fetish for watching women urinate, which was his principal source of sexual arousal, and which he presumably did act upon sometimes. (He was reluctant to talk about this). His main complaint, however, was that he was tortured by the compulsion to say sexually obscene and violent remarks to those around him. The effort of resisting his demonic side showed as a stiffness in talking, his lips being pursed with tension, whilst his eyebrows were knit together much of the time.

This particular man was sufficiently sophisticated intellectually to rationalise his symptoms, and expressed no guilt about them. Another Anacardium patient, however, was deeply ashamed of his alter-ego. He was far less intellectual than the former, and had not managed to rationalise his obsessive thoughts and impulses in the same rather clinical way. When I saw him initially he was acutely distressed by the struggle going on inside himself, and fearful of going insane. He also reported having had the same obscene compulsions for as long as he could remember, but they had intensified following the stress of separating from his wife. With treatment his perverse subpersonality gradually became weaker and less insistent, although it had not entirely disappeared by the time he stopped coming to see me.

### Divine Inspiration

The division within Anacardium's mind is more stark when the contrast is between not a demonic side and a normal side, but between a demonic side and a divine side. A recent patient of mine was an example of this more classic split between good and evil. He was a pleasant, rather nervous young man who was referred by a counsellor with 'emotional problems'. He first told me that he was often depressed, and he frequently thought of suicide. He then went on to say that he had a fear of women, that they always tried to manipulate him, and hence he avoided them. He said that he had a fear of sex, and said it was because he thought of sex as impure. At this stage he could have been almost any constitutional type, particularly if his symptoms were the result of sexual abuse in childhood, which often results in suicidal depression, fear of the gender of the abuser, and an aversion to sex in general. However, my patient then began to speak in more religious terms. He said that he felt 'called by God' to bring light to others, and that he felt very close to God. This contrast between suicidal depression and divine inspiration alerted me to the likelihood of a relatively insane constitutional type. My patient then said that he had had a breakdown a few years previously, in which he felt he was 'surrounded by spirits' (Kent: 'Delusions - sees dead persons', 'Delusions- sees devils'). After this experience he felt as if he were half divine and half demonic (Kent: 'Delusions of being double'). He felt guided and protected by one of the spirits, but felt that others were urging him to do obscene things. I gently coaxed him to reveal more, taking pains to make it clear that I understood what he was saying, and was not surprised or alarmed by it. He said that he had an urge when walking down the street to swear at passers by. He also would have fantasies of dousing everyone in a crowded street with petrol and setting them on fire. A voice would say 'Kiss them' as he passed strangers in the street. This contrast between divine and demonic was very distressing to my patient. It made him feel in danger of eternal damnation, and even the smallest moral decision became like a life and death struggle for supremacy between his two wills. For example, he used to work as a taxi driver, and when he came across a customer who was waiting for another taxi which was late he would agonise over whether or not to 'steal' his colleague's customer. He felt that his every action was significant, and was either righteous or accursed, and furthermore, that everything that happened to him in his life, from the smallest detail to the largest, was either a reward from heaven or a punishment from hell.

I gave this man Anacardium 10M and he said a few weeks later that the obscene impulses had faded to faint thoughts that were easily dismissed, and that his depression had lifted. He was still rather obsessed with good and evil, but was clearly less distressed and more in touch with reality. Such cases may never become completely sane, but with the help of the similimum they can remain sane enough to avoid the excesses to which their constitution is prone.

### Violence

I have not come across an Anacardium patient who admitted to acting out his violent impulses, but the potential is clearly there. Kent lists Anacardium under several violent rubrics, which implies that the Anacardium patient does not always resist his violent impulses. My ex-taxi driver said that he wished he could shout at women, and added that women respected a man who shouted at them. This matter of fact statement led me to believe that such a man was easily capable of great cruelty should his grip on reality slip just a little further.

### Paranoia

Kent lists Anacardium under several paranoid rubrics, including 'Imagines being persecuted'. The only clear evidence of this that I have seen is the fear of women that the above case involved. Most relatively insane types are prone to paranoia, and it seems that Anacardium is no exception. A milder form of anxiety is often seen in Anacardium people in the form of a lack of self-confidence (Kent: 'Lack of self-confidence'). One patient who responded to the remedy said initially that he was usually too afraid to speak up when in a group, except when he was feeling divinely inspired, when he felt supremely confident (Kent: 'Mania').

### Mental Fogging

Most of my Anacardium patients have complained of some degree of mental confusion. Some say that their memory is very poor (Kent: 'Forgetful'), whilst others say that they find it difficult to concentrate on reading or even on television. This is hardly surprising, given the conflict going on inside Anacardium's psyche. It is rather like the failure of communications which may occur in a country that is experiencing civil war. A couple of my Anacardium patients were quite sane and had no psychotic features. In these cases the principle symptom was a mind wrestling with indecision over difficult choices in life. One man came to see me specifically because he felt so stressed about having to decide upon some direction in life. He had previously worked as a salesman, which he found unsatisfying, but when he came to consider the choices available to him he entered a peculiar agony of anxiety and indecision, which was very intense. His whole appearance was one of intense distress, and he talked about his difficulties in making choices as if he were being tortured. This kind of intensity of distress associated with talking about problems is seen in Aurum, but Aurum does not have the same degree of indecision, and my patient was not depressed as such. He said he had always had difficulty in making decisions, and though he was engaged to be married, he was tormented by the thought that there may be 'someone else out there' who was his real soul mate. He was a very intense man, with very serious interests, and I initially gave him Natrum Muriaticum, which did not act. He then told me that as a child he would lie awake at night praying to God not to let him be possessed. This made me realise he needed a psychotic remedy, and in view of his indecision I gave Anacardium 10M, which greatly calmed his distress, and enabled him to make some rational decisions about his future. I have had one more case where the only indication for Anacardium, apart from a few weak physicals, was this intense agony of indecision. It seems that the more integrated Anacardium person is still torn between two wills, but this takes the form of severe indecision, rather that a battle between good and evil.

### Physical Appearance

I have seen too few Anacardium patients to say much about their appearance, but one common feature was a rather tense face, a reflection of the internal struggle that is the essence of the type. The general appearance is usually one of intensity, which shows particularly in the eyes.

# Argentum Nitricum

*Keynote:* Impulsive, erratic mentality

$A$rgentum is one of those remedies that the student homeopath learns early on in his training; a remedy for phobic states and pre-exam nerves. It is consequently doled out liberally for these conditions, without result in many cases. Only when the remedy fits the patient constitutionally will it help in cases of agorophobia or extreme anxiety, and since it is a relatively uncommon type, the majority of such cases will respond to more common remedies, such as Sepia and Arsenicum.

## The Eccentric

To identify Argentum one must learn to recognise the strangeness of the type. There is a strangeness or eccentricity about the Argentum individual that is usually apparent almost immediately, especially in the case of Argentum men. Argentum people are very open and forthcoming in most cases (rather like Phosphorus) and do not try to hide their eccentricity during the interview. As with all true eccentrics, it is the mental or intellectual aspect of the personality that is 'off-centre', rather than the emotions. The healthy Argentum mind is extremely sharp, and given to lateral thinking, rather than the more common linear, logical type. It makes connections easily between perceptions that would remain unconnected by the average intellect, such as the price of coffee and the state of the environment. The more healthy the Argentum individual is psychologically, the more likely it is that these connections have some validity. As Argentum's mind becomes weaker, they become less reliable, and brilliance deteriorates first into eccentricity, and then into frank delusion. (A similar progression can be seen in some Sulphur individuals.)

The average Argentum individual is a mental rather than an emotional type. In other words, he lives more in his head than in his feelings. It can be a strange and wonderful place to live in, rather like Alice's wonderland, or Los Angeles. Most Argentums enjoy exploring the world of their intellect. They tend to become interested in the unconventional, and in matters that are at the cutting edge of intellectual discovery, and owe their acceptance and application to the future; matters such as the colonisation of space, biorhythms and underwater birthing. Argentum is fascinated by such subjects, and is liable to share his opinions and discoveries enthusiastically. His childlike enthusiasm is infectious, lightening the mood of the homeopath in the same way that the brightness of a contented Phosphorus can. Argentum's eccentricity is particularly evident in male members of the type. The majority of Argentum women I have treated were relatively mental as opposed to emotional, but they did not have the eccentricity that is so typical of the men. For this reason, female Argentums can be more difficult to identify. They still have the typical fears of Argentum, and also the impulsivity, but they otherwise come across as far more 'normal' than the men.

Argentum's mind is mercurial in every way. Quick of perception, but lacking endurance, it tends to flit from one focus of interest to another. At best this produces a mind that has an enormous breadth of knowledge that is reliable and penetrating. At worst it results in superficiality and a scattered mind that cannot be relied upon (Kent: 'unable to fix attention').

Unpredictability is a key feature of Argentum. Kent says that Argentum is 'irrational and does strange things and comes to strange conclusions'. In the healthy individual this irrationality takes the form of impulsively doing or saying what amuses him, or what he wants to do, without the usual regard for what other people may think. Argentum often has a sharp wit, and may suddenly jump upon the words of one he is listening to make a pun out of them. His playfulness is something like that of Phosphorus, but is more intellectual. Even Argentum's dress sense tends towards the unconventional. Several of my Argentum patients have worn bright harlequin-like colours that were quite out of keeping with the prevailing conservatism of the British. (The colours were generally well matched, indicating a sense of style and aesthetic appreciation—a method to the madness.) One Argentum patient actually worked as a clown, busking in city malls. He wore a harlequin suit at work, curiously reminiscent of the colours worn by some of my other Argentum patients.

### The Unstable Mind

Like other predominantly mental types, Argentum's pathology appears first on the mental rather than the emotional level (Kent: 'the intellectual feature predominates, the affections are disturbed only in a limited way'). The first sign of a deterioration in Argentum's mental functioning is often an increase in the frequency and the strangeness of mental impulses. Even relatively stable Argentum individuals are prone sometimes to strange impulses which they know are irrational. For example, an Argentum schoolteacher may suddenly get the impulse to write a swear word on the blackboard, or to tip an inkpot over a student's head. In the vast majority of cases these impulses are resisted, although they can be powerful and require all the individual's will to resist them.

One impulse of Argentum is very common and is characteristic of the type. This is the impulse to jump when looking down from a height, whether it be a top storey window, or from the railings of a bridge. The impulse can be so strong that the individual avoids these circumstances for fear that they would jump (Kent: 'impulse to jump'). This impulse occurs in the absence of any suicidal desire , and is quite inexplicable, both to the patient and to the homeopath. It is just one of those strange impulses to which Argentum is subject.

Not surprisingly, the individual subject to these strange impulses sometimes thinks he is losing his mind. In many cases the impulses come only occasionally, and are easily resisted. In these cases the homeopath may only be able to gather the impression of a generally impulsive character, since the more peculiar impulses are either absent or are not mentioned. (In these cases it is worth asking the patient specifically whether they are prone to any peculiar thoughts or impulses.) However, in cases of deeper pathology the characteristic impulses can become intense, as can the fear of mental breakdown (Kent: 'fear of insanity').

With deepening pathology Argentum's mind becomes less and less reliable. Concentration becomes difficult, words are misplaced, and the memory becomes patchy and vague. The individual is aware of this mental deterioration, and it usually causes alarm. The feeling of alarm causes thoughts to crowd in upon each other, leading to a feeling of hurriedness (Kent: 'hurry, while walking'). Whenever Argentum feels nervous he becomes hurried, rather like Lachesis and Medorrhinum.

As Argentum's mind becomes more and more erratic, fear becomes a major problem. Argentum individuals can develop all manner of fears. A particularly characteristic fear is an anxiety felt when looking up at tall buildings. Many Argentum people feel this to some degree, even when their minds are reasonably stable, and when it is found it is a reliable confirmation of the remedy type. Some patients cannot say what the anxiety is about, but many say that they are afraid that the tall buildings will fall on them. This reflects the shaky foundations of the patient's own mind (just as Thuja's dreams of falling reflect his guilt and fear of punishment).

Another common fear is claustrophobia (though Natrum Muriaticum is needed for this phobia far more often than Argentum). Again the patient has a sense that the walls will fall in, and so this is closely related to the fear of high buildings.

In such a state of fear the patient naturally feels that the world is not a safe place, and this can give rise to feelings of paranoia (Kent: 'fear—of people'). I remember one very classic Argentum case, a young man who was so nervous on seeing me that he would stop speaking every few seconds in midsentence in an attempt to gather his wits enough to continue. If anyone walked by the door, he thought they were listening to us, and would suddenly end the consultation and walk out in a state of great agitation. Within a few days of taking Argentum Nitricum 10M he was much calmer, and was able to speak about himself without fear of eavesdroppers. His paranoia was actually a somewhat realistic sense that if people were aware of the chaos in his mind, they would think him weird and reject him. This particular patient also demonstrated a trait that I have seen only a few times in Argentum people, which is listed in italics in Kent's repertory for Argentum - a sense of excessive remorse (Kent: 'Anxiety—with guilt'). He apologised frequently for taking up so much of my time, and often said that he was a bad person. (This was in part referring to his past sexual promiscuity.)

Agarophobia is another characteristic fear of Argentum. It may be mild, causing anxiety only in wide open spaces, or severe, preventing the patient from going out at all. (Agarophobia is liable to occur in any individual who feels that his mind is breaking down, since wide open spaces produce a sense of exposure and vulnerability.) Fear of immanent death is also seen sometimes, as is fear of disease (cf.Arsenicum).

Argentum is one of the principal remedies for anticipatory anxiety (Kent: 'Anxiety anticipating an engagement'). It is as though the already shaky mind cannot cope with the uncertainty of not knowing how a coming task or event will turn out. The event may be as little as meeting an old friend, or visiting the doctor with a minor complaint. Argentum's imagination is liable to run riot in these circumstances, usually imagining the worst. Like Lycopodium, Argentum may become anxious when he thinks that something is expected of him ,or when he has to perform in some way. At such times anxiety can become extreme, accompanied by palpitations and diarrhoea. This is related to a characteristic expectation of failure, which is often unrealistic, at least in the more healthy Argentum individual. At such times encouragement from a friend can bring enormous relief, an example of the impressionability of the type, which results from a lack of mental stability.

When fear has risen to a state of panic, Argentum individuals often become very needy, and may beseech those that they trust for help and reassurance. In keeping with the erratic, uncontrolled nature of the Argentum mind, the individual may develop totally unrealistic expectations of others, thinking that they can save him from himself. The open, desperate and beseeching quality resembles that seen in frightened Phosphorus individuals. Indeed there are considerable similarities between the two types. Both are impressionable, although this characteristic is seen in Argentum mainly when he is in a state of fear, whereas it is generally the normal state for Phosphorus. Furthermore, both types can lose mental clarity under stress and feel that their mind is failing them, giving rise to panic.

Phosphorus' mind is generally less sharp and less analytical than that of Argentum, and more sensitive to environmental influences. Argentum is more liable than Phosphorus to develop specific phobias when stressed, and is distinctly more impulsive, and more prone to bizarre ideas (Kent: 'Strange notions and ideas come into his mind. A strange idea comes into his mind that if he goes past a certain corner of the street, he will fall down and have a fit, and to avoid that he will go around the block'.) For Phosphorus the primary weakness is a lack of boundaries to the personality, whilst for Argentum it is the erratic quality of the thinking processes.

### The Social Animal

Some Argentums are sociable, whilst others tend to be loners. Most are relatively open, often to the point of appearing innocent, again like Phosphorus. Argentum has a bright, childlike curiosity, and tends to lack social inhibitions. He is liable to strike up conversations with strangers, using cues in the immediate environment to lead into topics which interest him. For example, if it begins to rain whilst he is standing at the bus stop, he may comment to the stranger next to him, "I knew it was going to rain. I've noticed that the birds in my garden don't sing in the morning when it's going to rain. How do you think they know?" Because of his very eccentricity, Argentum may find it hard to make friends. He is not particularly shy, unless he has become fearful in general, but he may have difficulty finding friends who are not put off or intimidated by his strange ideas, and forthright manner (Kent: 'Indiscretion'). On the other hand, he may be appreciated by his friends and partner for these very qualities.

Unlike Phosphorus, Argentum tends to be independently minded. The Argentum wife is liable to have interests of her own, and will not mind that her husband does not share them. She is her own person, with her own opinions, likes and dislikes, and she will not depend upon others unduly for her sense of identity. The relatively healthy Argentum individual knows what she thinks, and is liable to stick doggedly to her views, (Kent: 'Obstinate') rather like Sulphur. Like Sulphur, most Argentums enjoy expressing their ideas, but they are seldom as loquacious as a Sulphur in full flow. However, when Argentum becomes fearful, her thoughts may become obsessive, and her conversation will then reflect this (Kent: 'Talks on one subject'). Also it is when Argentum is anxious that she feels the need for company, and the need to talk (Kent: 'Company, desire for' and 'Desires to talk to someone'). Those Argentum individuals who do become loners do not usually do so out of choice, but rather because they have been unable to find a comfortable niche in society where they feel accepted.

I have found Argentum to be roughly equally common in both sexes. In partnership Argentum tends to be romantic, and the libido is usually high.

Argentum is a fascinating constitutional type. It is easily missed when the pathology is mainly on the physical plane, since the more unusual mental features which are well known may be absent. The mentally healthy

Argentum individual is bright, quick-witted and somewhat eccentric, and is more intellectually orientated than the average Phosphorus, and less ego-tistical than the average Sulphur.

## *Physical Appearance*

Argentum generally has a slim, wiry physique. The complexion may be fair or dark. In keeping with the intellectual nature of Argentum, the facial fea-tures tend to be angular rather than rounded, and the eyes often have a sharp, electrical quality about them. The face tends to look younger than its years, and there are often fine wrinkles or 'laughter lines' radiating from the corners of the eyes. The face is generally broad, reflecting the openness of the personality. Argentum's dress-sense is often quite unconventional.

# Arsenicum Album

*Keynote:* Physical insecurity

To understand the Arsenicum individual, one has to understand the 'anal-retentive type', to use a Freudian term. (It is no small coincidence that neat arsenic is a powerful purgative.) According to Freud, the anal-retentive type has become stuck emotionally at the stage in early childhood (known commonly as the 'terrible twos') when the child has learned to say "no", and punishes the parents by refusing to cooperate, especially by retaining his stool defiantly. The adult anal type is always saying no, resisting, and holding his anger in. To quote Freud, the anal type becomes 'orderly, parsimonious and obstinate. Parsimony may appear in the exaggerated form of avarice; and obstinacy can go over into defiance, to which rage and revengefulness are easily joined'. In these few words Freud summed up most of the characteristic negative qualities of Arsenicum. If we look to Kent's repertory we find Arsenicum listed under the following rubrics; Obstinate, Fastidious, Avarice and Rage. (It is ironic that Freud himself was almost certainly Arsenicum constitutionally, judging from both his appearance and his character).

## Fastidiousness

When I was a child, my aunt, on meeting me, would check my fingernails for dirt before asking me how I was. If my nails were too long, she had her scissors at the ready, and would set about trimming them with all the authority and zeal of a priest performing a sacred rite. Indeed, to my aunt, cleanliness was next to godliness. My mother tolerated the uninvited manicures. What did irk her somewhat was Auntie's habit of walking up to the mantelpiece on entering our house, and running her finger along the top, looking for dust.

Arsenicums try to create order in their environment in an attempt to allay anxiety. They are the most fastidious of all the constitutional types (excluding the more pathologically obsessive fastidiousness of some Syphilinums and Veratrums). Nux is the only other remedy listed in the repertory under the rubric 'Fastidious', but Nux is really concerned more with efficiency than orderliness, hence he is often tidy at work, but not at home. (Natrum and Causticum should be added to the rubric 'fastidiousness'.)

Arsenicum individuals have an attention for detail that is unsurpassed. They often choose meticulous occupations, such as accountancy, manicurist and fine craftwork. Arsenicum is a perfectionist at work, particularly with regard to the final appearance of the product, whether it be a bookshelf, a ledger sheet or a painting. All the i's will be dotted, all the t's crossed. Natrum is also a perfectionist at work in many cases, which results in some homeopaths confusing the two types. There are subtle differences between the two in this regard. Natrum is very self-critical, and feels guilty or a failure when his work is not perfect. This is really a compensatory mechanism for his sense of being unworthy. Arsenicum, on the other hand, is motivated more by a fear of chaos and physical disintegration. He feels anxious but not guilty if the work is not perfect. Furthermore, Arsenicum imposes his meticulous standards upon those around him, whereas Natrum generally applies them only to himself (and sometimes his family).

As one would expect, Arsenicum's attention to detail is usually expressed in the clothes he wears. Here we see two types of Arsenicum. One is pragmatic but lacks flair. His clothes are immaculately clean and smart (even his casual clothes look freshly pressed) but rather staid. The other type is equally tidy in appearance, but always looks chic as well. Hering referred to this type of Arsenicum as the 'gold-headed cane patient'. The separation of Arsenicum individuals into these two sub-types occurred relatively early in homeopathic history, the former being labelled (somewhat unkindly) the 'drawhorse', the latter the 'thoroughbred'.

Arsenicum is just as meticulous at home as he is at work. I once shared a flat with an Arsenicum man, who would always scan the kitchen with eagle eyes as he walked through, on the lookout for any dish that I may have failed to put away. In particular he had a habit of reminding me each day to hang the wash cloth up to dry after using it, and he would become distinctly annoyed if I overlooked this. After several months of politely pointing out every minor transgression of mine, he eventually exploded with rage one day when I didn't have time to wash the dishes before going out. Months of smouldering resentment poured forth, taking me totally by surprise.

The latter incident illustrates Arsenicum's tendency to feel resentful when his own high standards (high in a material sense) are not adhered to by others. Since most people are not as fastidious as Arsenicum, circumstances which generate resentment are liable to occur every day, producing in many cases a kind of sourness, as the accumulated resentment trickles out little by little.

The fastidiousness or attention to detail that is so characteristic of Arsenicum sometimes applies not only to the ordering of physical things, but also to speech. My Arsenicum aunt, for example, would correct sloppy grammar and pronunciation just as zealously as she removed dirt from fingernails. Her own syntax and pronunciation were immaculate—Arsenicum tends to practice what she preaches.

The more integrated Arsenicum individual learns to accept a more relaxed standard, and is less prone to resentment, but this does not come easily, and the perceptive homeopath will notice subtle ways in which even the more relaxed Arsenicum client attempts to impose order upon the environment.

### *Physical Insecurity*

The insecurity of Arsenicum (which drives him to control his environment) is on a more physical plane than that of Natrum Muriaticum or Pulsatilla, who are looking for emotional security. In addition to fastidiousness, it manifests as an unrealistic fear of poverty and destitution, leading to the characteristic frugality, or downright meanness, of Arsenicum when it comes to spending money, especially upon others. Arsenicum people tend to keep a tight hold on the purse strings, out of a fear that they will not have enough to get by on in future. It also leads to a tendency for the Arsenicum individual to collect or hoard almost any spare item that may one day come in useful. Bits of string, paperclips, scrap paper and empty jars will all be carefully saved and put tidily away for future use. "Waste not, want not" and "If you look after the pennies, the pounds will look after themselves" are sayings that in all likelihood were coined by Arsenicums. Dickens' character Ebenezer Scrooge is a beautifully faithful portrait of the more extreme kind of Arsenicum miser. To Scrooge financial correctness came before all else, eclipsing all considerations of the heart. In true Arsenicum style, Scrooge attempted to justify his meanness on moral grounds, condemning the irresponsibility that led other people into debt. He was not only mean, but also obsessively punctual, and totally unrelenting when imposing his standards upon others. However, even Scrooge had a heart, and like him, many Arsenicums learn to modify their tight fiscal control in favour of more humane considerations.

Hypochondriasis is another expression of the physical insecurity of Arsenicum (Kent: 'Delusions of illness'). The fear of illness can lead to an obsession with personal hygiene (though not to the extent seen in the closely related Syphilinum), and also with diet. The hypochondriacal Arsenicum individual may take a cupboardful of dietary supplements each day in an attempt to ward off sickness, and is likely to subscribe to every health magazine on the market. One common obsession is with regular bowel habit. In keeping with Freud's description of the anal-retentive type, the Arsenicum individual may become overly concerned with her bowel habit (and that of her children) even in the absence of constipation. (This obsession appears to be more common in Arsenicum women than men.) Old ladies who are addicted to purgatives, and who eventually end up in hospital with potassium deficiency, are often Arsenicum types.

When the Arsenicum patient is sick he is likely to take it very seriously. His concern with treating minor ailments like colds enthusiastically with vitamin

C, inhalations and even bedrest may appear to be nothing more than prudence, but underlying his 'sensible', thorough approach is the fear of serious illness and ultimately of death. The more anxious members of the Arsenicum family will experience very real fear on catching a cold or developing a cough; the basic Arsenicum fear of physical annihilation.

Some Arsenicum people are so hypochondriacal that they end up 'doing the rounds' of doctors and therapists, rejecting each one in turn because they fail to recognise the deadly disease that the patient is sure he has. Cancer is a particularly common fear amongst Arsenicums. The slightest symptoms may convince the anxious Arsenicum that he has cancer, and send him to the doctor to be saved if it is not too late. Ironically, the Arsenicum individual really is more prone to developing cancer constitutionally than most other types. One could argue that the constant fear of deadly disease eventually manifests just that in the body, or alternatively that the Arsenicum individual realises, at least subconsciously, that he is more prone to cancer than most.

Even relatively well balanced Arsenicums have a fear of death that haunts them from time to time. They may feel uneasy at funerals, when hearing of the death of someone whom they were not particularly close to, or when the subject of death comes up in conversation. Death is the ultimate uncontrollable unknown, and the very thought of it generates anxiety in the security-conscious Arsenicum mind. Similarly, Arsenicum has a fear of being alone in the dark, and a tendency for ailments and anxieties to intensify at night, particularly in the small hours, when the unconscious mind is more accessible, and chaos knocks on the door. (It is interesting that Syphilinum, a remedy type very close to Arsenicum, has just the opposite—a love-affair with all things deathly.)

## Anxiety

Arsenicum is one of the principal 'anxious remedies'. In the relatively well balanced individual anxiety may not be a big problem. It may surface occasionally as an irrational fear that finances are running out, that the spot on his arm is malignant, or that his children have some serious illness. Most Arsenicums are well in control of their life, and can absorb a lot of stress before their defence mechanisms break down. Consequently a great many Arsenicum patients will not come over as anxious in the consulting room. The younger ones in particular are likely to appear confident and fearless. It is only when life has dealt Arsenicum a few heavy blows that he begins to fall prey to anxiety in a big way. Until then he usually gives an impression of confidence in public, and this impression is not misleading (as it often is with Lycopodium and Natrum Muriaticum). Arsenicum is closely related to both Nux Vomica and Sulphur, and shares the self-confidence of these types to some extent. However, under continued stress Arsenicum will develop anxiety to a far greater extent.

Since Arsenicum individuals tend to be self-disciplined and in control of their lives, (rather like the Kalis and the Natrums), they are liable to break quite suddenly when they can no longer cope with stress. When this happens it is generally called a 'nervous breakdown'. Anxiety suddenly becomes overwhelming, and the person ceases to function rationally. In the case of Arsenicum the anxiety will generally focus upon the characteristic fears of illness, death and poverty, as well as free-floating fear, particularly when alone and at night. However, a really anxious Arsenicum can become afraid of just about anything. (There are fourteen rubrics for Arsenicum in Kent's repertory in black type or italics under the heading 'anxiety'.)

The most obvious thing about a very anxious Arsenicum person is his restlessness. (Kent: 'Anguish-driving him from place to place.) He becomes extremely agitated, and cannot keep still for a moment. The doctor is faced with a patient who paces up and down, wringing his hands and despairing of relief. Unlike an agitated Phosphorus, an agitated Arsenicum is very hard to reassure. If you tell him that everything will be alright, he may stop his pacing for a moment and say "Oh Doctor, do you really think so?", and then return to his despair and his agitation as if nothing had been said. Like Aconite, he may think that he is about to die, and nothing will persuade him to the contrary (except a high potency of Arsenicum). Sometimes this state of fearful agitation is seen in those who really are dying. In these cases a dose of the remedy can bring about a peaceful end.

Some anxious Arsenicums develop a fear of being poisoned. This form of paranoia is commonly seen in senile patients, who most probably resonated to the energy of Arsenicum all of their life, but did not display this characteristic until their mental health had deteriorated towards dementia. Many highly poisonous remedies have this fear of being poisoned as part of their remedy-picture, therefore, it is not surprising to find it in Arsenicum, which for centuries was the most popular poison in Europe.

## Suspicion

The paranoia of the agitated Arsenicum is an exaggeration of the suspiciousness seen even in relatively healthy cases. Typically the Arsenicum patient will make very sure of the qualifications and the competence of the therapist before agreeing to proceed with treatment. Having ascertained that you are a medical doctor as well as a homeopath, she may go on to enquire, "How long have you been practising?", and, "Have you ever done any harm with your treatments?" If you tell her that you are going to give her arsenic, you will have to work very hard to regain her trust!

The suspiciousness of Arsenicum is simply another expression of the physical insecurity of the type. Arsenicum people are cautious by nature. They will scrutinise a business proposal very carefully with their highly discriminating intellect, searching for hidden dangers. Generally they will favour practical security over emotional satisfaction, when an opportunity for the latter may endanger the former. The Arsenicum father, for example, is liable to be even more suspicious of his daughter's boyfriends than most, especially if the relationship is 'serious'. He will generally be more concerned with the financial prospects of his potential son-in-law than the question of whether his daughter will be happy with the latter. Arsenicum's suspicion is basically a desire for assurance that nothing will endanger the physical security of himself and his loved ones. In contrast, Natrum is far more worried about protecting emotional security.

### Down to Earth

Arsenicum is one of those types that combines a sharp intellect with a sound practical sense. Like Nux, practical realities are important to Arsenicum. He may enjoy an abstract intellectual discussion, but only if he has first fixed the tap that was leaking, and paid the rent. The Arsenicum boss will be exacting of his subordinates with regard to practical details, noting every instance of wastage or inefficiency. Similarly, the Arsenicum employee will be both meticulous and conscientious, and furthermore will usually possess a higher than average ability to make practical improvisations and adjustments. (Sulphur is a great ideas man, but Nux and Arsenicum will get the job done.)

Many Arsenicum people make use of their practical skills by becoming craftsmen (and women). Mechanics, carpenters, gardeners and artists are some of the practical occupations favoured by Arsenicum. The image of the careful craftsman, diligently producing quality work, is one of the more positive expressions of the Arsenicum persona. Natrum Muriaticum, Silica and the Kalis all tend to be conscientious at work, but Arsenicum combines this with practical ability more than any other type.

Like other down to Earth types, Arsenicum people usually derive a great deal of pleasure from the physical senses. In this they most resemble Silica, since their sensual enjoyment is coupled with a high degree of discrimination or sophistication. Hence Arsenicums tend to appreciate fine cuisine, fine music and fine art. Arsenicum may be diligent in his work, but he usually likes to find time for life's finer pleasures as well, and does not begrudge himself a certain amount of indulgence.

### The Aristocrat

The traditional separation of Arsenicum into two sub-types is justified in my experience. There are those that are more earthy and practical, and those that are more refined and intellectual. The latter has been traditionally called the 'thoroughbred', since he (or she) tends to have long elegant body lines, and refined facial features. This type tends to have an aristocratic air, regardless of his actual status in society. All Arsenicums are proud people, but the aristocratic type often takes this as far as being contemptuous of his fellow man (Kent: 'Contemptuous, Critical, Censorious').Only those who are as refined as he thinks he is are given the time of day. The sneer of distaste at an undignified sight or comment is one of the thoroughbred's favourite weapons. I have noticed that many of the more contemptuous Arsenicum people that I have come across actually have an anatomically upturned nose (especially the women), as if centuries of disdain have been bred into the features.

The aristocratic Arsenicum individual is even more concerned with appearances than his more earthy brothers. He will choose the finest clothes to wear, his hair will be immaculate, and his home will be filled with delicate pieces of art. Discrimination is the keynote of the thoroughbred, in both the positive and negative aspects of the word. Whatever is crude is rejected, whether it be a person or a necktie. Naturally, most people would find it difficult to be around such a person. Confident assertive types like Sulphur and Nux Vomica would be most able to withstand the criticism that a discriminating Arsenicum is likely to dish out from time to time. On the other hand, Silica and Ignatia will share Arsenicum's love of refinement, and Natrum Muriaticum tends to be a perfectionist, and hence may live up to the refined Arsenicum's expectations.

Even the less refined Arsenicum tends to have a great concern for appearances. I have noticed that those Arsenicums who are relatively poor materially have a tendency to exaggerate what they do have, in an effort to avoid the stigma they themselves attach to poverty. One such patient of mine had never worked for a living. He had a relatively minor physical disability which enabled him to obtain a disability allowance, upon which he lived in meagre conditions. During the consultation, however, he would often refer to how high his standard of living was, considering his low income. He was clearly concerned with compensating for the lack of prestige which he felt as a result of his lowly social status.

Another Arsenicum patient of mine had once been wealthy, but had since fallen upon hard times. She always wore her finest clothes when she saw me, and preferred to talk about her previous life of wealth and status, rather than facing the reality of her present situation. Most (but not all) Arsenicums seek wealth and prestige, either through their own efforts, or through marriage, and a great many find it.

Because the refined Arsenicum is so discriminating, he may become rather 'precious', in the sense of being too refined to tolerate normal everyday living conditions. This is particularly true of those Arsenicums who are both refined and hypochondriacal. To protect themselves they exclude all 'gross' influences from their lives, and in the process they tend to exclude most people as well. I remember one such man who was an interior designer by profession. He was tall, and thin in the extreme, and he always wore very dignified clothes, particularly double-breasted suits and cravats. He was in his fifties, and had never found a woman who could live up to his exacting standards. He spent a lonely life, looking for the companionship that had eluded him. He almost found it in the person of my Arsenicum aunt, but, alas, he was too precious even for her.

This preciousness that we see in some Arsenicums is a result of an excessive refinement. Like a thoroughbred horse, or a greyhound, the body and mind are so finely balanced that they easily become temperamental and highly strung. If they don't have exactly the right conditions they become sick, either physically or emotionally. In this case the most likely emotional disturbance would be anxiety.

A precious Arsenicum man tends to appear effeminate, since he is anything but robust. His main interests are likely to be the arts, health and diet, all of which he tends to be rather obsessive about (Kent: 'Mood—finicky). Silica, Ignatia and China may also become so refined that they become oversensitive. Nevertheless, none of these three types has the same 'precious' quality that we see in some Arsenicums, which reminds one of a spoilt or overprotected child. This is because, in addition to refinement and hypochondriasis, selfishness or self-obsession is a prominent feature of Arsenicum.

### Determination, Anger and Selfishness

As I have said previously, Arsenicum is closely related to Nux, and shares some of the latter's determination. Arsenicum tends to be one-pointed in his activities. Whatever is dear to him he will pursue thoroughly, and he will become angry if someone tries to prevent him from doing so (Kent: 'Obstinate"). All but the most anxious Arsenicum individuals are independent by nature. They make up their own mind and then stick to it. Silica is also like this, but Arsenicum has more will-power and confidence than Silica when it comes to expressing his viewpoint, and implementing his desires.

The one-pointedness of Arsenicum is accompanied by a certain degree of inflexibility in most cases. This may result in a lack of openness to the opinions of others, and an intolerance of different attitudes and lifestyles. I came across this once in a newly acquired acquaintance who was unable to accept that at the time I was a vegetarian. She would lecture me on the selfishness of expecting others to accommodate my idiosyncrasy, positively indignant that I would not eat her meat, although she knew in advance that I was vegetarian. I soon discovered, from chatting to her husband, that she was obsessively clean, and had an irrational fear of death, which confirmed my suspicion that she was Arsenicum constitutionally.

Selfishness is a characteristic that may be possessed by individuals of any constitutional type, even the angelic Phosphorus. There are, however, different ways in which selfishness manifests, according to constitution. Thus Sulphur tends to be lazy, and will neglect his family in favour of his pet enthusiasm, whereas Ignatia is often spoilt, and reacts petulantly when she feels ignored. The selfishness of Arsenicum is more global, in that it tends to manifest as a general tendency to put self before others. This is particularly true of Arsenicum men. The women tend to be less selfish, but will still tend to put themselves and their family before others to a greater extent than other constitutional types. This lack of generosity is related to the physical insecurity of Arsenicum. It is as though Arsenicum feels that he cannot afford to be generous, either physically or emotionally; he may need whatever he has in future.

At the extreme end of Arsenicum's range there are individuals who are cold and cruel, who seem to have no feeling at all for others, and a great deal of sourness and anger indeed. The police-officer Javert in Victor Hugo's 'Les Miserables' is an excellent example of this type. His life becomes an obsessive vendetta, dedicated to pursuing a criminal who has broken his parole. In typical Arsenicum fashion Javert justifies his meanness with an attitude of moral superiority. He is as pious as he is cruel, although his piety is really a love of orderliness, rather than a love of God. Faced with the increasingly obvious natural goodness of his quarry, he eventually commits suicide rather than face the fact that his rigid, by-the-book morality is merely an instrument or vehicle for his hatred.

Just as any constitutional type can be selfish, so any type can be unselfish as well. Not all Arsenicum people are especially selfish. Some are generous and philanthropic, deriving pleasure from helping others. The more generous Arsenicum is often to be seen in the role of a benign authority figure. Scout masters and school teachers are the sort of roles which allow Arsenicum to help others, and at the same time teach the qualities of self-discipline and orderliness that are so dear to them.

Irritability is another characteristic that may be possessed by any constitutional type, but it is certainly more frequently encountered in some than others, and Arsenicum is one of the more easily irritated types. (Arsenicum is listed in Kent's repertory in italics or black type under five separate irritability rubrics.) Arsenicum is most liable to become irritated by untidiness, inefficiency and waste. All of these refer to the material plane of existence, which is usually Arsenicum's principal focus. The more sophisticated Arsenicum individual learns to hide his irritation and anger most of the time, but this is not achieved without considerable cost. Many Arsenicum men in particular carry around with them a volcano of smouldering anger, which one day may erupt when the irritation is too great to ignore. Then the years of accumulated bitterness may pour forth, in either physical or verbal aggression (Kent: 'Rage', 'Malicious', 'Sudden impulse to kill'). In the mean time, the effort to suppress anger and irritation results in tension, a problem for a great many Arsenicum individuals.

## *Relating*

Arsenicum individuals usually make loyal and dependable partners. They are quite capable of being affectionate, though not overly so. Given the propensity for loneliness of the type, a mate is often the sole source of intimacy for the Arsenicum individual, and family life can become a highly valued focus for the person's whole life, providing a haven of comfort and security in a world that is perceived, at least to some degree, as being hostile. The relationship may at times be strained by the fastidiousness and critical tendency of Arsenicum, but Arsenicum people can provide less practical partners with a sound grip on material realities. It is usually the Arsenicum partner who keeps a check on finances, and prevents the more spontaneous Sulphur or Phosphorus mate from taking foolhardy risks. One quality that Arsenicum demands in any relationship is respect. He or she will give to the relationship as long as the giving is mutual. Arsenicum has too much self-respect to allow any spouse to dominate or take advantage.

Arsenicums usually make devoted parents, taking their parental duties very seriously, and feeling genuinely concerned for their children's welfare. They are not likely to be indulgent parents, and they may err on the side of being disciplinarian at times. In such families it is preferable that the spouse is a softer, more indulgent type, to provide balance. Some Arsenicum parents have a tendency to value the child's material prospects in life more highly than his emotional fulfilment. In other words, like many parents, they may impose their own value system upon their children. This naturally produces rebellion in children, and can leave the less flexible Arsenicum parent feeling unappreciated, and wondering where they went wrong.

On the positive side, children who have an Arsenicum parent usually know that they can rely on him or her to be both honest and consistent, and such children will grow up knowing what integrity means, and honouring certain values which give life stability and meaning. Often the Arsenicum parent will provide a model of community service, helping out neighbours in practical ways, recycling the rubbish, and setting up neighbourhood watch schemes. Arsenicum enjoys making a practical contribution to the community, and is often active in opposing new developments which threaten the harmony and environmental integrity of the neighbourhood. In this way his innate conservatism is a positive asset to the community.

Arsenicum people often value the extended family as a source of support and social enjoyment. Within this familiar circle they tend to be at their most relaxed, and are often both jovial and relatively warm. Although Arsenicum individuals tend not to be very expressive of tender feelings, they will always 'be there' for their family in times of stress, and can make excellent counsellors when family and friends are in trouble, since they are sensible, intelligent and have a strong sense of values, as well as a desire to help those that are close to them.

When dealing with people outside the family, Arsenicum individuals tend to be polite, but a little aloof. They may be open, in the sense of being willing to talk about themselves, and even share their feelings with others, but still a barrier remains in most cases. This is the same kind of distance that the Kali individual tends to maintain between himself and others. It is mainly unconscious and unintentional, and it may leave Arsenicum wondering why he or she cannot get close to other people. This emotional distance is usually more pronounced in Arsenicum men than women, and it results from the individual living more in his rational, highly discriminating intellect than in his heart, and from constantly making judgements of others.

Arsenicum women are often quite sentimental, and sensitive to the feelings of others, particularly to another's suffering. They are likely to respond with anger as well as sympathy when they see someone being abused, and are frequently quick to offer practical help at such times. The Arsenicum woman tends to be very protective of her family, and relates easily to others who are seeking to protect their own emotional security from outside interference. For example, an Arsenicum woman is likely to be very supportive of a friend whose husband is having an affair. This is not only because she has high morals, and because she loves her friend, but also because she knows how devastated she would feel in the same situation. She is likely to feel angry and even bitter towards her friend's husband for threatening something as sacred (and reassuring) as marriage.

Arsenicum women are just as determined as their male counterparts, but they are usually more expert at using guile to achieve their goals. Such women are often adept at getting their own way without seeming to assert themselves, using subtle leverage to manipulate their partner. Arsenicums of both sexes can be scheming, but the women do it more gracefully! Similarly, the Arsenicum woman may impose her will upon friends and acquaintances with the judicious use of veiled threats. When the conversation is drifting in a direction that she does not approve of (e.g. towards favouring her husband's preference for a drink before dinner) she may give a look to the speaker for just one instant that is so penetratingly cold that he changes his words. The 'attack' may have been so swift and surgical that he does not even realise what has happened.

The security-consciousness of Arsenicum women often results in a reluctance to move far away from the parental home. Like Natrum women, they find the proximity of their parents reassuring, and also are liable to feel guilty if they cannot be there for them in times of need. Arsenicum men also tend to be very diligent in caring for elderly parents, and they are liable to expect their own offspring to do likewise.

### *Physical Appearance*

Physically, Arsenicums tend to divide along the lines of the thoroughbred and the drawhorse, with considerable overlap between them. Both types have a taut, sinewy body, and bony facial features. The refined type has a slim body, with long bony fingers. The women tend to be 'petite', with small delicate facial features, and the men often have narrow aquiline noses, giving a Roman or hawkish appearance (Kent: 'Nose-pointed'). The refined type has fine hair, which is usually straight.

The more earthy type has a short, muscular or stocky body, with short strong limbs and a less refined facial appearance, which still tends towards boniness. The eyes often have a kind of hollow look about them, being set back a little in their sockets. The hair is more likely to be black than that of the refined type (which is often light brown), and is thicker and coarser.

# *Aurum Metallicum*

*Keynote:* Loathing of life

It's not much fun being an Aurum individual. One of the nicest things about treating Aurum cases is seeing some lightness enter their lives after taking the remedy. Like the gold from which the remedy is made, there is a great heaviness about Aurum, a heaviness that in most cases has been there since early childhood. When a patient reports that he has been depressed all of his life, think of Aurum. For the Aurum individual, some degree of depression is a normal state of being. They do from time to time enter into deep and seemingly hopeless depressions, but even in between these episodes there is a feeling of a dark cloud continually hanging over them.

### The Sensitive Heart

The Aurum child grows up sensing that love is only forthcoming from his parents when he does his best to please them. Often the parents were very exacting, expecting the child to excel at school, or at whatever they were good at, or had wanted to be good at but were not. Such parents reward the child when he succeeds, and punish him whenever he does not fulfil their expectations. The Aurum child is extremely sensitive to criticism (Kent: 'Oversensitive', 'Ailments from scorn'), since criticism from his parents implies that he has not pleased them, and hence is not loved by them. In order to avoid the pain of rejection, the child learns to do his best at all times. This produces a seriousness and a lack of spontaneity in the Aurum child, which usually progresses to feelings of depression and despair even before the child becomes an adult. (Exactly the same dynamics occur in the childhood of many Natrum Muriaticum children, and the results are similar, but less severe.)

### Isolation and Relationship

The emotional pain that the Aurum child experiences as a result of highly conditional parental love (or sometimes no love at all), is severe, and results in a protective walling off of the heart. Only by shutting down the emotions can Aurum avoid the hurt that is always there inside. Aurum learns early to be independent, to rely on nobody but himself, and to show no signs of weakness. In relationships he is inaccessible, never giving totally of himself, since that would open up the old wounds that never heal. This is one of the loneliest of constitutional types, combining great sensitivity with fear of rejection. Aurum is listed in black type in Kent's repertory under the rubric 'Forsaken feeling'. All Aurums were abandoned by their parents emotionally to some extent, and the feeling of being totally alone in the world never really leaves them.

When Aurum is in a romantic relationship he will sense that there is a chance of being loved for himself and hence of healing the wounds within. This will produce a struggle inside between the urge to protect himself, and the desire to be loved. He may gradually open up to his partner (the vast majority of Aurums are male), and if the relationship continues to go well the old walls of deliberate isolation will break down, and something of a healing may take place. In such cases Aurum will become a devoted partner, and will value the relationship above all else in his life. He will also become a devoted father in many cases, and will strive to avoid the mistakes that his parents made. Not all Aurum relationships go so well. Sometimes Aurum will succeed in finding a reasonably satisfying relationship, but will take out his anger on his children. Aurum usually has a great deal of anger inside, as a result of the 'neglect' that he experienced as a child. Despite finding a loving relationship, the anger may remain, and come out in bursts of explosive temper from time to time. (Aurum is listed in Kent's repertory in black type or italics under eight separate anger rubrics.) Since he is a sensitive man, and has known a great deal of emotional pain, he is liable to feel very guilty after these outbursts of temper (Kent: 'Remorse').

Another danger for the married Aurum individual is that he falls into the same type of behaviour as his parents. (His father may very well have been Aurum himself.) Aurum will usually grow up with a tendency to strive very hard to prove himself, and he may not be able to stop himself from pushing his children in the same way as he pushes himself. For all types of people, the sins of the fathers have a habit of being visited upon the sons.

Like Ignatia and Natrum Muriaticum, Aurum is listed in Kent's repertory in black type under the rubrics 'Grief' and 'Ailments from disappointed love'. It is not difficult to see why this should be. If Aurum does finally manage to open his heart and share the much needed love of another person, he has made himself very vulnerable. If he should then be left by his partner, either through separation or bereavement, the pain that he will feel is immense. At such times there is a danger of Aurum entering into a profound depression. (This applies to the loss of any loved one, not just a partner.)

### *The Driven Man*

As I have said previously, the Aurum child learns to do his best in order to win parental approval. This often results in a life-long struggle to be seen to be successful by society. It is very important for many Aurums to have a prestigious position socially and professionally, and for this reason they often become workaholics. The typical Aurum takes few holidays, and is likely to spend half his holiday working. Aurum is probably the second most ambitious constitutional type. Only Nux Vomica is more universally ambitious, and there are great differences between the two types. Unlike Aurum, Nux is generally open, gregarious and optimistic. One could say that Nux is a natural leader, a born achiever who is full of self-confidence and has no self-doubts. Aurum on the other hand becomes ambitious as a reaction to parental pressure, and in order to compensate for the lack of self-worth that he feels deep inside his heart. (Natrum Muriaticum can become a workaholic and a perfectionist for exactly the same reasons as Aurum, but is generally not so ambitious. Indeed there are too many similarities between Natrum and Aurum to list. Basically one could say that Aurum is like Natrum Muriaticum, only more so. Most of Natrum's characteristics are present in Aurum in a more extreme form. Thus the lack of self-worth is greater, the tendency to isolation stronger, and the depression deeper in Aurum.)

In their struggle to be somebody important, Many Aurums are seduced by wealth, and the influence and respect that it brings. For some Aurums it is enough to be wealthy. They do not become workaholics, since their wealth brings them all the sense of self-worth that they need. If such a person loses his wealth, he loses all of his self-respect, and this is another potent stimulus for depression in Aurum. Many of the stockbrokers who threw themselves from the top windows of their skyscraping empires during the great Wall Street crash of the Thirties must have been Aurum individuals. It is interesting that potentised gold can bring relief to the sufferings of those who seek refuge in great wealth. Many a reclusive millionaire would do well to exchange a little of their solid gold for its homeopathic equivalent.

Aurum individuals usually have a strong analytical intellect, and appear cold and detached, particularly at work. They are liable to be very exacting with employees, expecting the same high standards from them which they expect of themselves, and allowing a minimum of leisure time. At work Aurum is totally one-pointed, allowing nothing to distract him from his goals. As a result, he often rises to executive positions quickly. Kali Carbonicum, Arsenicum and Nux also tend to be very focussed at work, and often very exacting of their employees, but all of these types are more relaxed and human at work than Aurum, who resembles a robot in comparison, not the dry automatic robot that some Kalis resemble, but the driven, unstoppable machine that features in films like 'Robocop'.

### Rage

Aurum is a very controlled person. He is one of the least spontaneous of all constitutional types. This can be seen in his body, which has a tense, rigid quality to it, like steel, and in his movements, which tend to be precise and staccato like a robot. Aurum tends to sit bolt upright in his chair. This rigidity is largely the result of controlling an enormous reservoir of anger. Aurum seldom loses his temper, but when he does, it is very powerful (Kent: 'Violent-vehement'). More often he bottles his anger inside, adding to the existing tension. Like Natrum Muriaticum, Aurum can feel hateful and resentful towards those who have offended him. He tends to be oversensitive to criticism, since it reminds him of his mortification as a child when he was rejected by his parents. This is probably why Aurum is listed in the repertory under the rubric 'Intolerant of contradiction', since this is a form of criticism or rejection.

A few Aurum individuals manage, through introspection, to identify the childhood family dynamics which gave rise to their impoverished sense of self-worth. In these cases one of two things can happen; on the one hand they may reject their parents' value system, and often that of the established society as a whole as well. In this case a deep bitterness usually remains, and the individual may decide that the world is a jungle, to be subjugated by force or manipulated by guile. I remember one such case, a young man who was thrown into a deep depression by bankruptcy. At one time he had been a millionaire. He had gained his wealth through bank-fraud, and he told me that he had suffered no pangs of conscience at the time, since the system was utterly corrupt, and hence was fair game for criminal exploitation. Although he could see that it was not a healthy way to make a living, he was tormented by the temptation to return to crime, since it was the only way he knew to earn the vast sums of money that he needed to feel good about himself. When he talked of the power and respect that he felt when he was rich, his eyes lit up and came alive for the only time during the interview. The rest of the time he sat rigid and motionless, his face mask-like except for the brief moments when he broke down and cried.

On the other hand, the Aurum person may seek a genuine healing through psychotherapy, and those forms of therapy which allow the subject to contact and express deeply suppressed feelings of anger and sadness that originated in childhood are particularly helpful in allowing the Aurum individual to break out of his prison of isolation and unhappiness, and find some genuine self-love. I was privileged to be present during the therapy of one Aurum patient, a man in his mid-thirties who was struggling to regain a sense of connectedness with other people, having withdrawn behind a mask of cool detachment. His father was a wealthy businessman, who despaired of his son's lack of material advancement. During therapy he contacted enormous anger towards his father, which he was able to release harmlessly in a safe environment. After this release he found that the barrier that he had erected between himself and others was noticeably softer, enabling him to make more intimate contact. (This confirms to some extent the psychoanalytic view that depression results from the internalisation of anger.) Even without psychotherapy, the remedy in high potency can bring about a great lightening of Aurum's burden, and a reduction in the frequency and severity of depressive episodes. The combination of homeopathy and deep psychotherapy can remove the very basis of Aurum's malaise.

### The Blackness

The depression of Aurum is usually diagnosed by psychiatrists as 'endogenous' or 'organic', a recognition of the constitutional susceptibility of the type towards deep depression. When depressed, Aurum falls into a pit of despair, self-loathing (Kent: 'Reproaches self'), self-recrimination, isolation and increasing mental paralysis. Nothing is blacker than the despair of Aurum. It is silent, without weeping for the most part, and the patient will continue to function efficiently in the world until the last moment, when he will either slip into hysterical weeping and be unable to collect his thoughts, or he will commit suicide. Aurum is far more likely to kill himself during a suicide attempt than other depressive types like Natrum Muriaticum and Ignatia, who are often seeking to attract some help by taking an overdose. Aurum is more likely to use some violent method like jumping off a bridge or driving his car into a brick wall (Kent: 'Jumping from a window'). It may be that these more violent methods resonate with the rage that underlies Aurum's depression.

Suicide is often viewed as an attractive option by Aurum. Like the haunted central character of Herman Hesse's 'Steppenwolfe', the Aurum individual may see death as a comforting thought, an escape route to fall back on if life becomes too painful. Even in the absence of serious depression Aurum may think fondly of death. One Aurum patient told me that the shadow of death had been with him throughout his life, as a kind of familiar friend, a constant backdrop to the rest of his experience.

Some Aurum people court death by engaging in dangerous pursuits like rock-climbing and motor racing. Treading the tightrope between life and death the Aurum individual often feels most alive and carefree (as does the wild Staphysagria). When he does descend into the depths of depression, suicidal thoughts arise. At such times dicing with death can bring some relief, and the depressed Aurum will often take a fast car ride to escape from himself.

During a crisis of depression, Aurum may drive himself at work, and also physically, in an attempt to hold himself together. One depressed Aurum patient of mine would take icy-cold swims in the early morning, as if trying to shock himself out of his depression. He would follow this up with a gruelling physical work-out in the gym, and since he could not face food, he became extremely gaunt and grey. Fortunately, a couple of doses of Aurum 10M brought him out of his depression, and put an end to his asceticism.

Although Aurum is a constitutional type, some depressed patients slip into an Aurum state who do not normally resonate to the Aurum wavelength. Many of the profoundly depressed patients in psychiatric wards would benefit from the remedy, including the female ones. All of the typical features of endogenous depression are found in the remedy picture. These include flat emotional expression, despair of recovery, sense of wretchedness (and hence of deserving punishment) and slowness of thinking. It is hard to reach the patient in such a state. They sit totally absorbed in their own tormented thoughts. If you ask a question, they will stare blankly for a few moments before replying, and they may be unable to clarify their thoughts sufficiently to tell you what they are feeling. Or they may suddenly break down and weep uncontrollably (Kent: 'Weeping, involuntary').

Aurum's depression is full of intensity (Kent: 'Anguish'), a torture that results in increasingly insistent suicidal urges. One elderly man who had been depressed for many years sat in my consulting room talking of nothing but suicide, berating himself for his failed previous attempts, calling himself a coward. The tension inside was tremendous, indeed he said to me "I'm not depressed, it's this terrible tension inside, like my head will blow off. I think suicide is the only option." Then he slammed his fist on the table, exclaiming in an anguished voice, "Damn it! I can't go on, I'll have to end it." I have never seen such intensity in a Natrum depression. After a few doses of Aurum Metallicum 10M he was a different person. He still felt somewhat depressed, but the intensity of his suffering had abated, and so had the suicidal thoughts.

Night-time is the worst period for Aurum. At night, and also in winter, the descending darkness intensifies its reflection in Aurum's psyche. It is likely that many of those who suffer from seasonal depressive illness would benefit from the remedy.

Being very much a syphilitic type, Aurum has a strong tendency to become obsessive mentally. In particular he is liable to go over and over past traumas, especially those in which he blames himself in some way. Aurum will frequently blame himself when things go wrong, and hence he will often torture himself with repetitive thoughts of regret and feelings of remorse. Natrum Muriaticum and Causticum also do this, but not nearly to the same extent as Aurum. Nobody is as obsessive about the past as Aurum.

Aurum's remorse will sometimes take the form of religious despair. Some Aurums resort to prayer at an early age as a means of seeking refuge from their own mental prison, and may become quite obsessive about praying, spending hours each day alone in their room in prayer. (The other type that does this is Veratrum.) When these religious Aurums fall into deep depression, a major feature is a sense of being damned (Kent: 'He imagines that he is wholly evil, is not worthy of salvation').

Another aspect of Aurum's depression is obsessive worrying. Particularly in the early stages of Aurum's depression he may mentally exaggerate all the problems he has, seeing relatively minor problems collectively as a mountain of trouble that there is no way to avoid, and being unable to stop worrying about them. This is just an exaggeration of Aurum's usual pessimism, which is loath to recognise anything positive unless it is solid and dependable (like gold).

Aurum is an uncommon constitutional type, and it should not be given routinely for deep depression, which will require Natrum Muriaticum far more frequently. In my practice I see at least two hundred Natrums for every Aurum case. When the pre-morbid personality appears to be Natrum, this should be given during deep depression, unless specific features of the case point to Aurum, including the generals and physical symptoms.

### *Physical Appearance*

Aurum people tend to have compact, muscular bodies. They appear rather stiff and rigid, as a result of muscle tension, which is a result of their struggle to contain powerful subconscious emotions. Their faces are usually rather gaunt and angular, and the expression is generally stiff, again due to muscular tension. Most of the Aurums I have seen have had very dark or black hair.

# Baryta Carbonica

*Keynote:* Immaturity

Baryta Carbonica is one remedy which is most easily understood by comprehending its essence, which runs through the whole remedy picture. All Baryta individuals have some aspect of the personality which has not matured fully. Sometimes it is just one isolated aspect, such as social skills, whilst at other times it is several. Some Barytas have a global underdevelopment of the personality, one that affects all aspects, resulting in a clearly immature individual.

## Origins

The Baryta child's slow development is often accompanied by a history of birth trauma, especially asphyxia, such as occurs when the umbilical cord is wrapped around the neck, preventing adequate oxygen from reaching the brain. In some cases there was physical trauma to the head during birth (or subsequently) resulting in a haemorrhage into the brain. Sometimes there was no physical insult at all, but childhood conditions were unstimulating or neglectful, resulting in slow development both physically and mentally/emotionally. A fourth possibility is that one or both parents were Barytas, and passed on their traits to the child, both genetically and by conditioning.

## Mental Retardation

Cases of gross mental retardation often belong to the Baryta type. The Baryta baby appears dull and relatively unresponsive to stimulation. Milestones such as smiling, standing and walking are delayed, as are subsequent complex skills such as talking, writing and social development. These difficulties remain to varying degrees as the child gets older, manifesting in a variety of ways, including poor concentration at school (Kent: 'Concentration difficult'), decreased comprehension, dyslexia, and behavioural abnormalities. The latter are usually of a passive kind, taking the form of dullness (unresponsiveness), extreme shyness and oversensitivity. Stubbornness is also a common Baryta trait. Like his close relative Calcarea, Baryta has a tendency to dig in his heels and say no when asked to do something. This is partly due to insecurity. Baryta feels instinctively that he is not properly 'equipped' to deal with the complexities of the world, and one of his strategies is to resist change of any kind.

Some Baryta children are of normal intelligence, but have difficulties with speech, writing or social interaction. Because of their intelligence, they have more insight into their condition, and tend to suffer more than those of diminished intelligence. One such child was brought to see me at the age of fourteen, suffering from severe acne. His speech was thick and hesitant, giving an impression of stupidity, (Kent: 'Speech slow'), yet he conversed intelligently, and was of above average ability at school. He complained of being ridiculed and bullied at school, and had been nicknamed 'Brain' by his schoolmates, being fully aware of the cruel irony of the term. Since his acne was severe, I felt it wise to commence with relatively low potencies of Baryta, which were very effective in improving the skin condition. Unfortunately, he did not continue to come for long enough to receive the high potencies which probably would have helped his speech disorder.

It is remarkable that individuals with longstanding brain damage can recover a great deal of function after the remedy is taken. I was once consulted by a man suffering from post-viral syndrome, who told me that much of the stress in his life was generated by his young son, who was severely retarded, and needed constant attention. I suggested that he bring in his son for treatment, which he did. The boy clearly fitted the Baryta picture, and was given three doses of the 10M potency. As an experiment (and unbeknown to me) his father decided to obtain a school report on his son just prior to treatment, and another one three months later. The differences in the two reports were striking (the school was not aware of the child's homeopathic treatment). The second report described a remarkable improvement in the child's condition. Not only was he far more capable and attentive at his lessons, he was also for the first time reliable enough to be given small errands, such as fetching the milk. Baryta appears capable of reactivating arrested development in all the different aspects of physical and mental functioning.

### The Dull Child
Dullness, or lack of interest, responsiveness and enthusiasm, is the principal characteristic of many Baryta children, particularly adolescent boys (Kent: 'Dullness-children'). These children often have no organic brain dysfunction, and no impairment of intelligence. They are just dull, apathetic, reluctant to talk and stubborn. (Kent: 'Averse company', 'Indifferent', 'Mood-indolent', 'Children-indisposition to play', 'Indisposed to talk'). Such children are extremely difficult for the parents to handle, since they will not cooperate, and are not interested in doing anything. In the consulting room they speak single monosyllabic answers to questions, and wear a dull, heavy expression, like someone who has the flu and is depressed. I treated one such boy, again for severe acne, and whilst his skin was undergoing an aggrava-

tion his parents said that the remedy had done miracles for his temperament. For the first time in years he was animated, polite and cooperative, and had regained an interested in his hobbies. This change was evident in the consulting room, where his expression was now cheerful, and his speech far more willing.

These dull Baryta children must be differentiated from Calcarea and Sulphur types, who can appear very similar, both physically and temperamentally. In Baryta the dullness is generally more constant and impenetrable. The dull, lazy Sulphur child will become animated when he is pursuing a pet interest, such as a particular game, or an idea, and then lapse into indolence when it is over. Furthermore, Sulphur has more self-confidence than Baryta. The Baryta child is not only dull, but also shy (Kent: 'Timidity'). In the consulting room he will avert his eyes from the gaze of the homeopath, usually looking down at the floor. The dull Sulphur child is not afraid, but simply bored and defiant. He will look at you without fear when questioned, but his answers will still be short and often evasive, since he is not interested in cooperating

Calcarea children sometimes become apathetic and uncooperative, but seldom to the same extent as Baryta. The dull Calcarea child is usually still quite a social animal, enjoying the company of his friends, but appearing sullen at home, usually because he is feeling defiant towards his parents. There is some shyness, but not nearly to the same extent as Baryta, who will remain suspicious of a stranger long after Calcarea has accepted him.

Another child who may be mistaken for the dull Baryta child is the dull Natrum Muriaticum child. The dull Natrum child appears sullen and will also answer in monosyllables. However, when he can be coaxed into speaking, he is more articulate than Baryta.

### Lack of Refinement

As one grows up, one usually becomes more sophisticated, both intellectually and socially. This refinement is often lacking in Baryta individuals, and this relative crudity of appearance and manner may sometimes be the first impression that strikes one about a Baryta individual, especially an adult Baryta. Whilst Calcarea is generally earthy and uncomplicated, Baryta can be crude and totally lacking in social graces. One Baryta young lady that I knew would always have food stains on her clothes. She was not stupid, yet she tended to dribble when she ate, and did not seem to notice the mess that she made. After a dose of Baryta 10M she not only stopped dribbling her food, but also began to wear attractive clothes, in place of the shapeless assortment of garments that she used to pick up from charity stores. Such is the power of the remedy to accelerate all aspects of development.

Social skills are often the last to be mastered by Baryta, who always retains some degree of shyness (Kent: 'Averse to strangers' company'). I remember one young man who struck me immediately as being of the Baryta type, before I had taken his history. First of all, he had the heavy facial features typical of Baryta, with ridges above the eyes that gave an almost ape-like impression. He was very sociable, but something about his manner told me that he was not at ease in company. His speech was unusually loud, and punctuated by frequent guffaws of bellowing laughter, which was often inappropriate. Similarly, his responses to what other people said were exaggerated. If I said that I was tired, he would commiserate with me as if I were dying, whereas a touch of irony in my voice was greeted with peals of laughter. He was clearly still in the process of learning to refine his rather crude social skills. Some Baryta adults succeed in developing quite mature social skills, but still retain a certain nervousness in company, which might reveal itself as nervous laughter, or as being too keen to please.

### Emotional Immaturity

Many Baryta individuals are well developed intellectually and socially, but remain immature emotionally. Shyness is one aspect of this emotional immaturity. The Baryta child is so shy that he hides behind his mother for the whole interview. The Baryta adult may not go that far, but there is usually a desire to hide when new situations come along, particularly in the presence of strangers. This shyness can be crippling socially, preventing Baryta from leading a normal life, and especially from daring to approach members of the opposite sex. Most Barytas receive more than their fair share of taunts and ridicule as children, and this leaves them with a constant fear of being laughed at (Kent: 'Imagines being abused'). All young people are afraid of making fools of themselves when approaching members of the opposite sex whom they do not know, but Baryta's paranoid fear of being laughed at can make such approaches impossible.

Barytas tend to enter romantic relationships later than other people, partly because of their shyness and fear of rejection, but also because they are likely to be slow in developing an attraction for the opposite sex. This is yet another example of the slow development which is the essence of the type.

When Baryta individuals do find someone with whom they can feel at ease, they are often childlike in their trust and openness, sharing all their fears and all their dreams. They are likely to become very attached to such confidantes, regarding them with affection bordering upon devotion. Being so vulnerable, Baryta is very sensitive to reprimand, and may easily feel rejected by an innocent remark.

The adult Baryta individual struggles to hold his own in a world that seems ruthless and bewildering. Often he will find a protective niche to shelter in, such as a safe job, and a room in a relative's house. The more confident

Baryta may find a devoted partner, who can provide the reassurance and security that he needs.

Baryta is one of the more fearful remedy types. Apart from shyness and fear of ridicule, other childish fears are commonly seen, including fear of ghosts (in adults), fear of travelling far from home, and fear of loud noises. New challenges, such as a change in residence, or a job interview, are likely to be met with apprehension, although they may be carried off without this showing unduly. Many Barytas gradually acquire a degree of emotional maturity, eventually catching up with their peers at the age of thirty or forty. In these cases an inquiry into the pace of development of the patient's personality may guide the homeopath to the remedy, even if the patient now appears relatively mature. (There will almost certainly be some vestigial signs of immaturity, but these may not be noticed in the interview.)

### Earthiness

Like Calcarea, Baryta is a very earthy type. One expression of this is a love of eating, that sometimes amounts to pure gluttony. One teenage Baryta girl whom I treated admitted that she regularly stole food from the fridge at the college where she was studying. When I asked her why she did this, she replied innocently, "Because I wanted it". She was not short of food herself, and it was always the delicacies like ice-cream and biscuits that she stole. She illustrates another aspect of Baryta's childishness; an inability to take responsibility for her actions.

Another expression of Baryta's earthiness is a sound practical ability in many cases. Many Baryta individuals do well in practical occupations, such as carpenter or gardener. I am reminded of the late Peter Sellers' hilarious portrayal of Chance, the gardener in the film 'Being There'. Chance is taken in by wealthy sophisticates who accidentally run him over in the street. Mistaking his pronunciation of his name as 'Chauncey Gardiner', they interpret his constant references to the care of the garden (which is the only thing in life he feels familiar with) as profound philosophical metaphors. Eventually his charming reiteration of simple practical truths wins him the Presidency of the United States, without him having any idea how he got there. The fictional character of Chance, the gardener, is an excellent portrayal of the Baryta type, whose naive simplicity wins the admiration of his more complicated countrymen.

Despite the relative simplicity of the majority of Barytas, some do develop sufficient confidence and sophistication to achieve positions of responsibility in society. These more developed Barytas are especially likely to be missed by the homeopath, who is more likely to give them Calcarea or Sulphur. They usually have a few traits that still point to some isolated areas of arrested development, such as speech impediments, an inability to perform mental arithmetic, or an isolated childish habit, such as mixing their food on the plate. If the homeopath is alerted to the possibility of Baryta by the physicals, or by one of these isolated personality traits, then a history of the childhood and adolescent personality will usually reveal further Baryta features, such as late developmental milestones, the need for special tuition in certain subjects at school, or extreme shyness.

### Senility

Old age is sometimes referred to as a second childhood. Those elderly people who become senile tend to revert to childish modes of thinking and behaviour, and in these cases Baryta Carbonica can arrest or reverse the process. All the features that we see in the younger Baryta may develop for the first time during senile dementia, including dullness, mental retardation, confusion, and childlike emotional behaviour (Kent: 'Senile dementia', 'Absent-minded', 'Dullness-old people'). One particular feature of Barytas of all ages, but particularly senile Barytas, is a tendency to worry over inconsequential matters. Since the world is too complex for them to comprehend, they become focussed upon small matters, such as which brand of tomato sauce they should buy, and may worry over making the wrong choice (Kent: 'Irresolution about trifles'). The demented Baryta is most likely to suffer from suspiciousness of other people, or a fear of being watched, and may isolate himself for this reason. He is also likely to become childishly dependent upon others, not only for practical support, but also for emotional reassurance. Childishness is the main impression one gets from the senile Baryta individual.

It may be difficult in cases of senility to differentiate Baryta from Sulphur and Lycopodium, both of whom can become childish in their old age. The senile Sulphur person tends to display a degree of self importance, or even delusions of grandeur, and will boast about his (usually imaginary or greatly exaggerated) achievements. He is also likely to retain an obsessive intellectual interest in certain subjects, and to prattle on endlessly about these in a way not seen in Baryta. Lycopodium becomes very forgetful and confused when senile, but then so do the other two types. Lycopodium is liable to remain more intellectually sophisticated than Baryta despite his senility, and like Sulphur he is liable to become bossy or even tyrannical. Baryta, on the other hand, is more passive, although stubbornness may be a feature.

### Physical Appearance

Baryta is not a common type. Outside institutions for the elderly, or for retarded children, the homeopath will not come across it often. The physical characteristics will help in alerting him to the Baryta patient. Physically there are two body types that are commonly seen. The more numerous is the stocky type, who has heavy facial features, a large body, and thick wavy hair. Hirsutism is common in the females of this type. There is a tendency to put on weight, especially around the buttocks and hips. Ridges are sometimes seen above the eyes, and the eyes tend to have a wary look about them. The lips are generally thick, reflecting a sensuous nature, and the fingers and toes are short and thick, reflecting the unrefined, physical nature of the majority of the type. The other, less common physique is the puny, underdeveloped Baryta. These people are very short and thin, with small faces that are usually lined, and have small eyes with puffy bags or wrinkles beneath them. They give the impression of malnourished, wizened looking elves.

## Baryta Muriaticum

This relative of Bartyta Carbonica is almost as common as the latter. As one might expect, it shares aspects of both Baryta Carbonica and Natrum Muriaticum in both the physical and mental features. From a physical point of view, the patient often presents for treatment of epilepsy, which Baryta Muriaticum suffers from far more often than Baryta Carbonica. Mentally, the Baryta Muriaticum person has the same slowness of intellect that one sees in the Carbonica, and is usually shy and socially immature, but not to the same extent as Baryta Carbonica. He tends to be more sensitive emotionally, in both positive and negative senses of the word. Thus he is not only more easily hurt than Baryta Carbonica, but he is also more sensitive to the feelings of others, and like Natrum Muriaticum he will usually take pains to avoid hurting another's feelings. He has a richer inner life than Baryta Carbonica, and like Natrum he will tend to keep most of his feelings to himself. Since he is sensitive and also somewhat slow mentally, he is more likely to suffer from depression than Baryta Carbonica. One Baryta Muriaticum patient whose petit mal responded well to the remedy was a very gentle soul, who worried a great deal before he started a new job. He tended to get depressed because he was too slow to keep jobs, and also because he was too shy to meet girls. His intellect was capable of understanding subtle concepts, but it was slow in execution, and he would easily forget what he was ordered to do. He felt more confident after taking the remedy, but it did not stop him from being a shy and rather slow Baryta.

# Belladonna

*Keynote:* Mania

Belladonna is a rare type; even rarer than related types like Stramonium and Veratrum Album. It is principally known as an acute remedy for fever, and inflammation, especially when the fever is accompanied by delerium. This gives us some indication as to the nature of the Belladonna constitution.

## Metaphysical Interests

Belladonna is the only one of the constellation of potentially psychotic types where the individual is as likely to be sane as insane, and unlike my Stramonium or Veratrum patients, most of my Belladonna patients were relatively sane, but with individual traits which pointed towards the potential for psychosis.

One typical Belladonna trait which straddles the worlds of the sane and insane is an interest in metaphysics. I have seen this in every one of my Belladonna patients. In both sane and insane patients it appears as an obsession with matters spiritual and psychic. All of my Belladonna patients have professed to have psychic abilities, and this has been accompanied in each case by an obsession with understanding non-physical realms of reality. During a Belladonna fever a patient is delerious, and has hallucinations of spirits, angels or demons (Kent: 'Sees devils, phantoms'). The patient who is constitutionally Belladonna is also prone to visions, hallucinations and psychic phenomena. In the sane Belladonna person abilities which also occur in more stable types, such as precognition and astral travel, are more liable to occur than visions and hallucinations. In such cases there is generally a great fascination with these abilities, and other psychic matters. It is difficult for the homeopath to judge to what extent such abilities are genuine, as opposed to imaginary. One sane Belladonna patient had taken part in a class which investigated psychic abilities amongst students, and had found that his psychic abilities far exceeded the other students in the class. He said that he thought about metaphysical matters much of the time, and that he considered the human mind was capable of virtually anything.

Belladonna individuals often sense that they have power of a magical or psychic kind even when they have not had direct evidence of it. Two of my Belladonna patients said that they believed they had power to heal others, but had not tried to do so. Another said that he was sure with a little practice he could learn to move objects by will (Kent: 'Delusion-that he is a magician'). He said this knowledge scared him, but it also fascinated him. This is reminiscent of Mercurius' fascination with magic, and also have the delusions of grandeur of Veratrum and Platina. However, I have never seen Mercurius profess psychic abilities to any great extent, and the sense of personal power of Belladonna is far more restricted than that seen in the latter two types, which is why it is seen in sane or relatively sane individuals.

## *Violence*

All of the Belladonna individuals I have treated have been male. Belladonna is such an assertive, fiery type, like Sulphur, that this does not surprise me (Kent: 'The mental symptoms are all active, never passive'). As with all fiery types, violence is a big feature in the Belladonna mental picture. Here we come to an apparent contradiction in the Belladonna psyche. Most Belladonna people describe themselves as both open and warm-hearted. One schizophrenic Belladonna patient described himself as 'a hugga hugga love machine'. This is not really surprising, however, when one considers that fire is both warming and destructive. All fiery types have both passionate and destructive elements in their psyche, and both of these elements are more extreme in the unstable types like Belladonna and Platina, than in more stable fiery types like Sulphur.

Belladonna has an explosive temper. He may bottle it for a long time if he is relatively sane, but from time to time it will explode and do damage. Belladonna individuals are liable to make the most of a sudden brawl, and they may be instigators. One Belladonna man said that he had a fear of robbers breaking into his house. This put me in mind of Natrum Muriaticum, but he then explained that he was afraid that if anyone broke in he would bash them to death. Another Belladonna man said that as a child he had bashed his sisters head against a wall, and did not realise he had done wrong until he had been severely and repeatedly lectured about it. It is this remorseless aspect of Belladonna's violence that separates it from the rage of more stable types like Nux and Natrum Muriaticum.

Belladonna individuals who are relatively sane are not only prone to explicit violence. Like all fiery types they tend to be bossy and domineering, particularly with those they are close to. Being an unstable type, Belladonna tends to feel a little unsure of himself with strangers, and may appear shy or withdrawn. However, with those he knows well he tends to be both opinionated and assertive.

Those Belladonna individuals who are relatively insane are the most prone to rage. They enter into manic states, which include blind fury, as well as other aspects of excitation such as religious inspiration and sexual arousal.

## *Mania*

Belladonna has a particular profile of insanity, which overlaps with the profiles of other potentially psychotic types like Anacardium and Stramonium. One major aspect of Belladonna's insanity is visual and auditory hallucinations (Kent: 'Delusions—sees spectres, spirits', 'Delusions—hears voices').One young man came to see me to get off major tranquilizers, which he had been taking for years for paranoid schizophrenia. He was a pleasant, extroverted man who was passionate about his metaphysical interests, and his belief in his abilities to heal people. He wanted to set up a healing centre, but he was quite unstable, and incapable of any regular work. He stared with a manic intensity as he spoke, and frequently cracked up in loud peals of laughter (Kent: 'Loud boisterous laughter'). However, he looked dejected when he spoke of the side effects of his medication, which robbed him of his sense of inspiration, and he cried when he told me that nobody loved him, and that even his sister treated him with suspicion. He heard many voices in his head, and had names for them all. Like many psychotic people, he had a subtle understanding of psychology, and he used this to identify the voices in a way that made them appear more normal. Thus he called one voice his higher self, since it spoke of his spiritual mission to heal, and reminded him of his spiritual origins, whilst another he called his alter-ego, since it was evil and tried to convince him he was worthless and damned, and might as well give up trying to be stable. Others he called his ego and his guides. He was prone to both beautiful and horrible visions, which he interpreted as true perceptions of heavens and hells, and he had a strong desire to teach others about these other worlds.

Like other potentially psychotic types, Belladonna is prone to paranoia. My young schizophrenic patient would feel that others were plotting to kill him when he was in a manic phase, and also, more realistically, that he was going to be taken away. He railed about the cruelty and insensitivity of the mental health system, saying that it treated him like an animal. It was his warmth and openess which led me to prescribe Belladonna, along with his metaphysical, rather than religious interests. On a regular dose of Belladonna 10M he was able to stop his tranquilizers, and he stayed relatively stable for several months. When he started to get more manic I would up the frequency of the dosage from weekly to daily or even hourly, and this would calm him down. Unfortunately, after several months of successful treatment he became convinced that he no longer needed treatment, and so he relapsed and was admitted to hospital.

## *Summary*

Belladonna is the most liable of the potentially psychotic types to remain stable and sane. He possesses all the fiery qualities of inspiration, enthusiasm, anger and assertiveness, all of which become magnified in the insane Belladonna individual. There is usually an obsession with matters metaphysical and psychic, and a belief in possessing psychic powers. In contrast, the other psychotic types tend to have overtly religious hallucinations and beliefs, although there is some overlap here.

The sane Belladonna suffers from an erratic mind, which will not concentrate easily, but whic appears gifted at lateral thinking, and hence problem-solving. (This is also true of Mercurius and Argentum Nitricum, and some of the more sane members of the other potentially psychotic types.) There is a tendency to daydream, instead of focussing on the task at hand. Belladonna's fantasy is likely to be quite fantastic, like science fiction or Lord of the Rings. He is a relatively bossy, assertive type, who does not suffer from depression to any great degree, and tends to have uncompromising views.

The insane Belladonna is subject to hallucinations, as well as moments of ecstasy, rage, sexual arousal and intellectual inspiration. He also experiences paranoia.

Confirmatory features for Belladonna include a history of hyperactivity in childhood, a tendency to inflammatory conditions, and strong body heat.

### *Physical Appearance*
Belladonna men tend to be stocky and muscular (Kent: 'Vigorous, plethoric'). The face is often broad and the lips are generally quite thick. The hair is usually dark and wavy.

# Calcarea Carbonica

*Keynote:* Inertia

Calcarea is prepared from the oyster-shell, and its origins tell us much about the psychology of the type. The oyster is one of the less dynamic creatures of the sea. It prefers to stay safely inside its shell, clinging to a rock for security. Inside its shell it is soft and amorphous, and its activities revolve around assimilating food and digesting it.

The Calcarea individual is slow, solid, down to earth, plodding. Whilst more fiery types like Lachesis and Sulphur look for excitement and glory, Calcarea is content to stay at home and watch television, preferably with someone to cuddle, and a good supply of high-calorie nibbles. Each remedy type expresses its need for security in a different way. For Lycopodium security is sought through the approval of others. For Aurum it is wealth and prestige, whilst Pulsatilla simply needs to know that she is loved. For Calcarea, security means the familiar. Change is threatening to her (I find that about three-quarters of the Calcareas I see are female), and is avoided by simply staying put. Hence Calcarea may stay in the same job for twenty years, despite having the ability to take on something more demanding. She may remain in the town of her birth for her whole life, venturing further afield only for holidays (usually to popular, well-catered for resorts on the beaten track), and always glad to get back home.

This conservative tendency can be seen in many areas of Calcarea's life. Calcarea children in particular are wary of new experiences. They will be slow to experiment with new foods, slow to make new friends (though sociable with existing friends), and reluctant to consider different philosophies and points of view as they get older. Like Arsenicum, Calcarea tends to be very concerned with material security. As a result, both types have a tendency to be hypochondriacal, and to worry about the future, and what might happen to them in a material sense (Kent: 'Fear that something will happen'). There are, however, considerable differences as well in this regard. Whereas Arsenicum will try to control his environment by being precise, fastidious and frugal, Calcarea simply avoids change, and within the confines of familiar circumstances is able to relax and be indulgent to a far greater extent. Security is Calcarea's principal concern, and once this is reasonably assured, she will enjoy life, without needing a great deal of excitement, wealth or prestige.

## *Simplicity*

Calcarea is an uncomplicated person. Being orientated primarily towards physical reality, and to the satisfaction of sensual appetites, and the equally natural enjoyment of family life, she avoids the soul-searching of more introverted types like Natrum Muriaticum, and the intellectualism of Sulphur, Lycopodium and some Natrums. Calcarea is simple, homely, down to earth and pragmatic. Her simplicity is refreshing, since it is natural, like that of Phosphorus (although quieter as less brilliant). Even the most intelligent of Calcareas have a natural, unpretentious quality, and a love of the simple pleasures in life, such as eating, drinking, going for walks and making love. Most Calcareas are content as long as they have security, friendship, and the freedom to live a little luxuriously from time to time, not by spending vast sums of money, but by savouring the simple luxuries like a hot bath on a winter's day, or a fireside chat over tea and crumpets. I have a Calcarea friend who manages to eat and dress extremely well despite a meagre income. Food and clothes are two of her principal sources of pleasure, and most of her money goes towards them.

It is Calcarea's connection with her physical senses, and with the Earth, that enables her to maintain this simplicity. Calcarea is one of the more sensuous types (like Pulsatilla, Medorrhinum and Baryta), deriving a great deal of pleasure from the senses, without requiring the sophistication that more refined types like Silica and Arsenicum enjoy. Most Calcareas overindulge in food, since they find it so enjoyable, and being sedentary by nature they usually become overweight before long. Here they differ from overweight Natrums (who outnumber fat Calcareas by about twenty to one), since they are liable to be relatively unconcerned by their size. Natrum has a tendency to feel ugly and unlovable, and this tendency is only exaggerated by obesity. Calcarea, by contrast, is often quite content in her obesity, since she is less conscious of her appearance, especially when she is secure in the loyalty of her spouse.

Like other earthy, sensation-orientated types, Calcarea is often good at practical tasks, and many will have artistic abilities as well. They are unlikely, however, to risk making a living from such a precarious pursuit as art, preferring to keep it as a hobby.

Calcarea's pragmatic, no nonsense approach to life is put to good use at work. Whilst the closely related Sulphur is often bored or lazy at work (unless it also happens to be his passion), Calcarea is generally steady and reliable. She may not be fast, but like the tortoise, she will get there in the end, usually without making any mistakes on the way. Furthermore, she is likely to be affable and uncomplaining as an employee (and will generally accept a relatively low wage, as long as she is happy with the work). Calcarea is certainly not a workaholic, although she may at times work long hours to help out her boss, or stand in for a colleague. For herself, she would prefer to work shorter hours and enjoy her leisure. Although she may take pride in her work, her main focus in life is usually her family (and this applies to Calcarea men as well). A weekend at home with the family sounds more attractive to the average Calcarea than to most other types, and Monday morning is not usually looked forward to with much enthusiasm.

### Parochialism and Pettiness

Every positive quality has its flip-side. Sulphur is inspired, but oblivious of practical realities, whilst the Kalis are logical, but lack imagination. In the case of Calcarea the virtue of simplicity is accompanied in many cases by 'smallmindedness'.

Calcarea's interests usually revolve around the satisfaction of the needs and desires of herself and her family. This can give rise to a certain clannish mentality, which could be roughly expressed as, "You're O.K. if you're one of us." Since Calcarea's focus is on the family, and on practical everyday concerns like what to cook for lunch, she is liable to miss the broader picture. Kent was characteristically blunt about this in his Lecture Notes; 'Calcarea leads to little ideas, it compels the mind to littleness, to little ideas, or to dwell on little things'. (Kent was probably a Sulphur, and hence exactly the opposite.) This is true in many cases. Calcarea is likely to be more interested in what he is going to have for dinner, or in whether his local football team is winning, than in more collective concerns like international politics, or more abstract notions like philosophy and ethics. This is not simply a matter of intelligence. Even the more intelligent Calcareas tend to be more interested in local than in national or international concerns, and in practical matters rather than abstract theory. Thus a Calcarea person who is concerned about the environment will act locally by helping to recycle waste, but will probably pay little attention to global ecological issues like the preservation of the Amazon rainforest.

Not all Calcareas are interested purely in personal and domestic affairs. Some have a wide general knowledge, and take an interest in a great many subjects, from the mundane to the philosophical. Calcarea is often a collector, and some Calcareas collect information rather than antiques and toy cars. The way they do so is interesting. Unlike Lycopodium and Sulphur, who often study subjects avidly and thoroughly, Calcarea tends to 'graze' on information. Over the years she may gradually make her way through a great many factual books (dotted in between fictional ones most likely), absorbing a good deal of knowledge effortlessly. And because she is interested in the little details of life, as well as the 'big picture', she may store away a huge repository of little known facts, such as the proportion of fat in a camel's hump, or the name of President Reagan's astrologer. Then in conversation, these little gems will come out when the appropriate subject is being discussed, and Calcarea's friend will marvel at the widespread knowledge possessed by this apparently rather simple, uncomplicated person.

Kali Carbonicum also tends to collect a mine of detailed facts, and to slip them into the conversation when appropriate. These two types have quite a lot in common, both physically and mentally. Both are very earthy, practical, no-nonsense types, and both have a tendency to worry over little things. However, Calcarea tends to be more relaxed, less formal and less rigid than the Kalis. Also, Calcarea is not pedantic about the facts she has learned, whereas Lycopodium and Kali can be.

I once knew a Calcarea lady of about forty years. She had married, had children, separated, and then entered a kind of second adolescence, in which she caught up on all the years she had missed out by marrying young. She dressed very trendily in the fashions of teenage girls, and she looked more like thirty than forty years old. Her face was squarish, with an open countenance, and she had fine wrinkles radiating out from the corners of her eyes, which looked like laughter lines. Her body type was on the endomorphic side, but she was not obese, although she took no regular exercise. From my point of view, the most characteristic feature of this lady's personality was that she loved to chat. She could chat to anybody, about anything, and chat and chat until the cows came home. She would test my patience by chatting through good movies (usually to my wife). Whenever any new subject was raised, she would have something to say about it. Her comments tended to be serious and factual, but not pedantic. She was particularly well informed regarding activities (political or recreational) in her own area, but could usually find something to say about virtually any topic. I eventually gave her Calcarea 10M when she came to see me in a panic one day. Her ex-boyfriend would not leave her alone, and it was upsetting her so much that she was feeling anxious and tearful all the time. Being a mild and generous soul, she had at first been too soft in her treatment of this unwelcome 'ex', but she was eventually forced to shut the door in his face. Within a day of taking the remedy she was calm again, and had stopped obsessing about how to handle the situation.

My Calcarea friend was certainly more 'mental' (as opposed to emotional or practical) than most Calcareas, but she was not intellectual, in that she did not analyse to any great extent the information she gathered. I have never come across a really analytical Calcarea, and this is in keeping with the impression Calcarea gives of being a predominantly practical, earthy type, despite the fact that she may have above average intelligence. (In contrast, Kali Carbonicum and Lycopodium both tend to analyse information a great deal, as does Sulphur, another great collector of facts.)

Most Calcareas do take an intense interest in the personal. On the positive side this makes them attentive listeners and loyal friends. It also tends to make them interested in gossip, and in such details as the colour of the Queen's dress, or Fergie's latest hairstyle. (Calcarea is often fascinated by Royalty, as is Natrum Muriaticum.)

Calcarea is a sensitive type (Kent: 'Oversensitive'), and when her feelings are hurt she is most liable to resort to pettiness. If she feels insulted or rejected she may behave childishly, resorting to juvenile tactics of revenge. For example, she may close the door in her husband's face, or reveal embarrassing personal details about the person she is angry with to mutual friends. This kind of petulant behaviour is particularly seen in Calcarea children and adolescents, especially in the girls.

### *Hospitality and Homeliness*

Calcium is the principal element in the bony skeleton. Like the bones of the skeleton, the Calcarea individual performs a stabilising or even structural role in the body of society. Calcareas are the 'good eggs', the salt of the Earth, solid, dependable, with sound common sense, and a generous heart for anyone who is accepted into their wider family. The stranger may be treated with some caution, but once he has demonstrated his good intentions, he is allowed into the oyster's shell, to enjoy the homeliness and comfort of its interior, and the pearl of love and loyalty that Calcarea extends to those she trusts. In this sense Calcarea resembles Natrum Muriaticum, but the latter is more wary of letting people in, more guarded, and then more emotionally intense towards confidantes.

When one reads of olden times, and of the characters who populated our villages and towns two or three hundred years ago, one gets the impression that Calcarea was the commonest type in those days, and this may have been so. The image of the matronly inn-keeper's wife, extending hospitality to all and sundry, keen to gossip, and not above a bit of bawdy fun, is one that for me encapsulates much of the essence of Calcarea. It is common knowledge that people living in rural areas, although initially wary of strangers, are most hospitable once they invite you into their homes. I suspect that Calcarea is more common in the countryside, where it is still possible to live a simpler life, and also more common in third-world countries. As society becomes industrialised, and more sophisticated, Natrum Muriaticum becomes more and more common, taking over from Calcarea as the principal type. (We will examine this further in the chapter on Natrum.)

Both male and female Calcareas have a love of home, and a nurturing tendency which makes guests feel like part of the family. Calcarea, unlike Natrum, is not likely to stand on ceremony with strangers. There is a simplicity about Calcareas. You know where you stand with them, and if they trust you, they are likely to be chatty and pally, rather than intense and overbearing. (A good example of a relaxed and refreshingly straightforward Calcarea can be seen in the film 'L.A.Story' in the character of the English journalist played by the actress Victoria Tennant who falls in love with the wacky weatherman played by Steve Martin) Most Calcareas are good at looking after others, without falling into the trap of neglecting themselves. Unlike Natrum, another nurturing type, Calcarea usually feels worthy of love and happiness, and is able to receive just as easily as she gives. In a relationship the Calcarea partner will generally be very supportive of the other, both verbally and practically. Calcareas are good at remembering the little things which show that they care, such as birthday presents, cups of tea, and bunches of flowers. In fact, Calcarea tends to indulge whoever he or she loves. The Calcarea partner is generally loyal, devoted and dependable, without losing her (or his) sense of identity. Here Calcarea differs from Pulsatilla, and from some Natrum, Phosphorus and Staphysagria partners, who completely lose themselves in their attempts to please the other.

The Calcarea parent will be just as supportive and indulgent as the Calcarea partner, but in a relaxed way. Family life comes naturally to Calcarea, and children are generally nurtured without being smothered , and are allowed to fly the nest without much fuss. The Calcarea mother will most probably worry about her children after they have left home, but she will not stand in their way. It is as though Calcarea still has a 'natural psyche' which instinctively knows what is best for her family, without having to think about it. Just as birds accept and even encourage their young to fly the nest when the time is right, so Calcarea parents perform their natural role, and then step out of the way when the children are old enough to fend for themselves.

Households in which one or both parents are Calcarea are generally teeming with life. Children are given a fairly free reign, and pets are usually favoured, both by the parents and the children. Many Calcarea households are veritable menageries, pulsing with the pregnant life of half a dozen pets, and a brood of unruly children. In such a chaotic home the Calcarea mother feels in her element, and the Calcarea father, although he may sometimes seek refuge in the pub with his mates, feels far more at home in such warm domestic chaos than he would in a quiet, tidy and controlled atmosphere.

The family is very important to Calcarea. Large family gatherings are typical, and Calcarea is likely to invite her ageing mother to move in with her family as she becomes too frail to look after herself. When away from home Calcareas tend to feel homesick (particularly the children). Calcarea children are more likely than most to tolerate or enjoy family holidays late into adolescence, when their peers are chafing at the bit and trying to get away from their parents. They are also more likely to remain in the parental home after they have left school and begun working. This is partly because they love the familiar and the comfortable, but also because one or both parents are liable to be Calcarea, and hence to be pleasant company. Unless she is particularly tense, Calcarea is generally easygoing, and does not put many emotional demands upon her loved ones. They can come and go as they please, and since she is not only undemanding, but also warm and indulgent, they are liable to enjoy her company. The Calcarea child will often stay at home until she gets engaged or married (often to her childhood sweetheart).

## *Sentimentality and Sensitivity*

Water is said to be symbolic of emotion, and the sea in particular is often associated with the subconscious mind, which is full of emotions from the past. It is appropriate then that those remedies that are derived from the sea (Calcarea, Natrum Muriaticum and Sepia) correspond to emotional personalities. Calcarea is a little less emotional than Natrum and Sepia, because she is so grounded in her senses, so down to earth and pragmatic. Nevertheless, Calcarea is still emotional, in the sense of being soft, nurturing and sentimental (Kent: 'Mildness'). Calcarea can easily be mistaken for Pulsatilla, since both are mild and nurturing by nature, as well as being similar in physical appearance (blonde and fleshy). The principal difference lies in Calcarea's earthiness, which prevents the constant flux of emotions that Pulsatilla is subject to, and makes Calcarea more stable, and less dependent on others. (Graphites lies somewhere between the two).

Most young children are sentimental to some extent, but the Calcarea child grows out of this slowly, if at all. Thus she is likely to retain and treasure her soft toys longer than most (eg. all of her life). The older Calcarea is sentimental about anniversaries, and enjoys sending and receiving greeting cards with intimate messages on, and holding onto certain items which remind her of past good times, and of absent friends. Most Calcareas have treasured photo-albums. (This kind of sentimentality is also seen in Pulsatilla, Natrum Muriaticum and sometimes in Phosphorus).

Calcarea's soft heart cannot bear to hear of cruelty (Kent: 'Oversensitive-hearing of cruelties'), although she is not prone to the kind of moral indignation that Causticum feels on coming across injustice, and she is not the type to rock the boat by campaigning for social rights. She simply winces at the thought of another creature suffering, especially as a result of cruelty, since she feels the pain herself to some extent, in the same empathic way as Phosphorus. I tend to think of Calcarea as lying midway between Phosphorus and Natrum. All three are sensitive, emotional types. Phosphorus is extremely open to the feelings of others, and is also just as open about her own feelings. Natrum closes off in order to protect herself, both from being hurt, and from feeling too much of others' pain. Calcarea, possessing a reasonably healthy balance, lies somewhere between openness and self-protection.

The contented Calcarea can sometimes be mistaken for Phosphorus, since she is simple and natural, enjoying life without too much introspection, and without pretences. It is when Calcarea is hurt that she can be mistaken for Natrum, since she will withdraw into her shell, and refuse to have anything to do with the person who upset her. At times like these Calcarea can be resentful and even bitter (Kent: 'Offended easily'). The main difference between an offended Calcarea and an offended Natrum is that the former will snap out of it far more quickly than the latter. This is in part due to the fact that Natrum will tend to bottle up her anger and frustration until the situation is dire, whereas Calcarea will speak up sooner and hence avoid being abused.

When Calcarea is upset she has a tendency to react irrationally, (Kent: 'He forms conclusions from his emotions rather than his intelligence'.) Again this is true of most of the emotional types, with Aurum being the most controlled, and Ignatia the least. Calcarea lies somewhere in between. She may cry when her husband forgets their anniversary, and in her sadness she may accidentally burn the dinner, or in her anger she may go out for the evening without leaving a note, but Calcarea tends to come back to her senses pretty quickly. She is sensible most of the time, and irrational only when upset.

Calcarea is listed in Kent's Repertory under the rubric 'Magnetised-desires to be'. This is because Calcarea is a passive type, and like many of the milder emotional types she enjoys being charmed, particularly by a member of the opposite sex. Calcarea girls are prone to developing crushes, and will hang on a heart-throb's every word. This susceptibility to another's charm can sometimes lead to broken hearts, but again Calcarea's sensible side usually sees to it that the moping doesn't last too long, and that the business of everyday life goes on.

### The Timid Oyster

Calcarea avoids feeling anxious most of the time by sticking with the familiar. One of the most characteristic results of this is underachieving. Calcarea tends to fear the challenges that would result from being successful, especially academically and professionally (Kent: 'right in the midst of his success he quits his business'). It is very common for Calcarea to embark upon a college course, or a work traineeship, and then drop out of it towards the end, despite the fact that she was capable of finishing with an average or above average pass. She will usually be unable to explain why she dropped out, or will rationalise her decision. For example, she may say that she dropped out of her art course because she was offered a good job, when in fact the job did not stretch her or make good use of her talents. Alternatively, she may abandon her work or studies when she enters a new relationship, justifying her decision by saying that she now wants to have more time for her man. In fact Calcarea drops out because she is afraid that she will not be able to cope with the increase in demands upon her time and her skills that worldly success would entail. Calcarea is not lacking in intelligence or skills. She is just afraid to use them fully.

Calcarea is one of those types that worries without cause about the future (Kent: 'Fear something will happen'). As usual it is the females who tend to worry more, but Calcarea men also have a tendency to fear the worst, especially when embarking upon something new. Similarly, the Calcarea parent will worry about the children having an accident, and will get agitated if they are a little late coming home. In general it is the little things which worry Calcarea, and unlikely future calamities.

When Calcarea does take on a new responsibility the fear of being unable to cope can give rise to general apprehension, and to all manner of irrational fears. (Kent lists Calcarea under fourteen separate anxiety rubrics and sixteen fear rubrics in either black type or italics.) The anxious Calcarea appreciates reassurance, and usually manages to regain some perspective before long. It is unusual for Calcarea to suffer from the kind of panic attacks and long-term anxiety problems which affect more nervous types like Argentum and Lycopodium.

### Dullness and Obstinacy

Like Baryta, the Calcarea child tends to be slow in developing, but unlike the former, he does usually catch up pretty quickly. For example, the Calcarea child may be very late in teething, or may start to crawl and walk a couple of months later than the average child. Speaking and learning to read may also be slow at first, and this initial slowness may give rise to later fears of overextending himself. The resemblance to Baryta extends further than merely slowness of development. Like Baryta, some Calcarea children are dull, unadventurous and apathetic (Kent: 'Dullness—sluggishness'). They may get into a rut in which they are only interested in watching television, or playing with a particular toy, and will resist all attempts to interest them in conversation and other activities. Some Calcarea children are like this all the time, whilst others go through dull phases. Naturally, a dull child may be suffering from a lack of parental interaction, or may be withdrawing into himself to protect himself from an unhappy atmosphere at home. This can happen to children of any constitutional type, but Calcarea will lapse into dullness and apathy more quickly than most others, and will react in this way to a variety of negative influences (rather like the oyster who hides in his shell). Calcarea is not so likely to become aggressive like Tuberculinum, but rather dull and obstinate like Baryta. One way to distinguish the dull Calcarea child from the dull Baryta child is to remember that Baryta children are far more shy than Calcarea children.

The Calcarea adult generally avoids the kind of torpor that children of the type sometimes fall into, but may nevertheless become dull, unimaginative, sedentary and routine-bound. With Calcarea it is often more physical lethargy than mental apathy that restricts life, but the one may easily lead to the other. This dullness resembles that of the apathetic Sepia, but is seldom as severe, and tends not to be accompanied by despair. Calcarea is relatively strong emotionally, and it takes a lot of misfortune to turn her misery into real depression. When Calcarea is miserable, she is more likely to cry softly than to howl, and to feel sorry for herself and indulge herself, rather than feeling wretched (Kent: 'Whimpering, low-spirited and melancholy'). She seldom if ever tastes the depths of emotional pain suffered by more introspective types like Aurum, Natrum and Ignatia.

Like Silica, Calcarea lacks stamina, both physically and mentally. Even the brightest of Calcarea individuals can have trouble completing prolonged mental tasks, and the attention span may be too short to concentrate for long, not because Calcarea is easily distracted like Phosphorus, but because the mind becomes tired (Kent: 'No ability to sustain prolonged mental effort'). Many a Calcarea student is plagued by headaches as a result of the strain of trying to concentrate. In order to get around this limitation, many Calcarea individuals learn to pace themselves when studying or writing, doing a little often rather than a lot at one time. (Silica also does this.)

Like Sulphur and Silica, Calcarea tends to be stubborn. This is not surprising in view of the tendency to avoid change. Since the familiar is reassuring, it is clung to. The Calcarea child is usually very good at saying 'No', digging his heels in like a donkey when he is pushed to do something. If you want to change the behaviour of a Calcarea, you are more likely to succeed by telling him to do the opposite of what you want him to do. For example, trying to rush a Calcarea may have the opposite effect. He is slow by nature, and will slow down even more if pressured.

Calcarea's stubbornness is sometimes expressed as prejudice, against certain individuals, whole sections of society, or concepts which are unfamiliar. The more Calcarea is afraid of change, the more she is likely to feel threatened by people or ideas which seem foreign, and hence the more liable she is to harbour prejudices. The more aware Calcarea individual may seem free of obvious prejudices, but careful observation may reveal more subtle ones, such as a distrust of people belonging to the Gemini star sign, or an assumption that poor people don't wash (Kent: 'Aversion to certain persons').

Like Pulsatilla, Calcarea is seen especially often in early childhood. In particular, small babies are often Calcarea constitutionally, before entering a Pulsatilla stage at about eighteen months, and then their adult constitutional type by about five years of age. Infancy is naturally a time of assimilation, when the principal activities are eating and sleeping, hence the resonance with the relatively passive Calcarea wavelength. Calcarea babies are usually very placid and easy to care for, except for their tendency to wake in the night crying. They are docile babies who enjoy other people, but will sit quietly playing by themselves as long as mother is near. They tend to sleep a lot in the daytime, and their tendency to wake at night may be related to a fear of the dark, and a fear of being alone, both of which may be manifested later on by Calcarea children.

## *Physical Appearance*

Physically most Calcareas have a characteristic appearance. The body is fleshy, with a tendency to obesity, and a soft layer of fat is present even in non-obese Calcareas. The hair in Caucasians is usually light brown or blonde, and the skin is pale and 'milky' in appearance. The complexion has been described as 'chalky', as if there were a thin layer of talc over it. This is in part due to a slight puffiness of the skin, resulting from the layer of fat underneath, and also to the fine, downy hairs that are often present. Like Pulsatilla, Calcarea often has a 'peaches and cream' complexion, being pale but with rosy cheeks. (In contrast, Silica, Syphilinum and Lachesis are usually pale without the rosiness, or 'cream without the peaches'.) The face is usually rounded and soft in appearance, but more cerebral Calcareas often have a broad, squarish face, with a wide mouth. (The fleshiness of Calcarea's face reflects her soft, emotional side, whilst its squareness reflects her earthy pragmatic nature. In contrast, the earthy Kali has a squarish face which is not at all fleshy, since he is not at all emotional.) The lips are generally full, reflecting a sensuous nature. Like Baryta, Calcarea's limbs and digits tend to be shorter and fatter than average, or else squarish and strong looking.

The actress Victoria Tennant is a good example of a Calcarea both in terms of appearance and of the roles she usually plays in films.

# Causticum

*Keynote:* The idealist

Causticum is a fascinating constitutional type. It is quite uncommon, and the Causticum personality has been described in only a sketchy fashion in the old materia medicas. Consequently, many homeopaths have only a vague impression of the Causticum mentality.

### Idealism, Empathy, and Injustice

The aspect of Causticum's personality that is almost entirely lacking from the old materia medicas is one of the most central, namely idealism. There are several idealistic types (Sulphur, Staphysagria, Phosphorus, China) and each has a different kind of idealism. Thus Sulphur dreams grand schemes designed to bring about an ideal world, but may do nothing practical about them, Staphysagria is often vaguely interested in all things spiritual, and is inclined to dream impractically about becoming a spiritual aspirant in India, whilst Phosphorus is inspired by the grand vision of other idealists, but is not always very discriminating. (China tends to be genuinely psychic and spiritual, but has difficulty adjusting to the harshness of the material world.) Causticum's idealism is based upon two factors; firstly a deep empathy for the suffering of others (Kent: 'Sympathetic'), and secondly a deeply felt sense of justice. No other type combines these two elements to such a great extent. A third element (which helps to separate Causticum from Phosphorus) is a highly analytical mind. These three elements often combine to produce a practical idealist—someone who actually does something concrete to try to realise his vision of a more just and caring society. (The majority of Causticums are male.)

A great many Causticum individuals have an interest in broad social issues, and feel insensed when politicians and others in positions of authority appear to restrict individual liberties. If you suspect that a patient may be Causticum constitutionally, it is often helpful to ask them if they react strongly to the news on the TV or radio. Many Causticums say that they feel so upset or angry when they listen to the news that they cannot do it too often. Typically the Causticum idealist will write letters frequently to newspapers and to politicians, attempting to right social injustices. Some focus on large issues such as racial discrimination, or the divisiveness of economic policy, whilst others campaign locally for the expansion of individual freedoms. A recent patient of mine came for treatment of muscular rheumatism, which crippled him with pain every time he caught a cold or flu, or was exposed to a cold wind. He seemed rather serious and withdrawn, and I wondered about Natrum Muriaticum as a remedy, but it did not fit his symptoms. Then he mentioned that he was in the process of campaigning to abolish the local laws which made the wearing of bicycle helmets compulsory. On further questioning he confirmed that he often wrote letters to the editors of newspapers about views he held strongly, and had had many of them published. He had also campaigned for aboriginal rights. It was then that I saw that he was a relatively introverted Causticum, and gave him Causticum 1M, which rapidly improved all of his symptoms, including a tendency to suffer from nervous tension.

It is important to differentiate between the Causticum campaigner and the Natrum Muriaticum campaigner. The former is what I call a natural campaigner, since it is Causticum's nature to fight injustice and the infringement of personal freedoms. Natrum, on the other hand, tends to campaign for more personal reasons. It is the Natrums who have suffered from various injustices, or from natural calamities or diseases, who tend to campaign on behalf of others in similar circumstances. When a Natrum's child dies of muscular dystrophy, he will start a charity and become passionate in its support. A Natrum who has been the victim of sexual harassment will start a campaign to punish the perpetrators of such harassment. In contrast, Causticum is more impersonal and more universally committed to justice and freedom. He does not have to have been a victim himself to campaign. It is his nature. The best investigative journalists are often Causticum constitutionally. Causticum is an intellectual, analytical type in the main, and is perfectly suited to exposing injustice and corruption in society through insightful writing. The controversial Australian journalist John Pilger is a classic example. Pilger's documentary style is thorough and uncompromising, so much so that he interests only the more serious student of political and social comment. His primary aim is to unmask corruption and official secrecy, in the interests of greater individual freedom, and a more informed, caring society.

Causticum is so dedicated to truth in many cases that he seems a bore to other people. All he wants to talk about is politics and social injustice, or about his ideas to change society. Consequently, he is liable to be a bit of a loner, since he is too intense intellectually and morally for most people. (His moral intensity is nearly always liberal rather than conservative.) Sulphur may also bore people with his passionate and endless intellectual theorising, but Sulphur is generally more in love with his ideas than with practical and disciplined attempts to bring about change.

Naturally, a great many revolutionaries are liable to be Causticum constitutionally. Their passion allied to their keen intellect attracts other less brilliant idealists into the fold. Karl Marx was probably a Sulphur, the intellectual giant behind the revolution who lived in comfortable society in London. In contrast, the young revolutionaries on the ground who were willing to die for their ideals no doubt included a good many Causticums. Causticum can become a little fanatical in his zeal, but without Causticum's fanaticism a great many revolutionary changes in society would never take place.

Not all Causticums are political activists. Even amongst the idealists (some Causticums are not idealists—see later) some prefer a more spiritual approach. I remember one elderly Christian preacher who came to see me with a case of vocal cord polyps which prevented him from preaching effectively. He was a warm and clearly inspired man, who exuded human generosity as well as 'reasonableness'. Like many Causticums he was an extrovert who was easy to get to know, and as keen to listen as he was to speak (unlike Sulphur). Much of his work involved running a centre for the homeless, which he enjoyed passionately, and he had set up similar homes in the United States before moving to England. This man had the warmth of heart of a Phosphorus and the intellect of a Sulphur, yet he did not have the ego of a Sulphur. I gave him a couple of doses of Causticum 1M and he returned two weeks later most grateful to myself and the good Lord for giving him his voice back. (It is remarkable how quickly polyps will recede with the correct remedy.)

### *Disillusionment and Grief*
It is not surprising that one so idealistic as Causticum is prone to become disillusioned when the world does not respond to his vision. The Sulphur idealist will brush off opposition and ignore indifference, and if one plan fails he will be ready with another the next week. Causticum is a little more sensitive. He will feel deeply aggrieved if his campaigning comes to naught, since he feels so deeply for the oppressed. Such 'unsuccessful' Causticums eventually sink into despair and bitterness.

I once treated a corpulent elderly gentleman who had the typical gaunt, deeply creased face of the Causticum who has fought and lost too many battles. His principal complaint was osteoarthritis, but it soon became apparent that he was depressed. It turned out that he had for many years campaigned for the local council to fund the establishment of a home for orphans, and had even moved from one area to another in search of a sympathetic council, but he had not succeeded, and the failure to realise his dream had broken his spirit. In the process he had lost his wife when she died, but he said that he had managed to soldier on without her because he had a mission to fulfill. Now he was about to give up, and the meaning had gone from his life. He wept openly as he said this, childlike in his innocence.

Thankfully, a few doses of Causticum 10M (which is safe to give in degenerative arthritis, but not inflammatory arthritis) restored his flagging spirits so much so that he felt ready to fight further battles, his sense of purpose renewed. Such is the power of the high potencies. Before his treatment he had been not only depressed and withdrawn (Kent: 'Mental exhaustion, hopelessness, despair'), but also very bitter with what he saw as the stupidity and blindness of the councils he had approached (Kent: 'the injurious effects of prolonged vexation'). Causticum should be added in black type to Kent's repertory under the rubric 'Indignation'.

Failure to realise his dreams is not the only stress which can lead Causticum to despair. Many Causticum people combine their social concerns with a rich personal life, and the loss of a loved one can be devastating for them. Causticum is one of only five remedies listed in black type in Kent's repertory under the rubric 'Grief'. We must not forget that Causticum tends to have a very warm and romantic heart, and is usually passionate about his loved ones. Hence the depth of his grief when he loses them. In fact the depth of Causticum's grief proves that Causticum is a more profound type than Phosphorus, who will bounce back more quickly despite an initial almost hysterical grieving, and more sensitive than Sulphur, who will also recover generally far more quickly than Causticum from a bereavement. Causticum's grieving is agonising, since the image and memory of the departed keeps recurring in the mind, and the sensitive heart weeps with every memory. Those Causticums who have some cause to throw themselves into will recover far more quickly from grief than the others, who will continue to pine for years in some cases.

### Obsession, Introversion, and Anxiety

Not all Causticums are extroverted and passionate. Most are idealistic, but some express their idealism quietly through writing, and are rather shy and withdrawn socially. In fact the introverted Causticum is just as common as the extroverted type, and like Lachesis, many are somewhere in between.

The introverted Causticum is far more prone to anxiety than his extroverted cousin. Female Causticums are more likely to be introverted and anxious, (but a good half of the men are too). It is important to remember that Causticum is a potassium salt, and it is thus not surprising that the more introverted Causticum individual shares many traits with the other Kalis. One of these shared traits is obsessiveness. The more introverted a Causticum individual, the more liable he is to become obsessive. This obsessiveness may be in the form of fastidiousness, as seen in Arsenicum and Natrum. Some Causticum people are extremely tidy, and will straighten pictures on the wall in strangers' houses. Others are perfectionists in their work.

The potassium salts all have a certain mental rigidity. In the more extrovert Causticum this takes the form of doggedly pursuing various causes. In the introverted Causticum there may be a problem with repetitive negative thoughts. Just as Lachesis must find an outlet for his powerful sexual energy, or become anxious, so Causticum seems to become anxious when he does not have an external focus for his mental energy. One expression of this is obsessive-compulsive disorder. After prolonged stress Causticum may start to obsessively check that doors are locked. He may also suffer from obsessive cleanliness and hand-washing, a syndrome more frequently associated with Syphilinum.

I once treated a pleasant old man (Causticum's pathological mentals tend to appear later on in life) who complained of writer's cramp. He told me that in the past he had suffered a nervous breakdown, which surprised me, since he seemed to be both open and relatively healthy emotionally. His nervous breakdown had consisted of compulsively going over past unpleasant experiences. Even years later he would still find it difficult to let go of these experiences. This habit, which one sees more often in Natrum Muriaticum, in combination with a relatively warm and open appearance, led me to Causticum, which not only cured the writer's cramp, but also greatly reduced the anxious ruminating over the past. This brings one to a contradiction in the mentals of the introverted Causticum. Such a person may appear open and easy to interact with in the consulting room, being able to talk about himself without inhibition or emotion, and yet he describes himself as introverted and quiet. Both impressions are correct. Even the introverted Causticums retain a certain openness and idealism when compared to the other Kalis. They are frequently incensed by injustice like their more extrovert cousins, and often take a keen interest in politics. Their views are generally liberal, and they do not have the social 'stiffness' that one usually sees in Kali Carbonicum or Bichromium. Neither do they have the defensive 'front' of the introverted Natrum. They come across as serious, intelligent, objective and humane, and this impression leads one to expect such an individual to have little trouble with anxiety. Yet they do suffer from anxiety.

One of the most characteristic forms of anxiety that the introverted Causticum suffers from is a sense of dread that something awful will happen (Kent: 'foreboding that something is going to happen'). This usually becomes a problem after years of stress, particularly as Causticum is growing old. Old age finds a lot of Causticums becoming more anxious and more withdrawn. The idealism of their youth is fading, and with it goes their self-confidence and their mental clarity (Kent: 'old broken down constitutions'). As anxiety increases it develops into this awful feeling that something terrible is going to happen. It is as if all the years of watching terrible things happen in society and being unable to change them produces a general expectation of disaster. This fear may take specific form as a fear that something will happen to himself or his family, and this can lead to suspiciousness or mild paranoia. It may also lead to a fear of death. Elderly Causticum individuals are often frail, timid and prone to confusion. They are very sensitive to the slightest adverse influence, such as excessive noise, or the slightest bad news, and little things can set their nerves off, resulting in trembling, agitation and a mild state of panic.

Causticum's nervous system thus becomes tense and hypersensitive as he gets older, particularly if he has had stress in his personal life, or with his health, and this deterioration may result in a downward spiral of ever increasing anxiety, leading eventually to despair. Very often the elderly Causticum becomes more anxious after the death of his or her spouse. The spouse was a steadying influence, and after losing them Causticum falls prey to foolish anxiety and ever increasing confusion. He may feel afraid when alone at night (Kent: 'Anxiety before falling asleep'), and may develop completely unrealistic fears, such as that he is going to be evicted, or that he has cancer when he does not. These fears are merely a reflection of the gradual disintegration of his faculties after years of tension.

### The Female Causticum
The majority of Causticum people are male, about three quarters of them. The female Causticum is generally of the introverted type, and is generally less idealistic and less analytical than the introverted male. She appears as a sensible, independent and anxious person, who is easily moved to tears, but is not intense emotionally. She is thus somewhat like the female Silica, but less refined and delicate, and somewhat like Natrum Carbonicum, but empathic and more broad-minded. There is also a close similarity with the female Kali Carbonicum, but the Causticum woman is less rigid and formal. Very often the physical features of the case are more useful than the mentals in identifying the Causticum woman, since the typical idealism is less apparent.

### Summary
Causticum is a difficult personality type to master both because it is uncommon, and because it has apparently contradictory aspects. Intellectual idealism is a key feature in the male Causticum, combined with a hatred of injustice. The extrovert Causticum is as warm and empathic as Phosphorus, but more intellectual and socially committed. He is as passionate and confident as Sulphur, but more sensitive and less egotistical. The introverted male Causticum is idealistic and analytical, and suffers from anxiety and also obsessiveness. The Causticum woman is generally sensible and anxious, with obsessiveness, and is somewhat introverted. Her intellect is generally keen unless she suffers from anxiety-induced confusion.

## *Physical Appearance*

Causticum tends to be slim and wiry physically. The face is angular, and tends to become hollow and gaunt with age, with deep facial creases. (The rock musician Bob Dylan is a good example. His lyrics are also typically Causticum in content.) There is often a greyish hue to the face.

# *China*

*Keynote:* Sensitivity

China is one of the most difficult constitutional types to come to grips with from the point of view of the personality. One reason for this is that it is a rare type, that is very poorly understood by most homeopaths. In fact, most homeopaths regard China as simply a local or acute remedy, not realising that it is a full constitutional type, with its own unique personality profile. Another reason for China's obscurity is the existence of contradictory elements in the persona of the China individual, such as timidity and criticism, and a third reason is the ethereal nature of many China individuals, which is too subtle to be grasped by the insensitive.

## *Sensitivity*

China is one of the most sensitive of all types (Kent: 'Extreme sensitiveness'). She has the emotional and the aesthetic sensitivity of Ignatia, but in addition there is usually a psychic sensitivity, and often an extreme physical/sensory sensitivity as well. One's first impression of a China individual is often one of sensitivity. She will approach you rather warily, and may remain wary until she knows you well, and even then, she will only reveal her true sensitivity if she is convinced that you are both understanding and sensitive (Kent: 'Timidity'). Naturally, those China individuals who have been subjected to trauma, particularly early on in life, are even more wary. I remember one such patient, a young woman of about twenty five years, who was especially wary of me during the initial interview. She viewed me with suspicion, as if I might harm her, and she was suspicious of my in-depth questioning, asking me why I wanted to know such-and -such. She was a highly intelligent woman, with a fine discriminating mind, and a love of truth and philosophy, who led a very isolated existence because she trusted few people not to harm her (Kent: 'Fear of people'). She was especially wary of men, and of doctors, since she had suffered previously from their insensitivity. I gradually learned that she had had an aggressive father who had terrified her, and had thus weakened the already delicate self-confidence that a China individual is born with. Her principal complaint was a delicate digestion, with numerous food sensitivities. After a course of China she was not only able to eat a far wider range of foods, but she had also gained a considerable degree of self-confidence, and felt better able to cope with a world that was no longer as threatening as it used to be.

There are two types of China individuals; the worldly and the other-worldly. Both are very sensitive, but whilst the former is principally sensitive to any form of aggression, the latter is also sensitive in a psychic sense. These ethereal Chinas are the most psychic of all constitutional types. They are generally fascinating people who are principally interested in spiritual matters, and they are all the more interesting because their spiritual interests are based on direct experience, rather than intellectual attraction. They are generally quiet, modest people who possess a great deal of wisdom, which they will not 'cast before swine'. One such lady, a young woman of about eighteen years, had huge dark Spanish eyes, and straight black hair that fell to her waist. She had an air of mystery about her, and she tended to speak in riddles if I tried to glean too much information about her spiritual experiences. Gradually I got to know her, and discovered that she was extraordinarily psychic. She said that she spent much of her free time in another world, an astral world which was as real to her as this one. She could go there any time she wished, and she had a boyfriend in that other world. In order to prove to me that she was serious she wrote a few lines of the script of that world, which was quite different from any script I had ever seen, and yet it looked both beautiful and coherent This woman was not insane or hysterical. She really did go to another world, one that she felt more at home in than ours. She found it hard to come to terms with the ignorance and brutality of this world, and she lived a protected life in a spiritual household. Eventually she moved out from this household and in with her new terrestrial boyfriend. The shock of this move was too great for her, and she consulted me in a panic. She had developed agarophobia with constant free-floating anxiety, and a fear that she would go insane. I gave her China 10M, and within a couple of days her anxiety was much more manageable.

The more psychic China individual can easily be dismissed as hysterical by homeopaths who are not aware of the reality of other planes of existence beyond the gross physical. There is much evidence that other dimensions do exist, and those homeopaths who doubt this would be wise to keep an open mind about such things, if only so that they can help their more psychic patients. The psychic China individual is a quiet, subtle person, rather than a hystrionic who is looking for attention. Those people who like to dramatise their psychic experiences are unlikely to be China constitutionally. They are more likely to be Natrum Muriaticum, Ignatia, or if they appear really 'over the top' Hyoscyamus.

The China woman (the majority are female) is most easily confused with either Ignatia or Thuja. The differences appear quite subtle. Ignatia generally has a stronger ego than China, and is rather more 'robust', in the sense that she is better adapted to coping with society's demands. Thuja is just as sensitive as China, and just as introverted, but tends to be more earthy, more in her body and more attracted to practical crafts. China is more liable to be philosophical than Thuja, and less practical (Kent:' theorizing, building air castles'). I have only recognised one China man, and he was most similar to Mercurius, being flighty, analytical and impish. He was, however, less grounded than Mercurius, having an ethereal beauty, and a passionate love of talking about spiritual matters.

## *Contrariness and Irritability*

The fire which inspires the more spiritual China person with meditative ecstasy and philosophical passion tends to be expressed as irritability in the more worldly China individual. The latter is still very sensitive, in the sense of fearful and suspicious, and also sensitive aesthetically and physically, but she is of this world. She is generally an analytical person, with a fine intellect, but lacks the self-confidence to make full use of it. She is also a rather willful person. Here we have a contradiction similar to that seen in Silica, a timid person who is willful. The worldly China woman tends to be more irritable and intolerant than Silica. Although she may lack confidence with strangers, and is generally on her guard in company, she can make her family's life hell with her moodiness and her tendency to criticise and blame. One such patient who responded to the remedy, a sophisticated woman of about forty years, was always complaining to me bitterly about how badly her daughter treated her. She eventually threw her daughter out of the house. I then saw the daughter at my clinic. She complained bitterly of her mother's selfishness and intolerance. More telling was her sister's report. Her sister got on well with her mother, but she also admitted that her mother was not an easy person to live with, because she was so critical. This critical aspect of China is associated with a selfish, self-obsessed streak. She will fly into a rage and persecute a member of her family, quite unable to see what she is doing. I came across such behviour in a young woman of about thirty years who consulted me for treatment of her moodiness. She would fly into a rage with her husband or her father-in-law, particularly premenstrually, and at such times she was quite beyond reason, exaggerating their faults and imagining slights and insults (Kent:'Delusions of being persecuted'). This behaviour used to surprise me, since most of the time she appeared gentle, timid and sensitive. She had an attractive impish face, with very large dark eyes (the introverted equivalent of Phosphorus) which shone with delight when she was happy, but stared in fear just as often. I did not see China as the remedy, and helped her moods more with psychotherapy than with homeopathy. After a couple of years I had moved to another part of the country, and she complained over the phone of blood and mucus in her stool, and told me that she had had a little blood in her stool for years, though she had never mentioned it before. At a distance I was able to see what I could not see close up. I gave her China 200c, and after a few days the problem cleared completely.

There is actually a continuum from the ethereal to the worldly China, with some China people in the middle. Thus some are quite intuitive, or even psychic, but also relatively skillful at dealing with the material world. The latter are never materialists in the sense that Nux or Lycopodium are, since they are too deep for that, but they may love fine things, and know how to obtain them. I once treated a very unusual woman of about forty years for chronic hepatitis. Her appearance was quite striking, with very pale face and black hair, large dark eyes and high cheek-bones. There was something oriental about her eyes, a feature I have seen several times in western China women. This lady had a rather dramatic persona, being prone to sweeping statements, especially of a critical nature. She reserved these criticisms for anyone and anything that displeased her, including the medical establishment, politicians, men, and her boyfriend (Kent: 'Contemptuous'). She was very psychic, and as I gained her confidence she told me more and more about her visions and prophetic dreams. Her psychic life dominated her daily experience, inspite of the fact that she was a mother. She spent a lot of time either praying or meditating, and thinking about her visions, and her work as an artist and a poet revolved around her psychic and spiritual experiences. Having grown up in a wealthy influential family, this lady appeared far more confident than other China women I have known, but it soon became apparent that her bold and rather aggressive exterior was a defense for a very vulnerable interior. She was sophisticated and had a highly discriminating intellect, and I nearly mistook her for Ignatia, but she was too psychic and too fearful. She was also more critical than Ignatia generally is, and her physical symptoms did not fit the latter, and so I gave China 200, which produced a brief aggravation of symptoms, followed by an increase in vitality. She is an example of a China individual who exibits traits from both ends of the China spectrum, being highly psychic and spiritually orientated, and also critical and socially skillful.

### *Dyslexia, Indecision and Ungroundedness*
It appears that China's psychic sensitivity exacts a price when it comes to rational thinking, or at least its verbal expression. Two of my China patients had suffered from dyslexia, and one tended to mix up his words when speaking. The latter, a charismatic young man with the looks of a god, would get flustered when speaking (Kent: 'Mistakes, misplaces words'). He would approach a sentence like a runaway locomotive and then trip up almost immediately, producing a stop-start delivery. This was especially true when he was speaking on his favourite topics—spirituality and philosophy. His enthusi-

asm, together with the subtle nature of the subject, led him to trip over words in his attempt to express so much with so little. In addition to his erratic verbal delivery, he was somewhat erratic in his behaviour, being rather unreliable and forgetful. There was a certain degree of scattering of his mind, and also a reluctance to be pinned down to commitments. He would spend his time partying when he should have been studying, and then would cram all night before exams. In other words, he was undisciplined and irresponsible, and yet he was very popular because he was both charming and well-meaning. The above description is quite close to Phosphorus and Mercurius, both of whom can embody the archetype of the irresponsible charismatic 'Divine child'. However, this man was too analytical to be Phosphorus constitutionally, and too ethereal to be Mercurius. He had when young experienced a series of terrifying episodes of expansion of consciousness to the point where there was no sense of individual existence, and these experiences confirmed for me the choice of China rather thsn Phosphorus or Mercurius. I gave him China 10M (which also fitted his past history of recurrent bronchitis and urticaria), and he reported later that he felt more grounded and able to concentrate on his studies after the remedy.

Not surprisingly in one who is so sensitive, indicision is sometimes complained of by China individuals. One young woman consulted me for this very problem. She was quiet, modest and very wise for her years. She said that she didn't know whether the perceptions she felt and the conclusions she came to about how she should live her life were coming from her ego or her intuition, and hence she didn't know whether or not to follow them. This is an unusually perceptive question in itself for a woman of twenty years of age. I did some Gestalt work with her, and it was clear to me and to herself afterwards that her intuition was very strong and reliable, and it was only self-doubt due to listening too much to other people which confused her. I gave her a dose of China 10M and a couple of weeks later she told me that she no longer had a problem with indecision. She was one of the China patients I referred to who had suffered from dyslexia. She had cured herself with the aid of educational kinesiology.

### Physical Appearance

China people usually have slim bodies with long delicate fingers, and long eyelashes. The face is angular and the more spiritual China individual has a rather triangular face with the chin as the apex of the triangle, reflecting the preponderance of spiritual rather than material interests. In both types the face is broad, reflecting a broad-minded nature, and the cheek-bones tend to be high, giving an elegant and somewhat oriental appearance. The eyes tend to be large and brown, and the hair is generally dark and straight, but is sometimes blonde. The lips are usually quite thick, reflecting a passionate nature, and the mouth is wide.

There is an impish quality to the face of many China individuals that results from the combination of wide eyes and angular face.

# Graphites

*Keynote:* Blandness

Graphites is not often thought of as a constitutional remedy, but there are people who resonate to this remedy throughout most of their lives, and this should not be surprising, since it is a remedy for chronic complaints. (Kent: 'It is as broad and as deep as Sulphur'). When a remedy is the similimum for a chronic state, it generally covers the totality of the patient's characteristics, and this is just as true of Graphites as it is of more familiar constitutional remedies.

One of the reasons that Graphites is easily missed as a constitutional type is that Graphites people have few if any striking features. They are quiet, unassuming, gentle, matter of fact people, who would be described as 'normal' and 'pleasant' by most people who know them. Another reason they are easily missed is that they resemble several other types, both mentally and physically. A great many Graphites cases are given Calcarea, Pulsatilla and Natrum Muriaticum (without much effect), since these types have many features in common.

## Simplicity and Gentleness

Graphites the remedy is made from carbon, and it is therefore not surprising to find similarities between the mentals and the physicals of Graphites and other carbon-containing remedies, particularly Calcarea Carbonica and Natrum Carbonicum. The carbon element appears to resonate with a down-to-earth kind of personality, and we can see in each of the above types a simple, matter of fact approach to life, uncomplicated by the intellectual pretensions of more sophisticated types, and yet level-headed in comparison with more emotional types like Pulsatilla and Ignatia. For this reason Graphites people have a kind of innocence. They are uncomplicated without being stupid, much as Calcarea people are. They tend to say what they think, and to be straightforward and free from guile, unlike Natrum Muriaticum, Sepia and Ignatia, whose subtle minds can deliberately manipulate others for their own purposes.

Graphites differs from Calcarea in being more emotional and a little more introspective and shy. Her shyness (the vast majority of Graphites people are female) and her softness resembles that of Pulsatilla at first glance, but she is generally a deeper, more subtle person than Pulsatilla. Once Pulsatilla knows you, she is generally extroverted and very playful. Graphites, on the other hand, remains a relatively quiet person even in familiar company. However, Graphites does have much of the soft maternal quality that is so typical of the Pulsatilla adult. There is an attractive softness to most Graphites people, that the homeopath can recognise straight away once he has seen it a few times. Such people are caring and empathetic, and will generally become distressed when confronted by another's suffering.

Graphites are gentle and sensitive, and yet more 'grounded' or down to earth than China, Phosphorus and Pulsatilla. They have less difficulty than the latter types in coping with the material world, since they have a good degree of common sense, and also quite often a keen intellect. As a result of their warm heart, allied to a sensible mind, Graphites women are often to be found in the caring professions. I know a mother and daughter who are both Graphites constitutionally. The mother is corpulent, jolly and very uncomplicated. She spends much of her time doing charitable work, looking after the elderly and the infirm for the pleasure of it. She does not take her work home with her, and always puts her family first, yet when she is at work she is there one hundred percent for her patients. The same could be said for some Calcarea helpers, whose cheeriness is understated but genuine. A third type who is often corpulent, cheerful and attracted to charitable work is Natrum Muriaticum. The latter differs from Graphites and Calcarea in being more intense emotionally, with a tendency to identify too much with those she is helping, and an inability to say no. Also Natrum's cheeriness is often in part a mask, hiding sadness within, whereas that of Calcarea and Graphites is generally just what it seems.

The Graphites helper's daughter is also a helper, offering massage and counselling at a nominal fee to those who need it. She is slim, more shy than her mother, and more introspective. I have treated her for ulcerative colitis, which gradually cleared up using Graphites in LM and 30C potencies. These two women illustrate well the two common subtypes of Graphites. The older Graphites (born before 1950) tends to be corpulent, jolly and uncomplicated, whereas young Graphites women tend to be more introspective, having absorbed more of the influences of the 'growth movement' of the last twenty years. (I have found this distinction between the younger and the older Graphites woman to be pretty consistent). Both types often have an artistic streak, and yet like Calcarea they will seldom abandon their first love —home life—to make their way as artists commercially. Graphites is a very feminine type, who seldom puts her ego or her intellect before her heart. Family life is generally her first love, the bedrock of her life, and she usually makes a natural and loving parent. It is when she has difficulties in her close relationships that Graphites suffers most. She is usually very dependent upon a few close relationships, and when these are absent or become stressed she will suffer greatly, as will Pulsatilla. She is more sensitive in this respect than

Calcarea (hence the ulcerative colitis, a condition probably unheard of in Calcarea individuals), and less able to cut off from her pain and make a go of a career than Natrum Muriaticum.

### Indecision and Moodiness

The Graphites individual does not share only her positive characteristics with Calcarea, Natrum and Pulsatilla. Her negative traits can also be found on the whole in these other types. Like Pulsatilla she tends to be content as long as her personal life is loving and secure, but she can be oversensitive to disharmony in her relationships, and she may become very moody when her parent or her partner does not behave lovingly towards her. Graphites may exhibit the whole spectrum of negative emotions when she is upset, and like Pulsatilla she is not able to hide them, even when she wants to. In a dispute with a loved one she may at first withdraw and brood with an intensity that imposes a dark heavy cloud on all around her. She will refuse to admit to being upset, hide her face, and just answer in monosyllables when spoken to. Then she will either find some solitude and cry, or begin crashing around the house, slamming doors and crashing pans and crockery, in an attempt both to announce her anger, and to defuse it. These outbursts of pique are very similar to those seen in Sepia, Natrum and Ignatia women when they lose their temper.

One of the reasons why Graphites crashes about without actually addressing her grievances to the other person, who is usually a man, is because she is afraid of confrontation. Graphites is a gentle, sensitive type, yet she can get frustrated enough to become very angry (Kent: 'Extremely fretful and impatient'), and when this happens she announces her anger tangentially, not daring to express it directly. When Graphites does express her grievance verbally, she generally breaks down into tears rather than shouting, in much the same way as Pulsatilla and some Calcarea women. These gentle types hate disharmony, and will generally forgive and make up very quickly, providing the other person will meet them half way. In contrast, Natrum Muriaticum, Ignatia and some Sepias are more assertive when they express their anger. They are quite capable of exploding verbally and even physically, unafraid of the response they may encounter. They are also less quick to forgive and may harbour grudges for a long time.

Like Pulsatilla, Graphites' emotions are generally close to the surface. They are more stable than Pulsatilla's, but will still become quite labile when problems arise (Kent: 'her moods are constantly changing'). She may become confused and despair with herself, because she is so up and down, one moment happy, and the next tearful and morose. And such times Graphites may entertain a lot of self-doubt, and even some self-condemnation. One

Graphites young woman whose premenstrual tension responded splendidly to the remedy described herself as 'very selfish' when she was feeling down, and yet she appeared to be a sensitive and generous person, and expressed no such sentiments when she was more herself. This low self esteem is similar to that seen in Natrum women, but is generally easier for the Graphites individual to overcome, since it is transient. Like Natrum Muriaticum, Graphites individuals are often very self-conscious in public, and they are more liable to blush than any other type when they are embarrassed.

Another result of Graphites' labile emotions is irresolution (Kent: 'She cannot make up her mind to do or not to do'). Her generally capable and sensible intellect becomes paralysed when she is at all emotional, causing her to agonise over the smallest decisions. At these times she may rely heavily on others to make up her mind for her. Even when she is not particularly emotional, Graphites may have difficulty deciding between two or more options. This is especially true of important decisions, such as which course to study or which job to apply for, since she lacks the confidence to take a risk. All the gentle, sensitive types suffer from indecision, which arises from fear of making 'the wrong decision', and the negative outcomes that may result (Kent: 'Fear of misfortune').

Whilst we are on the subject of fear, let us take a look at Graphites' fearfulness in general. Like most sensitive types, Graphites can be quite timid. Depending on her upbringing she may be shy of people, afraid of adventurous physical activities like sailing and rock climbing, nervous when her husband drives the car a little too fast, and oversensitive at night to the slightest noise. One Graphites patient admitted that she was forever waking her husband in the night to investigate little noises, which she feared were intruders. The same women had a fear when out at night in lonely places, not of attackers but of ghosts. (The fact that Graphites does not appear in Kent's repertory under the rubric 'fear of ghosts' should not put the homeopath off. Kent's repertory is by no means 'complete'.)

Probably the commonest fear one encounters in Graphites people is a general fear of the future. There is a tendency to be pessimistic, or rather, to fear the worst when considering the future, and this fear may sometimes inhibit action. The same fearfulness can be seen in Sepia, Calcarea, Arsenicum and Phosphorus. In the case of Graphites these fears are usually transient and do not dominate for long. When life is running reasonably smoothly Graphites individuals are generally quite carefree like Calcarea and Phosphorus, rather than forever on the lookout for trouble like Arsenicum.

Quite a common fear amongst Graphites people is a fear of losing their loved ones. Graphites people develop deep attachments to family and friends, and they are usually very aware of their dependence upon them. This can give rise to a nagging fear of 'what would I do if so and so died? How would I cope?'. Graphites is listed in italics in Kent's repertory under 'Grief', indicating that Graphites people suffer greatly from bereavement.

## The Graphites Man

Graphites men are at a distinct disadvantage in modern cultures. They are shy, and the masculine attributes which are so favoured by society are relatively weakly developed in most Graphites men. Graphites boys are generally soft and sensitive, and may be made fun of at school for being 'sissies'. They are liable to get on better with their mother than their father, and to take an interest in relatively feminine activities like cooking and gardening. The Graphites boy who has a traditional father who expects boys to be young men, who like football and don't cry, are especially disadvantaged. Such a boy will grow up feeling a failure in the eyes of both his father and society as a whole, since his positive (feminine) traits will receive no encouragement.

Graphites men are often painfully shy. They have, on the whole, a much harder time in childhood than Graphites girls, and hence they often grow up to be withdrawn and lacking in confidence. It is not unusual for a Graphites boy to be overfed by his concerned mother, who seeks to give him comfort through food. As a result, many Graphites men are obese, and this further adds to their lack of self-esteem. Typically, the young Graphites man is very nervous around the opposite sex, and may have great difficulty in overcoming his shyness sufficiently to form a romantic relationship. Being a very emotional, sensitive person, the Graphites man is often painfully lonely. His withdrawn nature does not allow him to easily compensate for his lack of a partner by developing his social life, as the single Natrum man often succeeds in doing. As a result, many single Graphites men are chronically lonely and depressed.

Those Graphites men who do form a stable relationship with a woman will usually want to get married. They make solid, dependable partners, who are affectionate for the most part, and sensitive to their wife's feelings. They also make caring and interested parents, who will put their family's needs before career or public expectations.

Graphites is an earthy type, and this is reflected in the sound practical ability of most Graphites men. They are generally handy, and will often follow practical and technical careers. They are not ambitious people, and they do not seek responsibility, but will perform their work honestly and reliably, year in and year out.

## Physical Appearance

Graphites tends to be quite rounded and soft in appearance like Pulsatilla, though there is sometimes a squarish look to the face. Older Graphites women are often obese, though their faces tend not to look bloated, but rather rosy and clear (since they do not suppress emotions). Younger Graphites women are often slimmer, but still soft and rounded rather than taut or bony. The lips are generally full, indicating a warm, sensuous nature. The complexion is generally either very smooth and soft, or else marked by eczema. Superficial tumours such as wens and moles are common. Obese Graphites are generally of dark complexion, and earthy in character, whereas slimmer Graphites are usually fair, and are deeper emotionally.

# *Hyoscyamus*

*Keynote:* Erotic psychosis

Hyoscyamus is a rare constitutional type, one of the family of remedies that correspond to manic and schizophrenic states (others include Stramonium, Belladonna and Veratrum Album). Since I have seen relatively few Hyoscyamus patients the following is only a brief sketch of the Hyoscyamus mentality.

The most common impression that the homeopath receives of a Hyoscyamus patient is that she is like Lachesis, only more bizarre. Four of the most characteristic features of the Lachesis mentality are also seen in Hyoscyamus; hurriedness (and loquacity), paranoia, jealousy and sexual obsession.

## Insanity

The Hyoscyamus individual, when not frankly schizophrenic, is skating on thin ice, and may fall through into insanity when stressed. Often the homeopath will sense very quickly that there is something bizarre about the patient's mentality. Their complaints may seem slightly unusual, (for example, she may say that her brain is clicking), and are likely to centre on the nervous system. One Hyoscyamus patient complained of attacks of sniffing, which she said occurred when her energies were blocked, at specific times in the day. She then obliged by going into a fit of sniffing in front of me, in a dramatic display that was clearly hysterical (Kent: 'Hysteria').

Most patients who are on the verge of a psychotic state are aware that there is something wrong with their thinking processes. The Hyoscyamus patients that I have seen usually complained principally about their nervous system and their mental processes. The more sane they were, the more fear they had of going insane.

## Shamelessness

Sexual obsession is a key feature of Hyoscyamus, in both the psychotic and the pre-psychotic individual. The patient will enjoy talking in a totally unselfconscious manner about her sexual life (the majority of Hyoscyamus patients who I have seen were women), often either boasting about how much she enjoys sexuality, and describing with relish a long list of sexual encounters, or lamenting the lack of them in her life. She is stimulated by talking about sex, and will bring up the subject again and again, especially if she sees that you are not shocked by her. Hyoscyamus individuals are subject to very powerful sexual feelings (Kent: 'Lascivious', 'Insanity-erotic'), which they will struggle with if they are relatively sane. Masturbation may be resorted to daily in an attempt to relieve the tension. The Hyoscyamus woman may be tortured by sexual frustration, and yet will resist infidelity when she is married, since she believes it is wrong. The closer to insanity she becomes, the less likely she is to resist her sexual urges.

There is a clear tendency in Hyoscyamus to want to expose the body sexually (Kent: 'Naked—wants to be'). I have not come across patients who expose themselves in public (apart from Hyoscyamus children and one demented hospital inpatient), but the Hyoscyamus women I have seen had a tendency to expose their sexual areas with the excuse of having some physical symptom or sign in these areas that they wanted investigated.

## Paranoia

Hyoscyamus is one of the most suspicious and paranoid of constitutional types (Kent: 'Suspicious', 'Fear of being poisoned', 'Imagines being abused'). Most Hyoscyamus people who consult homeopaths are not frankly psychotic, and many will tend to play down their more bizarre thought patterns in an attempt to avoid being seen as insane, hence their paranoia is often expressed quite subtly. For example, if the homeopath is not obviously sympathetic, she may feel that he is against her, and may even accuse him of being so. Or she may interpret a stern final electricity bill as evidence that the council is trying to evict her. Naturally, the more disturbed the Hyoscyamus person becomes, the more unrealistic are her paranoid fears. In advanced stages of pathology she may imagine that poison gas is being pumped into her house, or that the CIA is watching her. These frankly paranoid fears are accompanied by a great deal of anxiety, rising at times to sheer panic.

## Loquacity

Not all Hyoscyamus patients speak quickly and endlessly, but some do, particularly those who are on the verge of insanity. These people may easily be mistaken for Lachesis cases, but the content of the speech of the latter is generally not bizarre like that of Hyoscyamus. (Another type that may speak quickly, continuously and rather bizarrely is Cannabis Indica). Like Lachesis, Hyoscyamus speaks quickly, and changes track frequently, because her mind is being barraged by an endless stream of thoughts. Speaking quickly tends to release the pressure inside the head to some degree. It is difficult to keep such patients to the subject of your question, and also difficult to end the consultation, since the patient will continue to chatter, ignoring hints that the session is over. The homeopath may have to virtually leave the room himself to encourage the loquacious Hyoscyamus patient to get out of her chair, and she will continue to chatter at a rapid pace as she is leaving the room.

## Morbid Jealousy

Jealousy is a combination of attachment (or desire) and fear of loss. Any type can suffer from jealousy, but those types that are both anxious and highly sexed are most prone to severe or pathological jealousy, and these include Lachesis and Hyoscyamus in particular. Jealousy is pathological when it occurs in the absence of a likelihood of competition for, or loss of the loved one or loved thing.

In Hyoscyamus individuals feelings of jealousy can be so powerful that they totally dominate the life of the patient and her partner. The characteristic thing about the morbid jealousy of Hyoscyamus is that it tends to be accompanied by rage. A Hyoscyamus woman may appear entirely normal except when she is feeling jealous, when she is transformed into a biting, screaming, kicking maniac (Kent: 'Jealousy', 'Desires to strike'). At other times she manages to control her rage , but it is keenly felt nevertheless.

The jealousy of Hyoscyamus is not confined to sexual partners. One Hyoscyamus lady told me that as a child she was 'overwhelmed by jealousy' when one of her friends was stolen from her by another girl, and that this jealousy obsessed her at the time for several weeks.

## Religiosity

Some Hyoscyamus individuals adopt strongly religious attitudes (like Veratrum and Anacardium), and these religious beliefs become a vehicle for their delusions and even hallucinations (Kent: 'Religious turn of mind…they take on the delusion that they have sinned away their day of grace'.) As Kent points out, these religious Hyoscyamus people are apt to suffer from feelings of shame and fear of damnation. This is in part because they are subject to such strong sexual impulses. One of my patients, a pleasant but very nervous woman of about forty years, came to see me initially because she felt such a lot of anxiety, especially when she had to talk to people. I gradually learned that she was very religious, and was tormented by sexual thoughts, which she considered unclean. She told me that when she went into church she would have a vision of Jesus masturbating on the cross, and this disturbed her greatly, but also aroused her. After a few doses of Hyoscyamus 10M her anxiety and her loquacity were much reduced, and she became subject to more pleasant religious visions! It is interesting here to compare and contrast the religious Hyoscyamus with the religious Platina. Both have very strong sexual urges, which may become entangled with religious visions. In my experience, the chief difference is that Hyoscyamus' visions contain a degree of obscenity that is not common in those of Platina. This is in keeping with the theme of obscenity which runs through the type, from a fascination with faeces and urine in young and insane Hyoscyamus people (Kent: 'Speech illustrated by urine, faeces and cow dung') to the characteristic attraction of Hyoscyamus to sexual swear words. In contrast, Platina is more liable to have ecstatic visions in which she is the bride of Christ, or is making love with a nature spirit.

One very common form of religiosity in Hyoscyamus individuals is an attraction to 'New Age' ideas, such as aura-reading, crystals, etc. Like Natrum Muriaticum, Hyoscyamus is attracted to the psychic dimension of 'New Age' thinking, but is even more obsessive about it than Natrum.

## Rage, Mania and Delirium

Like Stramonium, Hyoscyamus harbours powerful sexual and violent urges in the subconscious mind, which may erupt dramatically during transient periods of insanity. In between these episodes the high sex drive is generally more apparent than the violent tendency, which is the reverse of Stramonium. Hyoscyamus individuals are prone to feelings of intense anger, but they are likely to control their rage unless they have entered a phase of frank psychosis, or have been rendered temporarily mad by jealousy.

Even during a psychotic phase it is my impression that Hyoscyamus displays more sexual interest, particularly exhibitionism, than violence. I once witnessed such an episode in an elderly lady who had been hospitalised for several years with a mixture of arthritis, heart failure and dementia. As she grew more confused she began to wander around the ward (Kent: 'Jumping out of bed'), muttering to herself, laughing, and taking off her dress. It was only when we tried to persuade her to return to her bed that she became violent, biting and scratching and screaming at the top of her voice. She was eventually given sedation, and screamed that she was being murdered by an injection of poison. This form of delirium is described in detail in the older Materia Medicas. It is characterised by wandering, muttering, laughing, singing (especially lewd songs) and sexual exhibitionism, as well as by violence when opposed. It is seen most commonly in elderly confused people, but may also occur in younger Hyoscyamus individuals during schizophrenic episodes.

In children the characteristics of Hyoscyamus are less disguised by social conditioning, hence the sexual and aggressive tendencies can be seen in the absence of delirium. Like Stramonium children, they tend to be hyperactive and disruptive, and may lash out violently when opposed, though less so than Stramonium. The Hyoscyamus child is prone to swearing (Kent: 'Cursing'), and is liable to totally ignore orders from his elders to stop his disruptive behaviour. Despite this kind of behaviour, Hyoscyamus children are often fairly well behaved in the consulting room. One such child, a boy of about ten years old, had been suspended from school for distracting his classmates, and for exposing himself in the lavatory. He argued somewhat unconvincingly that he had forgotten to put his pants back on .

I have come across small children who went into a Hyoscyamus state after being sexually molested. Children who are molested often become obsessed with sexuality, as well as aggressive and difficult to handle. One such child, who was only three years old when he was molested by his babysitter, became totally obsessed with sex. He would expose himself in the consulting room, utter sexual swear words, and try to touch his mother's sexual parts. He was also aggressive and would not obey any commands. In addition, he had become obsessive. He would only allow his toys to be put away in a certain order, and would throw a tantrum if his wishes were not followed. All this was in marked contrast to his previous normal personality. After a few doses of Hyoscyamus he gradually returned to his normal self.

A few of my Hyoscyamus patients showed no signs of bizarre mentality. In these cases the principal features were intense jealousy, feelings of rage, and panic attacks. The libido was very high, but there was no sign of exhibitionism, or of a compulsion to speak about sex. In these more integrated Hyoscyamus individuals the distinction from Lachesis is even more difficult. Generally Hyoscyamus is less extroverted than Lachesis (especially when she is relatively sane), and is more prone to rage and panic. Naturally the physicals and generals will help to differentiate the two.

### Physical Appearances

Hyoscyamus women tend to have one of two facial appearances. Some have plump, round faces, with quite thick lips. Others have squarish faces, with bright, beady eyes, which are often accompanied by fine lines radiating out from the corners. Many Hyoscyamus women are obese.

# Ignatia

*Keynote:* Emotional roller-coaster

Ignatia is not a very common type (I see about 50 Natrums for every Ignatia), but once the homeopath gets a feeling for the type it is unmistakable.

## Emotional Intensity

The most obvious characteristic of Ignatia is emotional intensity. All emotions - anger, sadness, joy love, fear, lust, are felt by the Ignatia individual with a degree of intensity not seen in any other type. For the most part Ignatia expresses her emotions (the vast majority of Ignatias are female), and hence is known by her friends and family to be a highly emotional person. However, there is some tendency to suppress unpleasant emotions, which grows as the Ignatia individual becomes less healthy psychologically. Like her more stable sister Natrum Muriaticum, she may sit on sadness for a long time, putting on a brave face to the world. Eventually, however, most suppressed Ignatias crack open, and when they do, the resulting avalanche of emotions is far more dramatic than that seen in Natrum (Kent: 'She is unable to control her emotions or her excitement').

Since emotions, as the word suggests, are moving and transient, Ignatia feels, and often appears to be very changeable (Kent: 'Mood—Alternating, changeable'). In most people the intellect filters and attenuates emotion until it no longer threatens the smooth continuity of the sense of self. In Ignatia however, the emotions are felt so intensely that they overwhelm the intellect, and so the person becomes, in effect, the emotion. Most Ignatia women are very expressive, and will soon let you know if they are furious, ecstatic, terrified or deeply depressed. (These extremes of emotion are seen in Ignatia almost as commonly as their milder forms.)

## The Healthy Ignatia

In their formative years, Ignatia children are extremely sensitive to their emotional environment. A few fortunate ones pass through childhood without being exposed to significant emotional trauma. These rare cases of emotionally healthy Ignatias exhibit all the positive characteristics of the type, free from the distortions of suppressed pain and anger, and the defence mechanisms that develop to avoid further suffering.

The well-balanced Ignatia is sensitive, passionate and refined (Kent: '...gentle, sensitive, fine-fibred women'). She feels deeply the beauty of the Earth, the depth of her love, and the thrill of achievement. Her intellect is usually sharp, but is not her dominant mode of experiencing herself and her environment. This is more emotional, intuitive and passionate. The healthy Ignatia girl is very open to the wonder of life, and more keenly perceptive than most (Kent: 'Senses hyperacute'). She is a deep person, who appreciates beauty, and thinks profoundly. She is liable to be a little quiet or even shy when young (Kent: 'Quiet disposition'), because she does not like vulgarity, and so she protects herself from the world to some extent. Like Silica and China, she will respond enthusiastically to those who are sensitive enough to understand her, and also to those who, though less sensitive, have demonstrated their good intentions. The healthy Ignatia is warm and affectionate to family and friends, and is more outgoing and spontaneous than other sensitive, refined types.

Most healthy Ignatias have artistic talent, and art is often an important interest to them, whether as artists or as lovers of art. Ignatia has a great deal of style, and seems to be able to look chic without trying. Less healthy Ignatias go out of their way to look good and to impress, but for the healthy Ignatia style and good taste come naturally, as part of her inherent refinement. It is no accident that French women are renowned for their sense of style. Many of them are Ignatias, as are many other women of Latin origin.

I remember one such healthy Ignatia, a music teacher and composer, who consulted me for treatment of hypoglycaemic symptoms. She was extremely open and vibrant, shining with an exuberant energy that enlivened me. Her interaction with me was enthusiastic and merry, punctuated by laughter, and the occasional tear when speaking of a past sadness. Her charisma and openness was reminiscent of Phosphorus, but she had more depth, and her ego or sense of identity was stronger. Her hypoglycaemic symptoms settled rapidly after a dose of Ignatia 1M, and she was keen to find out all about homeopathy at the second consultation. Ignatia's blend of sensitivity and passion gives her a vivacity that is closest to that seen in emotionally healthy Lachesis and Medorrhinum women.

### Free-Thinkers and Feminists

Ignatia can be said to be the most powerful of the feminine types. Healthy Ignatias have a natural authority which comes from an unusual degree of self-possession, coupled with a very sharp intellect. They are usually 'free-thinkers', who are attracted to the most profound and also the most progressive of ideas, and often they will pursue these academically and professionally. In my own practice I have come across three Ignatia women who all worked for radio, and all were involved or wished to be involved in making programs

which 'raised the consciousness' of the listener. One of these women studied Buddhism at university, and also became a Sanskrit scholar, and another
studied the cultural effects of Indian philosophy upon Indian women in the
eighteenth century. Like many Ignatia women, she felt impelled to speak out
for the rights of her weaker sisters, being something of a feminist. A great
many Ignatia women express feminist ideas, since they are as courageous and
as powerful as men (more than most men) and are outraged by the conde-
scension and domination that they see visited upon other women by men.

### Insecurity and Moodiness

The majority of Ignatias do experience some form of emotional trauma
during their early years. Ignatia is so sensitive that even relatively 'normal'
family conditions that appear to be harmless can generate insecurity. For
example, the child's parents may love each other, but have slipped over the
years into a habit of taking each other for granted, and expressing less of their
affection. This happens in the majority of couples, but it may be perceived
(albeit subconsciously) by the sensitive Ignatia child as a threat, since the
uninhibited flow of love that she needs is somewhat lacking. Ignatia children
are particularly susceptible to feelings of abandonment. It is a curious phenomenon that those individuals born Ignatias seem to attract circumstances
in their life which produce a lasting sense of abandonment. It may be that
they have been orphaned, and brought up by well meaning foster parents
who were nevertheless unable to understand the girl, or that one of the
parents was cold and unapproachable. Other individuals born into similar
circumstances grow into Natrum people. It thus seems that the constitutional
types have already been determined in utero, and subsequent conditions
serve only to produce more or less healthy examples of the type.

   Once the Ignatia child has been deeply hurt, she will never fully trust
again. A wall begins to form around the injured heart, a kind of callus which
becomes thicker and more rigid with every new trauma that life brings. At
first this defensive wall is expressed as anger and indignation, which wells up
whenever the Ignatia individual feels that she has been rejected, let down
or neglected (Kent: 'Anger-from contradiction'). The normally affectionate
Ignatia can become an Ice Queen at such times, saying as much with her tight
lips and steely silence as she does at other times with bitter curses.
Shakespeare probably had Ignatia in mind when he coined the phrase 'Hell
hath no fury like a woman scorned'. Like Sepia, Nux and Lachesis, the outraged Ignatia may resort to acts of vengeance (Kent: 'Rage leading to violent
deeds'), but more often, the offending individual is simply cut off from her
heart, and never spoken to again. Ignatia individuals are very black and white
(they actually wear these colours more than any others). They either love you
or hate you, and when they hate you they usually prefer to cut you off emo-

tionally, since the hate is really due to a deeply felt hurt which they would rather forget.

The Ignatia child expresses her insecurity as moodiness. She may be cheerful most of the time, but some small incident that would go unnoticed by a less sensitive heart will trigger that sense of being unloved that lies at the root of Ignatia's instability. It may be simply that her parents make a fuss of her sister on the latter's birthday, or that they do not give her the praise she expected for some achievement at school. At such times the Ignatia child is liable to sulk, withdrawing from those around her in a rather dramatic fashion, that is designed to punish as well as to attract attention (Kent: 'Moodsullen', 'Childish behaviour', 'Whenever she is crossed or contradicted she desires to be alone, and to dwell on the inconsistencies that come into her life'). When Natrum children are hurt they will quietly withdraw into themselves whilst maintaining a surface appearance that everything is alright. Ignatia, on the other hand, will turn her head away from her parents, storm off to her room, and perhaps announce, "Go away! You don't love me!", to the bewilderment of her parents, who have no idea what they have done to upset her so.

### Unrequited Love

During adolescence the Ignatia teenager is even more prone than her peers to intense and shifting moods. She is liable to develop crushes on boys, and eventually to fall madly in love with one of them. Most Ignatia teenagers are aware of their capacity for being hurt, and will avoid relationships until they feel sure their feelings are reciprocated. If they are then rejected by their partner, they will enter into a crisis of grieving that seems out of all proportion to the event (Kent: 'Ailments from disappointed love'). Of course, what has happened is that she has let down those defensive walls that have been protecting her heart for most of her life, and in that vulnerable state her abandonment has brought back all the suppressed pain of her earlier grief, when she sensed that she was not loved as a child.

During such crises Ignatia will break down and sob uncontrollably. She will lose all appetite, eating barely a thing for weeks (and vomiting when she does eat), as she dwells on the pain and the longing for the love that she has lost (Kent: 'In spite of her best endeavours, her grief has simply torn her to pieces'.) Any attempt to speak to her about her feelings will bring on floods of tears, and in her desperation she will say that she wishes she could die. Some Ignatias do take overdoses of sedatives or other tablets at such times, and may even kill themselves, since the pain in their heart feels unbearable.

Ignatia women often make a habit of falling for men who cannot return their love. The latter may already be married to someone else, or they may simply be incapable of loving freely. Kent comments in his Lecture Notes on

Materia Medica that Ignatia will fall for a married man, or for someone who is 'entirely out of her station'. All of us tend to attract situations in our lives over and over again which mimic the childhood dynamics between ourselves and our parents. It seems that this is the psyche's way of trying to heal the old wounds by 'rewriting the script'. Ignatia's habit of falling in love with unavailable men can thus be seen as a mirror of her childhood, when her love for her parents did not seem to be requited.

### Panic
During emotional crises Ignatia is often subject to feelings of panic. She feels vulnerable and out of control, and this generates a fear of going insane. It is wonderful to watch the speed with which the remedy restores stability and calm in these cases. A single drop on the tongue in the consulting room and the patient's expression changes within seconds from anguish to relief and wonder.

Ignatia can develop phobias when she is under stress. They may be directly related to some memory associated with the painful experience that precipitated the crisis. For example, she may have realised that her relationship was over whilst travelling on a bus, and thereafter be subject to anxiety when she rides on buses. She may not be aware of the origin of her phobia, especially as it may arise some weeks or even years after the precipitating event, when another stress triggers off the old subconscious memory. These phobias may gradually subside as Ignatia becomes more stable again, but sometimes they do not, a sign that the underlying grief has never healed.

### Grief
Ignatia and Natrum Muriaticum are the two remedies that all homeopaths think of first when considering the treatment of deep or prolonged grief reactions. The psychodynamics of the two are very similar, in that both types felt unloved during childhood (although this may have been unconscious), and their grief reactions are related to the old trauma of losing love, whether it be through bereavement or through rejection. Natrum is more controlled, and often grieves silently, whereas Ignatia usually loses all control when bereaved, at least initially. Ignatia will sob hysterically at first, in a kind of active shock reaction, followed by weeks of emotional volatility, in which outbursts of sobbing and also anger alternate with periods of silent (but very painful) grieving. Like Natrum, Ignatia tends to isolate herself when hurt (Kent: 'Consolation aggravates', 'Averse company'). She has been abandoned once, and dare not risk it a second time by seeking comfort from another. At times, however, she feels much worse when alone, especially in the acute stages of grief.

Any constitutional type can enter into an Ignatia state following a bereavement, or a separation from a loved one. The principal features are uncontrollable weeping, rapidly changing emotional states, nausea, vomiting and loss of appetite, with an unfillable emptiness felt in the stomach, and a sensation of a lump in the throat. Once the grief has become chronic, and settled to a background sadness which recurs only when the patient is reminded of the lost one, then Natrum Muriaticum is more likely to help. In other words, Ignatia is useful for the acute stages of grief, Natrum for its chronic effects.

One of the characteristic, but relatively uncommon manifestations of an Ignatia grief reaction is hysteria. 'Hysteria' in the medical sense means the occurrence of physical symptoms in response to emotional shock, and in this sense Ignatia is probably the foremost of hysterical remedies. (As Kent points out in his Lecture Notes, hysterical personalities who deliberately do outrageous things to gain attention will not be helped by Ignatia. They require remedies corresponding to more mentally unbalanced types, such as Moschus and Lilium Tigrinum.)

The hysterical reactions of Ignatia usually involve symptoms relating to the nervous system, such as epilepsy, muscle cramps, numbness and so on. I recently came across such a case, a young girl who suddenly developed fluctuating blindness, associated with rapid involuntary eye movements. She was investigated by eye specialists, and her symptoms were thought to be hysterical, that is, due to stress and having no organic cause. During the course of the consultation the girl appeared very sensible. She was mature for her age (12 years), and she was not able to explain why such a dramatic reaction had occurred . She had caring parents, and no obvious recent emotional traumas to justify her apparently hysterical blindness. Nevertheless, she did admit to feeling very tense for some months, and confirmed that her blindness was proportional to the degree of anxiety she was feeling. On talking with her parents it became clear that her father was obsessed with his business, and spent very little time at home. When he was at home his mind was still on his business, so the girl had very little real contact with him. Furthermore, her mother was suffering from a chronic illness which made her less able to be herself. On top of this, the patient had never been happy at her school, since she was sensitive and refined, whereas all the other children came from rough backgrounds, teased her for being a 'snob', and would not make friends with her. In other words, although there was no single traumatic event which could explain her symptoms, she was chronically starved of the kind of spontaneous love that only comes from parents who are relatively contented and relaxed, and this subtle, unintentional rejection was amplified by the less subtle treatment she got at school. A dose or two of Ignatia 10M rapidly cleared up the eye problems, and the stress was reduced by changing to a more genteel school, and by the father taking more time off from work to be with the family.

## *Bitterness and Masculinisation*

When Ignatia has been rejected by a loved one, (or merely perceives that she has been rejected), it is common for her to become bitter, or even vindictive. (Kent: 'Mortification', 'Quarrelsome', 'Anger-with silent grief'). At such times she is liable to throw up a smoke-screen of accusations about how unfairly she has been treated, how cruel the other person is, how selfish and uncaring, her indignation obscuring the truth that at some deep level she does not feel that she is lovable. Once again the circumstances in her life are confirming this belief to her. An insecure Ignatia is hypersensitive to any form of rejection, no matter how slight. If a social appointment she was looking forward to is cancelled at short notice she may bitterly resent it, and is likely to make her resentment clear. Winning back the affection of an affronted Ignatia is possible, but it requires first an apology, and secondly an obvious show of affection and respect, the two qualities she feels most in need of.

Those Ignatia women who have had particularly hard lives tend to become tough and bitter. The tougher they get, the more masculine they become. Still craving approval in some form, and yet no longer daring to be emotionally vulnerable, the tough Ignatia woman seeks to impress by dominating others. She is bossy, extremely touchy, and she has a temper that makes strong men tremble with fear. In order to feel important the tough Ignatia becomes ambitious, and sets her sights upon social approval. She becomes a determined career woman, battling to beat men in their own worlds of competition and intellectualism.

The more masculinised Ignatia becomes, the more she retreats into her intellect. Here she seeks to impress by becoming highly intellectual. Ignatia academics are often very proud of their credentials, and will make the most of the letters after their names. It makes them feel important, which is the next best thing to feeling loved. In our male-dominated society it is generally easier to gain approval through the intellect than through the arts or through practical occupations. Furthermore, by immersing herself in her intellect Ignatia can avoid the painful world of emotions, and being intellectual comes easy to many Ignatias, since Ignatia as a type is highly discriminating and usually has a fine mind.

The more masculine Ignatia woman can easily be confused with Nux Vomica, which although predominantly a male remedy type, does sometimes occur in women. The two are both determined, efficient, and aggressive, and many Nux women are also intellectually orientated. They both tend to wear masculine clothes, like suits, to wear rather 'severe' hairstyles, and to hold themselves in a tense, very upright posture. The homeopath has to delve a little to differentiate the two. Ignatia's strength is more brittle, since it is merely an armour acquired to protect a sensitive heart. Thus Ignatia is more defensive than Nux, and more liable to erupt at the slightest sign of opposition or disapproval. Nux is very confident in her self and her abilities, and hence can ignore the opinions of others to a great extent. The tough Ignatia woman will still look for love in many cases, and will still break down if she opens her heart and then feels rejected. (The physical appearances of the two types are quite different, which helps to differentiate them further.)

The other type that can be confused with the tough Ignatia woman is the tough Natrum woman. Here the resemblance is closer, since the psychology is very similar. The main difference is that Ignatia is more volatile. She is quick to erupt with either anger or tears, whereas Natrum will hide her feelings and control them. Both types look for approval through proving themselves in their career, but generally Ignatia is more attracted to the prestige of powerful, exclusive positions, whereas Natrum will be satisfied as long as she is seen as efficient and indispensable wherever she works.

## Prestige

The emotionally insecure Ignatia woman often works almost full-time on bolstering her shaky sense of self-worth. She will put herself out for a friend, as long as she can expect some reward, both in terms of vocal appreciation, and in terms of securing support for an uncertain future. Since she feels that she has been (emotionally) abused in the past, she is very wary of being taken advantage of, and she will usually make sure you remember if she has helped you out. Name-dropping is a favourite way for Ignatia to seek prestige. Ignatia is naturally charming, and often looks positively glamorous. Her looks, her refinement, and her gift for self-promotion often do bring her contact with the famous in society, and if she does not gain access to the elite of society as a fully fledged member, she will at least make the most of her famous contacts. I have known several Ignatia women who regularly slipped into the conversation their acquaintance with some celebrity or other, and one who even kept press cuttings of herself being photographed with famous clients.

Ignatia is generally a very sociable person. The healthy Ignatia delights in sharing her enthusiasms with others, and has an affectionate nature. The more vulnerable Ignatia often uses socialising as a means to attract approval and support. She often fills her diary with rendezvous, parties and soirees, maintaining contact with as many people as possible. At these gatherings she is positively charming, feeding off the admiration she receives, especially from the opposite sex. Ignatia is very dependent upon being appreciated, and will often fish for compliments when they are not forthcoming. (The characters that the actress Diane Keaton often plays are typical Ignatia types, and demonstrate this characteristic beautifully).

## Dramatism

Ignatia is one of the most dramatic of types. Many Ignatia women use this to good effect as actresses. Acting is in many ways ideally suited to Ignatia, since it rewards her natural qualities of emotional dramatism and vanity. To be dramatic, one needs an audience, and Ignatia learns from early childhood to use her audience to win love and approval, or to chastise for her unhappiness. Even when she is happy the insecure Ignatia dramatises her feelings in an attempt to get a response from whoever she is with, a positive response that says to her, "Yes, you are wonderful, and I love you." The insecure Ignatia boasts about her happiness, exaggerating it to make her appear special, and hence worthy of love. (Natrum Muriaticum and Phosphorus women also do this). When she receives praise, or even agreement, she will become rapturous, and will giggle with delight. (Giggling is very characteristic of Ignatia). On the other hand, the slightest negative response (or lack of response) from her audience leaves her dismayed, and then either depressed or angry. Ignatia longs to feel special to somebody, and much of her time is often spent on seeking approval.

## Refinement

Healthy Ignatias tend to be very refined. Ignatia's refinement is both intellectual and aesthetic/artistic. She is equally capable of subtle scholarly analysis and of delicate intuitive insight. In this she resembles Silica, and also some Sepias. Being such an emotional person, the healthy Ignatia is usually more interested in understanding the human condition (and the animal and plant condition), than in theoretical science which bears little direct relationship to her experience of life. Poetry, metaphysics and anthropology are areas that often interest her, as well as nutrition, health and esoteric science. She will tend to leave the 'hard science' of mathematics, physics, engineering and economics to the more purely rational types, and also to the more masculine Ignatias. She is perfectly capable of understanding them, but they do not appeal to her intuitive, feeling nature.

The healthy Ignatia is also refined socially. She will express herself politely and gracefully in most cases, and will have nothing to do with vulgarity. Because she feels deeply, her value system is clear, and calls for mutual respect and understanding. Like Silica, Ignatia combines delicate sensitivity with a strong sense of identity, and adherence to a high code of personal ethics. (Ignatia's sense of identity is actually stronger than Silica's on the whole, since it is not threatened by timidity and indecision to any great degree). Ignatia is usually fairly single-minded for all her delicacy, and she is liable to become confused and angry with herself very quickly if she compromises her own principles. Only when she has become toughened will she become more opportunistic, and adopt lower ethical standards. Even then,

Ignatia is usually true to her word, and demands that others be true to theirs, since she cannot bear to be deceived or taken advantage of. Ignatia's sense of integrity is so strong in many cases that she will become sick if she does not follow her own standards. I once treated a young woman for a severe case of panic attacks, associated with a remittent fever. Her symptoms began suddenly whilst she was travelling in a tropical country, and the mixture of psychological and physical symptoms made the diagnosis difficult.

She told me somewhat sheepishly that just before her illness started she was having a holiday romance with a man she had met on her travels. He was not particularly wonderful from her point of view, and she did not grieve on leaving him, but she did get sick. She felt very confused, but she confirmed that she had a steady relationship at home which she now realised was not worth jeopardising. It appears that her romantic fling had upset her sense of integrity so much that she had fallen ill. Her illness was eventually diagnosed as viral hepatitis, but I feel sure that the timing of her illness was no coincidence, and she intuitively understood this. Her panic attacks and her fever rapidly subsided after a few doses of Ignatia 10M, and she was left with tiredness, which improved on taking China.

### Physical Appearance

Physically Ignatia tends to split into two types, although there is a continuum between them. The more refined Ignatia is very slim, with long delicate bones. The more masculine type is heavier, and tends to gain weight easily. As Ignatia becomes more masculine, she tends also to develop more and more bodily and facial hair. Both types usually have a very dark complexion, although a few are redheads or even blondes. The face tends to be angular rather than rounded, and the cheek bones are generally high, which is one reason why Ignatias are often sought after models. The lashes are long and sensitive, and the nose is generally straight or aquiline, reflecting the strong and subtle intellect. One of the most noticeable features of Ignatia are her lips, which are very full, but delicately contoured like a bow, indicating both emotional intensity and refinement. Unlike Sepia, Ignatia tends to have thick curly hair, since she is more passionate. (The English comedienne Eleanor Bron is a good example of an Ignatia woman both physically and from the point of view of persona, as is the screen actress Barbara Streisand.)

# *Kali Carbonicum*

*Keynote:* Rigidity

Kali Carbonicum is by far the most commonly occurring Kali from a constitutional point of view. The only other one which is seen with some frequency is Kali Bichromium. These two have very similar personalities, being distinguishable mainly on grounds other than the mentals.

Kent remarks in his Lecture Notes that 'the Kali Carbonicum patient is a hard patient to study', and that the remedy 'is not used as often as it should be'. Kali is a closed type, and hence it is hard for the homeopath to get sufficient information about the personality to get a grip on it. The old materia medicas paint a very sketchy picture of the Kali personality, and as a result of this it is missed more often than not by homeopaths.

Most of Kali's mental characteristics can be understood as manifestations of the 'essence' of the type, which is rigidity. The first impression one gets of a Kali Carbonicum person is a certain formality, a stiffness that reveals a lack of relaxation of body and mind. Kali people have difficulty in really letting their hair down. This can be seen most clearly at parties and discotheques, where the spontaneous revelry of the other people can make a Kali feel even more inhibited and self-conscious. Even Kali's gait tends to be rather stiff, (and this stiffness is especially apparent if he dares to set foot on the dance-floor).

## *Conventionality*

Kali people come across as responsible, serious and conventional. A Kali friend once told me that all of his life he had found it difficult to have fun, because he was always so concerned with doing the right thing. Kalis are the most conventional of all types. Their fear of change sees to it that they resist the unproved and the unfamiliar. One of the most characteristic ways they do this is by doggedly 'sticking to the book'. A Kali Carbonicum employee will stick to the exact details of his job description, carrying out his duties as regularly as clockwork, and never sticking his neck out by doing something risky or unfamiliar. This can be seen most clearly in civil servants, petty bureaucrats, and others in positions of minor authority, such as traffic wardens. The Kali clerk will never bend the rules. It is more than his job is worth. (On the other hand, Kalis are very susceptible to public opinion, and to any threats to their own position, and hence could be coerced into secretly breaking the rules. Kali politicians, for example, would have to do secret deals like any other politician to remain in power.)

Kali's mental rigidity leads to an inability or unwillingness to adapt general rules to specific circumstances. For example, a Kali policeman may book a motorist for parking illegally, even though the motorist had pulled over because his engine had cut out. He does not do this out of malice, but rather because the law is the law, and he dare not be flexible in interpreting it, mainly because he is afraid of getting into trouble. Kali tries to avoid trouble by sticking to tried and tested formulae, be they the written laws of the land, religious codes, professional protocols, or the values handed down by his forebears. A good example of this is the kind of communist trade union official who loves to use very formal technical and political language, trying to justifying his pronouncements by borrowing the terminology of Marx and Lenin, in order to add weight to his position. On a larger scale, the rigidity of the Indian caste system, and the inhuman bureaucratic monstrosity of the old Soviet system, are examples of the rigid conservatism that is typical of the Kali mind.

I once worked with a homeopathic doctor who exemplified perfectly the Kali habit of sticking by the book. She was most afraid of attracting disapproval from her non-homeopathic colleagues, and one of the results of this was a fear of inducing aggravations in her patients. In order to avoid this, she used only the 30c potency when prescribing constitutionally. She was very particular about ensuring that her patients took all the orthodox medications that were indicated for their condition, as well as the homeopathic treatments she prescribed. Again, she did this to ensure that she did not endanger her position as a medical doctor. Her fear of getting into trouble was so pervasive that she practised quite the most conservative homeopathy I have come across.

Kali's attachment to clearly defined rules and regulations is similar to that seen in Arsenicum individuals, but there are subtle differences. Arsenicum generally has a stronger ego than Kali, and can be seen to pursue his principles of conscientiousness and propriety with zeal. Kali, on the other hand, is usually less confident, and sticks to the rules more out of self-protection than out of strongly held conviction. Arsenicum tends to be passionate and determined about his love of order, whereas Kali is sensible, logical and quiet about his principles. Both types tend to seek social approval, but Arsenicum tends to do it with more style, whilst Kali tends to appear grey and anonymous, more concerned with doing what is acceptable than with impressing people.

'Squareness' is a quality that is hard to define. It combines several characteristics, chiefly conservatism, inflexibility and excessive seriousness.

Arsenicum is often rather conservative, but does not seem nearly as square as Kali, since the former is more passionate and less rigid. For example, Arsenicum often dresses with some flair, whereas Kali's clothes are not only old-fashioned, but also frequently lacking in style. (Kali tends to play safe by wearing non-descript clothes in grey or brown.)

I was once sitting in with a prominent homeopath in California, when we considered the case of a young man suffering from post-viral fatigue. He worked as a Christian preacher on a university campus and was married to a quiet and sensible girl who shared his work. He himself appeared sober and responsible. During the interview no clear prescribing features were apparent, apart from the characteristic Kali anxiety felt in the stomach. The young man considered himself to be relatively open and progressive, and this may have been true in comparison with the other preachers in his church, but he was clearly less spontaneous and relaxed than most other young men of his age. The image of this conscientious, rather old-fashioned young preacher surrounded by a campus full of boisterous, radical students who were only a few years his junior brought to mind Kali Carbonicum. Natrum also comes to mind at such times, but young Natrums are not so stiff. The seriousness of many Natrums results from unhappiness which is hidden inside. Their eyes are evasive and somewhat watery, reflecting the emotions which they are attempting to keep at bay. Kali's seriousness is different. Kalis are generally so out of touch with their feelings that they come across as dry, mechanical and grey. There is no struggle with emotions (except occasionally with anxiety), no depression lurking inside. Rather there is a restriction of the life-force, which results from an almost total absence of emotional life. Like First Officer Spock of the U.S.S. Enterprise, Kali is efficient, logical and unemotional. However, even Spock had some feelings, and so do most Kalis.

I have come across many Kalis who embraced alternative forms of medicine and philosophy. If the homeopath simply judges from the patient's interests, he will fail to see the essence of the personality. It is not what the patient believes that is important so much as how he pursues his interests. No matter how unconventional the interest, Kali will pursue it sensibly, methodically, with intellectual thoroughness but little passion.

In my early days of homeopathic practice I sat in with a homeopath who exhibited many of the characteristics of the Kalis. He was polite, responsible, and very reasonable. In his history taking he examined every little detail of the patient's history, taking exhaustive notes which recorded hundreds of separate pieces of information. Faced with this plethora of details, he was often hard put to find a connecting thread, to make sense of the whole. In typical Kali fashion, he was very thorough, but found it difficult to see the essence of the case, since this does not require linear logic, but rather intuition. (In contrast, the Phosphorus homeopath would tend to get an overall 'feel' for the case, ignoring many of the details. These two types are polar opposites from a psychological point of view, though they share many physical features).

Yet another Kali homeopath I knew tended to take very little notice of the personality of his patients (since he was uncomfortable with emotions), preferring to base his prescriptions upon an electronic device (the Vega machine) which told him which remedy the patient needed. Many Kalis feel more comfortable with machines than with messy, unpredictable things like emotions.

## The Ultimate Rationalist

There is something two-dimensional about the Kali personality. Like a stick drawing, it lacks depth. It is no coincidence that the Kali salts are great skeletal remedies. Rigidity and structure is the very essence of the remedy. Take away the flesh and blood and we are left with a skeleton. The Kali mind is rather like a skeleton—rigid, dry and structured, lacking the flesh and blood of emotion and imagination. (Fortunately, even the skeleton is alive, and even the driest Kali has access to some feelings. But they are faint wisps compared to the feelings of most other people.)

Since they are unemotional, unimaginative people, Kalis live in and through their intellect. They are the most rational of all people. Like a computer, Kali will calculate the logical way to live his life, the logical way to plan his day, even the logical thing to say in response to his wife's complaint that he is so unemotional. Kalis tend to have a plan for everything, and they follow it to the last detail. Experimental scientists with their painstaking experimental designs are often Kalis, as are bank managers. Wherever cold logic and attention to detail is required, Kali will do well.

Kali is usually too busy following plans to have much fun. (Fun is an essentially alien concept to the average Kali). I once stayed at the house of a Kali friend and his family. One evening we all sat around and played the board game Cleudo, which involves making calculated guesses about the identity of a murderer, the murder weapon, and the site of the crime. To my amused astonishment, my friend drew up a complicated table, and earnestly set about recording every bit of information he could glean from the tactics of the other players. He used a kind of flow diagram to eliminate possibilities one by one, until he won the game, not by a calculated guess, but by a calculated certainty. His wife and children were forced to adopt the same tactics, since it was the only way they could compete with him. He was not a mean person, nor a fanatical person. He just didn't know any other way of functioning than through his intellect. He was not a closed person in the sense that Natrums are closed. He remarked that he didn't talk about his feelings because he didn't really have any.

Kalis have a very characteristic way of engaging in conversation. This involves considering the logic (or lack of logic) of whatever the other person says, and then analysing it out aloud. The more socially adapted Kali does this in a soft way, using humour to lighten the effect, but the logical analysis remains a central feature of all conversation. Again, Mr Spock of the Star Ship Enterprise illustrates this perfectly. Those Kalis who are less skilled socially can be quite painful to listen to, since their logical evaluations sound like university texts, and are delivered in a monotone which reflects a complete lack of passion. A Kali may describe his visit to a rock concert as if he were delivering a treatise on anthropology. The more relaxed Kali is a little less obsessively factual, but still comes across as 'earnest' in conversation, even with close friends.

Many Kalis are very quiet people, since they realise that they are unable to communicate in the more spontaneous manner of those around them, and keep quiet to avoid making a fool of themselves, or alienating the company they are in. When they find someone who is relatively intellectual, and interested in the same subject as themselves, they will venture forth in a serious debate on the subject.

Kali's tendency to be extremely rational in conversation resembles that seen in some Lycopodium men. On this point the two may be indistinguishable, but often the ultra-rational Lycopodium is too keen to get his point across, too self-assured, and has a tendency to talk on matters he knows relatively little about (to 'bullshit' his audience), whereas Kali sticks to what he knows. Sulphur also has a tendency to ramble on intellectually about his pet interests, and can be just as detailed in his analyses as Kali, but Sulphur is far more passionate in his speech, and in his interest.

The contrast between Sulphur's passionate idealism and Kali's matter of fact pragmatism is well illustrated by the difference in style between two U.S. presidents, Ronald Reagan and George Bush. Bush was initially discounted as a likely president, since he appeared so grey and anonymous in comparison with the flamboyant Reagan. When Bush did come to power he admitted that he didn't have what he called 'the vision thing', the committed idealism of his former boss. A similar and historically very close transition of power occurred in Britain, from the one-pointed determination of Mrs. Thatcher (Nux Vomica) to the reasonable, pragmatic approach of John Major, who in true Kali style was seen to be grey and lacking in charisma, but who could be trusted to be moderate, sensible and honest. Kali people are often trusted, since they appear so impersonal and responsible, and lack the powerful egos of more fiery types.

Like Arsenicum, Kali tends to be very practical. Physical security is very important, and this is one reason why he favours sound common-sense over flamboyant ideas. Kali tends to be a sceptic, dismissing theories that he can see no scientific proof for. As a result his world is very reliable, but also rather dull.

## Insecurity

Kali's insecurity is very similar to that of Arsenicum, being focused primarily on the material plane, and manifesting as a fear of illness (and death), poverty, and loss of social favour. Like Arsenicum, Kali is generally prudent with money. He is also likely to treat his body moderately, rather than going to the fanatical degrees of health-consciousness seen in some Arsenicum individuals. Indeed, many Kalis live a very sedate existence, which is routine-bound, and lacking in both exercise and dietary variety. The British television comedy series 'The Fall and Rise of Reginald Perrin' is a wonderful parody of the Kali executive who is utterly trapped by routine, logic, and the fear of stepping out and defying convention. Reggie ends up doing what every Kali secretly dreams of, rebelling against his rigid codes of behaviour, insulting people, making passes at women, and generally disinhibiting himself. Some Kalis manage to loosen up in a somewhat more gradual manner, becoming more flexible with the years. Very few break out in the radical manner of Reginald Perrin.

Kalis tend to worry too much, principally about practical matters. They also worry about their relationships with other people, since they are not good at social interaction, and yet feel lonely and insecure when alone. Like many other highly rational types (Lycopodium, Natrum, Arsenicum), Kali people are usually very concerned about their public image. Each of these types has a slightly different reason for seeking social approval. Natrum deep down feels unlovable and unworthy, and hence needs some affirmation of his worth from other people. Lycopodium feels inferior, a failure, and seeks to please and to impress in order to feel important. Arsenicum is not a people-pleaser, but values prestige for two reasons. First of all, it is a form of social insurance policy, to fall back on in times of need, and secondly it is pleasing to the Arsenicum ego. Once again, Kali resembles Arsenicum most closely. Kali is not a very egotistical type. Most Kalis are very modest people, who do not seek the limelight. It is to insure against loneliness, poverty and ill-health that most Kalis seek social acceptance. To be a social outcast used to be a threat to one's very survival in more primitive times, and it still conjures up the same fear today, especially in those who are not good at mixing socially.

## The Kali Entrepreneur

Not all Kalis avoid the limelight. I have come across several successful Kali businessmen who hit upon a 'recipe for success' and stuck to it, enabling them to amass large fortunes and a prominent public profile which they clearly encouraged. One was the owner of a 24 hour medical centre, and another the founder of a huge chain of electrical stores. These Kali business-men are workaholics who cannot relax and do nothing. They are driven both by a need to be busy, a desire for material wealth, and a desire for status. I treated the wife of one of these men, who told me that her husband could never relax, and worked seven days a week. He once tried taking off week-ends for the sake of his family, but he became so tense that he had to go back to work. It may seem strange that an ultra-cautious type like Kali should become the head of a business empire, but it is the Kali businessman's very caution, allied to his logic and discipline, which enables him to rise to posi-tions of prominence. He will first build up a small concern until it is running well, and then gradually expand and duplicate until a large empire is formed. With his attention to detail, and his apparent immunity to boredom, he will ensure that every aspect of his business is efficient before he is ready to ex-pand.

The Kali entrepreneur is quite a different person from the Nux entrepre-neur. The latter exudes confidence and is usually socially graceful, whereas the former is clearly uncomfortable talking to most people, and makes up in politeness for what he lacks in confidence socially. Since I have lived in Australia I have been both amused and surprised by the way certain Kali entrepreneurs use their own faces and voices to advertise their goods and services. These men have very little facility in communication, and come across in advertisements as both tense and unnatural, yet they saturate the airwaves with their faces and voices. I can only conclude that this is a Kali's way of making up in fame for what he lacks in personal confidence.

Most Kali Carbonicum individuals are a little timid, but I have seen a Kali entrepreneur behave quite ruthlessly when he felt one of his employees was a threat to him, sacking the emplyee with only a day's notice, and next to no explanation. The Kali entrepreneur, like other entrepreneurs, is obsessed with his business, and his relative lack of emotions presumably makes it easier for him to be ruthless when he deems it necessary.

### Anxiety

Like several other rational types, Kali people are generally very reluctant to admit to their weaknesses. They will often deny all fears and worries during the consultation, or will play them down as much as possible. I remember a very formal and upright university lecturer who came to see me for treatment of arthritis. She denied being an anxious person, but admitted that she did not sleep well, since she woke in the small hours to empty her bladder, and could not get back to sleep afterwards. When I asked her how she felt at such times, she admitted that she felt anxious, for no apparent reason (Kent: 'Anxiety on waking'). A couple of doses of Kali Carbonicum 1M not only greatly relieved her arthritis, but also enabled her to get straight back to sleep at night.

It is not really surprising that the Kali person suffers from anxiety, when one considers the rigid mental control which they enforce upon every aspect of their life. This control is both a result of insecurity, and a source of further anxiety, since the more rigid the person becomes, the more likely it is that their brittle defences will be broken by some unforeseen circumstance.

Kali people do generally manage to hide most of their anxiety for a long time, often for their whole life. It shows only as a certain tension or hesitancy of speech. Sometimes, however, they do suffer a breakdown. This is especially likely to occur after the loss of some important source of security, such as their job, or their partner.

If the Kali person does break down, the resulting mental picture is similar to that of the agitated Arsenicum. There is intense anxiety, especially when alone (Kent: 'Fear of being alone'), and especially in the small hours of the night. The patient is restless, irritable, and hypersensitive to noise, to physical discomfort, and to being touched. Even when anxiety is intense, Kali may give the impression that he is in control, and may continue to work fairly normally.

Relations with the opposite sex frequently cause Kali anxiety. This is in part because he feels awkward and self-conscious. The usual adolescent awkwardness with the opposite sex may continue well into adulthood, and may never disappear. Once Kali does establish a relationship, he is liable to be dutiful, but detached. Family life is an opportunity for him to lighten up a little, and it often makes the Kali person more confident and more relaxed.

Kalis are just as cautious as Arsenicums. They are slow to trust new ideas, and new acquaintances. This lack of easy trust was apparent in a patient of mine who sought treatment for hayfever. He was a psychologist, and was quite accomplished at analysing his own personality, and was open enough to talk freely about his anxiety problem. His physical symptoms were very clearly Kali Carbonicum, and his mentals were a good Kali fit, although Arsenicum could not be excluded entirely. A few doses of Kali Carbonicum 200 relieved the hayfever, but the improvement was shortlived. I then explained to the patient that a dose of 10M would be more likely to produce a lasting improvement in his hayfever, and would also help his anxiety. At this point he asked me to read out the section in my Materia Medica on the mentals of Kali Carbonicum, to convince him that it fitted his case. Having heard this, he asked what other remedies might be needed instead, and then asked me to describe in detail the personalities of these remedies. Then he phoned another homeopath, who was a friend of his, who discouraged him from taking Kali Carbonicum (because he was too 'liberal' for a Kali). Finally he took the dose, and entered into a brief period of melancholy, which lasted about a week, which he refused to attribute to the remedy (Kent: 'Obstinate'). After this he was noticeably less intellectual, and more in touch with his feelings.

The above patient's case contained an aspect of the Kali mentality that appears mainly during periods of anxiety; the tendency towards fixed repetitive thoughts, which come and intrude upon the patient without control. The thoughts may be profound or banal, meaningful or nonsense, but whatever they are, they cannot be exorcised from the mind (Causticum, another potassium salt, also has this symptom, as does Mercurius). Whilst trying to write a letter or listen to music, the thought 'All men must die' pops into his head, and cannot be erased. This is not the almost irresistible impulse to act of Argentum, but simply an irrelevant thought that will not go away. It is as though the Kali mind has gone a little mad, and cannot switch off one of its circuits.

### The Other Kalis

I have found that Kali Bichromium people are more often women, whilst the reverse is true for Kali Carbonicum. The personalities of the two are more or less indistinguishable, but the different gender distribution may explain why I have the impression that Kali Bichromium is a little softer and less rigid than the Carbonicum. In fact, Kali Bichromium sometimes resembles Calcarea Carbonicum, both mentally and physically, although she is usually a little more formal than the latter.

The other Kali types, Kali Arsenicum, Phosphoricum and Sulphuricum, are very rare as constitutional types, if they exist at all. I have not positively identified them, but if they exist, they would presumably combine typical Kali characteristics with characteristics of the other element, such as the sensitivity of Phosphorus.

### Kali Bromatum

This rare type is quite different from the other Kalis. I have only seen one case, but her mentals were so clear, and she responded so dramatically to the remedy, that I feel justified in including her case here. She was a young woman of about twenty five years, who came to see me for treatment of epilepsy and schizophrenia. She appeared quite sane, but shy and nervous. She was experiencing frequent grand mal fits, about two a week. I asked her about her schizophrenia, and she said that at the age of about fifteen she was playing hockey when she suddenly felt that the another girl in her team was against her and wanted to kill her. So, in self defence she whacked this girl on the head with her hockey stick, fracturing her skull. She was admitted to hospital with paranoid schizophrenia and given drug treatment for years afterwards. She was no longer on treatment, but still suffered from paranoid thoughts, accompanied by feelings of pure rage. She also suffered from extreme hypochondriasis, thinking that the slightest symptom was a sign of cancer. Although I was not familiar with Kali Bromatum, it was a simple matter to combine rubrics for epilepsy, hypochondriasis and paranoia and come up with the remedy. After a few doses of 10M her fits stopped completely, and she was even more pleased that she no longer got her 'silly thoughts'. In fact she felt so confident that she was looking for work for the first time in many years.

## Physical Appearance

Physically, Kali Bichromium resembles Calcarea, being fleshy in most cases, though the hair may be dark. Kali Carbonicum is usually thin and wiry, with dark or medium brown hair. Many Kalis have a thin, bony face that tends to maintain a rather stiff expression. The lips are usually thin, especially the upper lip, reflecting a lack of emotionality. Kali Carbonicum often has bags under the eyes, but the face is angular, unlike the rather full, rounded face of most Natrums. My Kali Bromatum patient was dark and petite, with large scared-looking eyes, rather like a China.

# Lachesis

*Keynote:* Sexual tension

The coiled serpent is a fine image for representing the Lachesis individual, whose remedy is made from the venom of the Bushmaster snake. In esoteric traditions the coiled serpent represents the kundalini energy residing at the base of the spine. This energy is said to be of a sexual nature in most people, but it can be made to rise up the spine, being transmuted as it rises into creative potential, and ultimately into spiritual experience.

The Lachesis individual is like a highly strung bow, taut with sexual energy, which must find an outlet if it is not to backfire upon its owner.

For many the outlet is sex itself. Lachesis people are highly sexed (Kent: 'Lascivious'), and when they make love they are very passionate. Sex is not only very enjoyable for Lachesis; it also relieves tension. Others sublimate their sexual energy into a passionate pursuit of art, career or spirituality. Lachesis is a very passionate type (Kent: 'Vivacious'), and whenever she thoroughly indulges in and expresses her passion, the result is both ecstasy and relaxation.

From adolescence onwards, the Lachesis individual vibrates with sexual energy. It gives her a passionate appetite for life, for excitement, and for stimulation. As long as this appetite remains satisfied, Lachesis will be fairly healthy psychologically. It is when the sexual energy is repressed, when it cannot find an outlet, that Lachesis develops physical and psychological tension. It may be that she has a partner who is not interested in sex, or that she has been without a partner for a long time, or that she grew up with a moral teaching that prohibited sex before marriage, and hence has remained a virgin. In these cases all will be well if an activity can be found which channels sufficient passionate energy to discharge the tension within, but if this does not happen, anxiety, restlessness and irritability will develop.

Lachesis' powerful sexual drive is tempered by a refined, sensitive nature. Less sensitive types like Nux and Sulphur may pursue their sexual appetites in a rather crude, unfeeling manner, but for many Lachesis individuals (especially the women) sex is usually reserved for romantic partnership, and is all the more passionate because it an expression of their love. When a Lachesis woman is in love her sexuality is heightened, and she will become very emotional if she is not able to make love frequently with her partner. If his libido cannot keep up with hers, she is liable to feel that he does not love her, and her frustration and hurt will provoke both tears and anger. A sexually frustrated Lachesis woman is rather like a spurned Ignatia; touchy and highly emotional. After she has made love she is calm again.

This theme of tension requiring discharge can be seen to run throughout the features of Lachesis, both mentally and physically. On the physical level discharges will ameliorate symptoms, particularly sexual discharges, and the discharge of menstruation. Vigorous physical exercise may also be used by Lachesis to discharge tension. On the psychological level talking is used as a means of discharging tension, hence the famous loquacity of Lachesis. The more sexually repressed a Lachesis individual, the more loquacious they will become.

## *Loquacity and Hurriedness*

Loquacity simply means talking a lot. Almost any constitutional type can have it. It is the way in which Lachesis talks a lot that is so characteristic. The repressed or tense Lachesis individual is often easy to spot on account of the speed with which she speaks. (For some reason the male Lachesis people I have seen tended to be far less tense than the women, and hence spoke more normally. I suspect that Lachesis men are less prone to a build up of sexual tension, since they are more likely to find relief in masturbation, and also more likely to resort to casual sexual encounters when they do not have a partner.) As sexual tension rises, Lachesis becomes more and more hurried, in thought, speech and action. At first she is able to speed up her activities without losing control. At this stage she resembles very closely the thyrotoxic patient (who is usually Natrum Muriaticum), whose continuous accelerated speech is quite exhausting to listen to, even though it is coherent. Such patients will ask the homeopath a question in the consulting room, and the moment it has been answered they embark upon another rapid barrage of communication, often ending in another question. In such consultations the homeopath says very little, unable to get a word in, since there are few gaps in either the patient's words, or in her thought processes.

As the tension increases further, it becomes impossible for the Lachesis individual to maintain orderly thought processes. The thinking becomes so accelerated that it gets jumbled, and this is reflected in speech, which becomes increasingly erratic. The faster the speech, the greater is the tendency to jump from one subject to another (Kent: 'Loquacious—changes subjects quickly'). At first there is some connection between one subject and the next, but as the speech gets faster, this connection gradually dissolves, until a kind of mania is reached, in which the patient jumps rapidly between unconnected topics.

Another characteristic of the loquacity of tense Lachesis individuals is the tendency for speech to gather momentum. Like a runaway locomotive hurtling down a hill, Lachesis' speech may start reasonably slowly, and get faster and faster until it is unintelligible in some cases. It is as if the pent up psychic energy has found a small outlet through speech, and gradually more and more of it gushes forth, widening the aperture as it flows.

Lachesis is generally a quick individual. Even the relaxed Lachesis has a quick mind, which can grasp a concept or a situation in an instant. Like a resting cobra, Lachesis may suddenly jump from inactivity into dynamic action when the situation demands (Kent: 'Quick to act'). The more healthy Lachesis individual has a kind of 'resting alertness', as if the nervous system were always primed and ready to go. (This characteristic of sudden and rapid change is seen throughout the whole remedy picture. On the physical level symptoms develop rapidly, as if from nowhere, and accelerate. Discharges, for example, start slowly, but accelerate rapidly.)

The more nervous Lachesis individual is in a hurry most of the time. The accumulated psychic tension finds some outlet through rapid activity, but irritability, impatience and anxiety usually accompany hurriedness, and Lachesis is no exception. As one would expect, the more assertive, egotistical Lachesis individuals are prone to anger and irritability when 'wound up', whilst the less assertive ones are more prone to anxiety.

## Appetite and Inspiration

Like other passionate types, Lachesis tends to be hungry for experience. For some this hunger is satisfied through the pursuit of external stimulation. Lachesis youths in particular can be hell-raisers, pushing against the confines of parental authority, and passionately embracing music, dance, alcohol and sex. Lachesis individuals have a Dionysian side to their character. In common with Phosphorus, Medorrhinum and Ignatia they can easily enter into ecstasy both through sensual gratification, and through meditative introspection (Kent: 'Ecstasy'). It is interesting to note how many aspects of the Lachesis type are traditionally symbolised by the snake. The snake has been used for thousands of years to represent the 'sinister' forces of lust, guile and sensual temptation, and also the 'higher' principal of wisdom. Each Lachesis individual chooses whether to indulge his sexual and sensual appetites freely, or to sublimate them into something finer and more spiritual.

The sensual side of Lachesis often leads to a love of alcohol and other stimulants, (Kent: 'Dipsomania'). The relaxed Lachesis will easily enter into a euphoric state with the help of drugs, whilst the tense Lachesis may come to depend upon them to unwind. In this sense Lachesis resembles Nux, and the more extrovert, assertive members of the Lachesis brood can easily be mistaken for Nux Vomica types. Both are quick, hedonistic, determined, and have a tendency to tension and temper. Furthermore, both types can be proud, calculating and vindictive. Kent was characteristically blunt about the more negative side of Lachesis in his Lecture Notes, but his comments about the 'self-conceit, envy, hatred, revenge and cruelty' of Lachesis could just as easily have been made about Nux. Sometimes the two cannot be differentiated on the mentals alone, and the physicals and generals must be relied upon to distinguish them.

The Lachesis type taken as a whole differs from Nux in being more sensitive, artistic and mystical, whilst Nux is more pragmatic. Many highly original artists are Lachesis types, and this includes performing artists such as singers and musicians. I once took the history of one such artist, a prominent producer and composer of 'New Age' electronic music. His music is so dreamy and lyrical that one would never consider Nux Vomica as his remedy. Furthermore, his house was full of exquisite designs from Eastern mystical traditions, and the air was thick with incense. His attraction to mystical tradition, as well as his prodigious creativity, brought Lachesis to mind, and this was confirmed by numerous other features of his case. For example, he hated flying, since the planes' air-conditioning never provided enough air for him.

Lachesis most closely resembles Ignatia and Medorrhinum, in that it is a 'deep' type, with profound and subtle feelings, and is also passionate (Kent: 'Vivacious'). Phosphorus, in contrast, is more superficial, more carefree, and less passionate, whilst Nux is not nearly so 'deep'.

Being a highly intuitive type, Lachesis is often attracted to philosophical ideas (Kent: 'Religious affections'). Lachesis usually has a keen intellect, which is used to make sense of the intuitive and imaginative insights to which he is prone. Because of the highly developed intuitive faculty, one does not come across many atheists amongst Lachesis people. (They are more likely to belong to one of the more purely rational types like Lycopodium and Kali Carbonicum).

It is important to realise that only the tense Lachesis individual is loquacious to any great degree. A relaxed Lachesis may be either introverted or extroverted by nature, but either way, he will not appear excessively talkative to the homeopath. In general the extroverted Lachesis is more hedonistic and sensual, and also more egotistic than the introverted Lachesis. The latter tends to be more philosophical, mystical and artistic.

The introverted Lachesis is something like the sensitive China individual. He is a visionary who seeks out quiet places to meditate upon the beauty of nature, or the meaning of existence. He is still passionate, particularly when in a romantic relationship, and he is liable to express his passion through music, poetry or imaginative writing. The introverted Lachesis can appear either timid or aloof in company, and there is often some truth in both of these appearances. Many Lachesis people are shy with strangers, and say little until they are more familiar. This is in part a reflection of the wariness of the type, which sometimes progresses to paranoia as pathology deepens. It is also in part a strategy which sensitive, deep-thinking people employ to assess whether or not the other person is perceptive enough to be worth talking to. The subtle Lachesis mind soon learns to avoid 'casting his pearls before swine'.

Wisdom is a quality that is very hard to define. Only those who are wise can recognise it. Others mistake learning for wisdom, especially those who are highly rational. No constitutional type has a monopoly of wisdom, but there are deeper types, those who are more intuitive on the whole, and these types are more likely to possess wisdom, which is an intuitive understanding of the internal workings of life, the hidden processes and patterns which underlie external appearances. The more introverted Lachesis individual often has a great deal of wisdom, but he is not liable to advertise the fact. Indeed those who are wise never do so. They do, however, express their wisdom to those they feel able to understand, both in conversation, and through their creative works. The serpent is a symbol not only of wisdom, but also of healing (witness the two serpents entwined on the staff of the caduceus, the ancient symbol of the healer). True healing, whether of oneself or of another, requires wisdom, and I have come across several Lachesis individuals who used their intuitive abilities to heal others through bodywork. Like other visionary types (Phosphorus, Medorrhinum, China), Lachesis often has the ability to feel the subtle currents of energy in the body, referred to by homeopaths as the vital force, and by the Chinese as the Chi. It is through the channelling of these currents that healers are able to affect the health (or vitality) of their patients.

### *Jealousy, Anger and Egotism*
Lachesis ranks with Hyoscyamus as being the most prone to intense feelings of jealousy of all the constitutional types. The more intense a person's desire, the more liable they are to feel jealous of others who have what the desirer wants. Thus we can understand Lachesis' jealousy as a natural consequence of his strong desire.

Sexual jealousy is the commonest form seen in Lachesis people, since sexual desire is usually their most intense attachment. In some cases this jealousy can be totally unrealistic, and can dominate the relationship to the point where it threatens its very existence. I remember one such patient, a middle-aged lady who came to me specifically for treatment of her intense jealousy, which was threatening her relationship with her husband. Not only could her husband not talk to another female without her creating a scene, he could not even watch television in the presence of his wife, since she felt overwhelming jealousy when a pretty woman came on the screen. It is interesting to note that she usually felt very sexually aroused when she was jealous. A few doses of Lachesis 10M greatly reduced her pathological jealousy, and probably saved her marriage.

Not surprisingly, intense jealousy can lead to intense anger, and this is not uncommon in Lachesis people of either sex. Lachesis' anger is sudden and intense in most cases, an eruption that is short-lived but powerful (Kent: 'Rage'). Jealousy is particularly liable to be the cause of Lachesis' anger, but it is not the only one. The more tense Lachesis individual can become generally irritable and demanding, and may become furious and vengeful when crossed (Kent: 'Malicious'). However, since tension in Lachesis is generally caused by sexual repression, this anger is ultimately a release of sexual tension.

The connection between sexuality and anger is seen more clearly in Lachesis women, for two reasons. Firstly, they are more likely to be sexually repressed. Secondly, a woman's sexual feelings tend to vary with her hormonal status, and this is especially true of Lachesis women. Many Lachesis women report that their libido is much stronger either at ovulation or premenstrually. At these times they are also more likely to be irritable, and to lose their temper. Lachesis women are prone to premenstrual tension, in the form of anger, oversensitivity to rejection, and weepiness. Their premenstrual tension is usually relieved by sexual intercourse to a marked degree, which suggests that it is due, in part, (or in whole) to sexual tension. Sudden mood changes are also seen in Lachesis women at the menopause, and after childbirth (Kent: 'Insanity—menopausal', 'Hysteria from suppressed discharges'). Anger is usually more prominent than depression at these times, as with Sepia women.

A minority of Lachesis people are distinctly egotistical (Kent: 'Haughty', 'Egotism'). They are usually the more extroverted type, and most are male. I once dined with one such person at a dinner party. He was a successful artist, with the typical Lachesis appearance of sharp, bony features, and red, freckled complexion. He spent the entire evening talking about his achievements and his plans for the future, showing very little interest in the lives of his fellow guests. He subsequently saw me as a patient, and when I asked him about his personality, he described how well-balanced, generous, sensitive, inspired and courageous he was. When I asked him if there was anything he would like to change about himself, he was stumped. He had many Lachesis keynotes in his history, and was given Lachesis 10M. When I saw him a few weeks later he reported a marked improvement in his physical complaints. I noticed that he was a great deal quieter than before, in the subdued state that often follows when very proud people take their simillimum in high potency.

Pride is usually accompanied by a tendency to become angry when criticised, and Lachesis is no exception. The proud, extroverted Lachesis is pleasant as long as he is the centre of attention, but will become bored when he has to take a passive role, and resentful if his own high opinion of himself is threatened. Not withstanding this, he is still unlikely to explode unless he has been sexually frustrated for some time, or is in the grips of jealousy. The greater the sexual tension, the smaller the trigger needed to release it, and the more violent the temper. The trigger need not have any direct connection with the underlying cause of the tension. Having said that, pride, particularly in a man, is very closely connected to sexuality, as is aggression. This is confirmed to some extent by the fact that most of the more proud constitutional types are also those with the strongest sex drive. Platina is an extreme example, being the most highly sexed, and also the most proud type of all.

Another theme running throughout the remedy picture of Lachesis is an intolerance of restriction. On the physical level the patient cannot tolerate tight clothing, particularly around the neck. Many of the pains of Lachesis are felt as being tight or crushing (like the grip of an anaconda), a reflection of the bound up tension inside. On the psychological level Lachesis is just as intolerant of restriction. He may be able to form a committed and intimate relationship (unlike many Lycopodiums and Tuberculinums whose fear of being tied down may prevent lasting relationships) providing that he is given plenty of space when he needs it, and is not told what to do by his partner. Many Lachesis people do remain single, either out of fear and shyness, or out of a refusal to have their freedom limited (Kent: 'Idea of marriage unendurable'). Lachesis becomes prickly when ordered about, and will soon express his anger at being restricted. Similarly, many Lachesis individuals find it difficult to adapt to the confines of a nine-to-five office routine. Not only do they need lots of fresh air; they also need the stimulation of doing something creative, and are more likely to work well on their own at home than in the confines of a highly structured environment. I once treated an artist for tenosynovitis. He was a sculptor, and his condition was interfering with his work. He was youthful in appearance, although in fact he was about forty five years old, with the typical Lachesis red hair and freckles, and lean hungry look. He told me that he often would work round the clock on a sculpture, and when I asked why, he said it was his passion, his joy in life. He had just left his wife and family 'to be free to pursue my art', He appeared to have no regrets and no remorse about leaving his family. In fact he couldn't contain his enthusiasm as he spoke about his plans to walk around Europe with a wheel-barrow, (with his new young girlfriend) offering to sculpt to earn his lodgings in each town and village. He was keen to be treated homeopathically, and took numerous swipes at the folly of allopathic medicine during the interview, in between philosophising and waxing lyrical about the deadening effects of conventional capitalistic business and nuclear families. By the end of the interview I had no doubt that he was a Lachesis constitutionally, but when he heard that he would have to give up coffee and cannabis he said he would come back when he was ready to do so. Like many Tuberculinum individuals, some Lachesis people are so addicted both to stimulants and to 'freedom' that they would rather die than be restricted.

This intolerance of restriction may explain the characteristic Lachesis aversion to being touched. This is often present in cases of physical pathology, where pain is greatly exacerbated by the slightest touch, but it can also occur on the mental level. When Lachesis is feeling tense, and particularly when he is feeling restricted psychologically, he will avoid being touched, and will feel more irritable when he is physically touched by other people (Kent: 'Aversion to being touched').

## Paranoia

It seems somehow appropriate that a remedy made from snake venom should have paranoia as a prominent feature of the mental symptomatology. As with jealousy and loquaciousness, this characteristic may be absent or very subtle in the more healthy Lachesis individual, and becomes more and more apparent as pathology deepens. The first sign of approaching paranoia may be a certain degree of suspicion (Kent: 'suspicious'). A tense Lachesis may begin to question the motives of others more and more, and to suspect that they are against him. The characters often played by the movie actor/director Woody Allen in his comical films illustrate this tendency beautifully. They often imagine that they are being discriminated against, or that the world in general is a dangerous place to live in. (For example, such a character may read an article about 'killer asteroids' on a collision course with the Earth, and then live in dread for weeks. He may buy a telescope in the hope of giving himself some advanced warning of the catastrophe, and even contemplate constructing an underground shelter.) Once Lachesis begins to feel unsafe, his imagination becomes his worst enemy. One very intelligent, articulate young Lachesis man told me that he was always afraid in company, because he imagined that the other people were thinking nasty things about him. This paranoia was in marked contrast to the confident, determined and independent way he appeared to live his life. Apart from myself, only his wife was aware of the extent of his fears, which were so strong that they put him into a panic inside when he was with strangers.

Most Lachesis people manage to keep their unreasonable fears pretty much to themselves. In some cases, however, paranoia becomes overwhelming, and the patient loses all perspective of reality ( Kent: 'Delusions of being pursued', 'Fear of being poisoned'). Assailants and plotters are seen in every direction, and the patient spends much of his time in terror, avoiding contact with others in an attempt to protect himself. This extreme form of paranoia can also be seen in Rhus Tox, Arsenicum and Hyoscyamus. The latter in particular can be very hard to distinguish from Lachesis, since it also has loquaciousness, jealousy and increased sexuality. In such cases the pre-morbid personality is usually more 'normal' in Lachesis than in Hyoscyamus, and during the paranoid phase Hyoscyamus is more likely to express ex-tremely bizarre thoughts than Lachesis, and to display sexual exhibitionism.

Apart from general paranoid tendencies, Lachesis has three very charac-teristic fears. Appropriately enough, one of these is snakes. The other type who commonly fears snakes is Natrum Muriaticum, but Lachesis' fear is usually more extreme, such that even the sight of a snake on television is enough to provoke palpitations and revulsion. Given the tendency towards palpitations, it is not surprising that Lachesis often has a fear that his heart will stop. This is also a reflection of the unpotentised remedy's ability to produce cardiac arrest in its victims. The third fear is also connected to snakes- the fear of suffocation. Several of the larger species of snake can suffocate their prey by wrapping themselves around its neck. Most Lachesis individuals cannot bear anything restrictive around their neck, and can also become panicky if their mouth and nose are partially restricted, such as when a mask is placed over the face. (Again, it is Natrum Muriaticum who is most often seen by the homeopath with this symptom, which is part of Natrum's claustrophobia.)

### *Physical Appearance*
Physically, Lachesis resembles Phosphorus and Sepia in being slim and lithe. There seem to be two main variants of the Lachesis physique—the tall and the short. Both are usually slim or even bony, although the women often have large chests. As with most sensitive, refined people, the fingers tend to be long and thin. The facial features are generally sharp, or even hawkish (like Arsenicum), rather than rounded. The lips tend to be thin, the mouth wide, not the clipped or absent lips of the emotionally shut down, but rather re-fined lips like a long bow, stretched out, but still classical in their shape. The hair is usually red, or brown with a reddish tint, but is sometimes black. The skin is pale and usually freckled. Curiously, the upper eyelids often droop slightly, giving a characteristic 'snake-lid' appearance. The actresses Maggie Smith and Vanessa Redgrave have typical Lachesis features.

# *Lycopodium*

*Keynote:* Impotence

Lycopodium is a big remedy. In terms of frequency in the populations of civilised nations it is second only to Natrum Muriaticum. Lycopodium is principally a male remedy, and about one fifth of men in civilised societies belong to the type.

Because there are so many Lycopodiums, there is a wide spectrum of different personalities within the type. The homeopathic student must learn to recognise all of them if he or she is to avoid missing the majority. A newly qualified homeopath once sat in with me at my practice. After analysing the case of a new patient we had just seen together, she said that the patient couldn't be Lycopodium, because he was sporty, and not very intellectual. He did not fit the 'standard' Lycopodium picture 'intellectually keen but of weak muscular power'. Nevertheless, the patient was a reasonably typical Lycopodium man, and he did respond to the remedy.

Impotence is a general term that means 'lacking in power'. The vast majority of Lycopodium people have a sense of impotency inside, even though they may appear to be relatively confident or even powerful individuals. They lack faith in their own abilities, and this lack of self-confidence can usually be traced back to their childhood.

There are two common scenarios in the home of the Lycopodium child. Firstly, there is the situation in which one parent, usually the father, undermines the child's confidence. He may expect the child to perform well at sports, and criticises more than he praises. This kind of father is apt to comment 'When I was your age I...' followed by yet another description of his great prowess as a child at anything from scoring tries to scoring with girls. Naturally, this kind of treatment soon produces performance anxiety in the child, who begins to dread any task he is expected to do well at. This anxiety only serves to weaken his performance, which then intensifies the growing sense of failure inside. Later on in life, the child is always struggling to prove that he is good enough. (A very similar dynamic is seen in many Natrum children. The latter, however, become perfectionists in their attempts to please their perfectionist parents. Unlike the Lycopodium child, such Natrum children believe in their abilities, since they tend to get positive reinforcement from their Natrum parents when they excel. The Natrum child senses that he is not good enough despite his excellent performance, since his parents' love is so conditional. The Lycopodium child, on the other hand, feels a failure because his performance is not good enough.)

The other common scenario is that the parent of the same sex is an unconfident Lycopodium, and the child acquires the same lack of confidence by example. The child may have more opportunity than his parents had, and also may receive more encouragement than they did, and as a result he may go on to achieve more in the world than his parents. Despite this, he will retain a nagging fear of failure, since he absorbed his father's fear by a kind of psychic osmosis during his formative years.

Whatever the childhood situation, the Lycopodium individual who is doing well in his work or in his partnership, will tend to have a constant fear in the background that his business will collapse, or that his marriage will fail. Again, there are similarities here with Natrum, who expects everything to go wrong just as life is working out well. The difference is subtle but important. Lycopodium secretly expects failure, whereas Natrum expects unhappiness. Lycopodium is happy as long as he is doing O.K., (happy and relieved), whereas Natrum is often unhappy inside despite his apparent success, since he felt unloved as a child even though he performed well.

Because of his fear of failure, Lycopodium suffers from anticipatory anxiety. Before an interview he will worry excessively about making a gaffe (Kent: 'He has a fear that he will make mistakes), and his anxiety will be felt as a queasy, churning stomach. Lycopodium usually performs better than he expects, since his sense of inadequacy is due not to his lack of ability or preparation, but to a 'no win' situation in his childhood. With time he may learn to ignore his anticipatory anxiety, and take on more and more challenges involving public performance, the very thing he originally dreaded the most.

### The People Pleaser

There's nothing like popularity for boosting self-confidence. The Lycopodium child learns early on to curry favour in order to be liked by his peers. He will copy the phrases and mannerisms that appear to please, give in to all sorts of demands, both from bullies and from others who are learning to get what they want, and generally try to be nice. Natrum children are upset when their special friends reject them. Lycopodium is upset if anybody doesn't like him; even a complete stranger. He develops an easy-going nature (Kent: 'Mildness') because he is afraid of confrontation, and would rather give way to keep the peace. In extreme cases this can lead to Lycopodium becoming a grovelling sycophant, whose frantic efforts to please are in direct proportion to his fear of punishment. And the punishment that he most fears is often social rejection.

In his efforts to remain popular, the Lycopodium man will go out of his way to please his friends. He usually has a number of good acquaintances, rather than a few close friends like Natrum. It is very characteristic of Lycopodium to put his friends before his family. Even though he is not all that close to his friends, he will do anything to keep in favour with them. In the process he will often neglect his family, since he can rely on their allegiance already. I once knew a tennis coach who was very affable, as most Lycopodiums are. He was married to a long-suffering Natrum wife, who saw very little of him. They had relocated from the city, where her family was, to a small country town, at his request. One day we were talking about country versus city life, and the wife made it very clear that she was unhappy away from her family, and had moved at his insistence. My Lycopodium coach replied that he could be happy anywhere, since he liked to be friends with everyone, and did not get too close to anyone. If ever he was invited to play tennis in the evening, he would always jump at the chance of socialising (and doing what he was good at—playing tennis), leaving his wife a virtual tennis widow. He eventually consulted me for treatment of chronic indigestion, which completely disappeared after a few doses of Lycopodium 10M.

Being a people-pleaser, Lycopodium is generally a diplomatic person. Even if he has no respect for another, his manner will usually be soothing and polite. This is one reason why Lycopodiums make such good salesmen. Car salesmen in particular are very often Lycopodium. There are many reasons for this. Firstly, Lycopodium has the smooth personal touch which makes people at ease, and hence more likely to part with large amounts of money. In most cases he genuinely likes people, and enjoys socialising with complete strangers. Even when he dislikes a person, he is good at disguising it, with a mixture of nonchalance and flattery. Furthermore, Lycopodium is a great opportunist. He is far more liable than Natrum to put personal gain before morality, and hence is suited not only to the selling of new cars with three year warranties, but also to the more shady dealing of second-hand car sales. Finally, most Lycopodiums love to impress, and the car is a great symbol of power and prestige. Even though it is not his own, the average Lycopodium salesman will derive a certain pride from extolling the virtues of a sleek powerful new machine, and will feel as if his virility has been questioned if the prospective owner decides that the engine is not powerful enough.

Game show hosts share many qualities with car salesmen, and they too are usually Lycopodiums. Unlike the more subtle politeness of a Lycopodium diplomat in the service of his country, the game show host is often nauseatingly nice to his contestants. He makes a special point of emphasising his popularity with his audience by being 'pally', friendly without being really intimate. This comfy 'pallyness' is typified by the veteran English game show host Bruce Forsyth, and his traditional greeting, 'Nice to see you, to see you nice'.

Although Lycopodium needs to please in order to feel secure, he will often find more elevated explanations for his friendliness. I once attended an 'encounter group', where one learns to explore the hidden motives of one's actions, and to achieve greater intimacy with oneself and others. There was a man of about fifty years on the course, who had boyish good-looks despite his age, complete with long hair and blue jeans. He had just come from another, more 'spiritual' course, where he had learned that he must love everyone. During our course, this man had great difficulty accepting the aggression that some of the participants were getting into and expressing. Whenever someone succeeded in contacting old sleeping feelings of anger, and expressed them, our Lycopodium peacemaker tried to rationalise with them, pointing out that whoever had made them angry was just looking for love. As you can imagine, this kind of behaviour did nothing but help the participants to get in touch with their anger, and our Lycopodium friend soon became very unpopular. Undaunted, he would stick to what he had learned, and announce to the group, 'I think we should love each other', at which point he was bowled over by a collective scream of 'Bull shit!'. He learned the hard way on that course that his friendliness had nothing to do with unconditional love, but rather was a plea for acceptance.

Another group of people who put their friendliness, and their ability to reason eloquently to apparently laudable use, are the American TV preachers. I am sure that a great many of these are Lycopodiums, particularly the more pushy ones who elicit donations from their flock with the same zeal that salesmen sell cars. These supposedly spiritual men use cynical emotional manipulation to part guilty people from their money, which is then spent upon women and fast cars. They are an example of the 'Charmer', the type of Lycopodium man who uses his ability to make people like him to live off them. Thankfully, most Lycopodium charmers have more morals and less power than these TV evangelists. (A few TV evangelists are liable to be Natrum or Sulphur.)

### Bravado

Bravado is seen more often in Lycopodium than in any other type. It is an attempt to cover up anxiety by acting confidently. Although the most fundamental essence of Lycopodium is impotence, a strong secondary element is inflation. On the physical level this inflation is seen in the gaseous distension of the abdomen, as well as in distended veins and haemorrhoids. These are examples of physical inflation secondary to weakness (of digestion, or of vessel walls). On the psychological level bravado is very similar, a case of inflation with nothing very substantial, secondary to a sense of weakness.

Not all Lycopodiums succumb to bravado. For simplicity's sake we can divide Lycopodium into three sub-types, which we could label 'the Wimp', 'the Strutter' and the average Lycopodium. In my experience the latter accounts for about half of the type, whilst the first two account for about a quarter each. The 'Wimp' (as I rather unkindly call him for the sake of emphasis) does not resort to bravado. His nervousness is undisguised and often quite crippling. He is the seven stone weakling who has sand kicked in his face, the coward who runs from the battle at the first sound of gun-fire, the fool who is so nervous in an interview that he spills his coffee all over his prospective boss's table. He has not learned to hide his fear behind the subtle defences of the average Lycopodium, or the cruder defences of the 'Strutter'. These 'Wimps' exhibit all the more obvious signs of nervousness described in the older Materia Medicas (Kent: 'Dreads the presence of new persons', 'Fear of undertaking anything', 'frightened at trifles'). They often find it difficult to express themselves, making mistakes with their words, or stuttering. They are the most given to attempting to please others, and they react to adversity with fear rather than anger. The tragicomic characters played by Jerry Lewis and Norman Wisdom are good caricatures of this type.

In direct contrast to the 'Wimp', the 'Strutter' counteracts his sense of impotency by exaggerating his masculine power. This may be done in a variety of ways. There are the physical strutters who go in for body-building and martial arts, so that they can kick sand in the faces of wimps (or at least look as if they would). A great many physical fitness enthusiasts are Lycopodiums, but those who go to extremes are often the strutters, who want to be seen to be strong. The physical strutter tends to be very proud of his sexual prowess, at least publicly. He will compete with his mates in this regard, boasting over a beer about his sexual conquests, and leering at pretty women. Since he overvalues the masculine, he undervalues the feminine, and this means that the strutter is a very chauvinistic man. He tends to think that women are there to look after him, or to sleep with, and that he is the boss. Needless to say, women married to strutters, particularly physical strutters, tend to have a rough time.

Strutters like to dominate others (Kent: 'Dictatorial'). Physical strutters do this with physical intimidation. If the dinner is not on the table when they get home, they are liable to shout at their wife, or worse. Since they are cowards, physical strutters tend to bully women and timid men, and seek to impress those with more power. They wear clothes which emphasise their muscular physiques, drive overpowered cars, and spend a lot of money on alcohol. When they come up against a confident intellect they are at their most defensive, since they cannot compete. Consequently, physical strutters tend to treat all but the most wimpish of professionals with respect.

Bullies are most likely to be either Natrum Muriaticum or Lycopodium constitutionally, since the bully has a deep sense of inadequacy inside. Like the Natrum bully, the Lycopodium bully is very keen to be liked, and will go out of his way to be nice to those who stand up to him.

Intellectual bravado (known colloquially as 'bullshit') is the principal defence mechanism of the intellectual strutter. The latter is not necessarily particularly intelligent or intellectual, but he thinks he is, and is able to impress some who are less intellectual than himself. A good example of this type is Colonel Manwaring in the British television comedy 'Dad's Army'. The Colonel makes the most of his position of petty authority, using it as a platform from which to wax eloquent and in the process put down those whose ignorance he can expose. Like all intellectual strutters, he uses rather pompous, flowery language, which is excessively elaborate. He prefers to use a lot of long words, rather than a few short ones, even though the latter would be more effective in getting his point across. As a result, most intellectual strutters are terribly boring. They deliver their pearls of wisdom (so they think) either with a preachy intensity, which is meant to imply grave importance, or with a flourish, as if to say, 'Hah! Look how clever I am!'. (This latter mode of delivery puts me in mind of Yul Brynner's film version of the King of Siam in 'The King and I'.)

The intellectual strutter is generally convinced that he is right about virtually everything, and will not entertain contradiction (Kent: 'Intolerant of contradiction'). He learns a little about everything, and then considers himself an expert in each field. Consequently, he is often to be seen butting in to conversations to correct statements that he considers are wrong. He may even do this to complete strangers (Kent: 'Disposition to contradict'). This tendency to thrive on exhibiting his knowledge is reminiscent of Sulphur, who also has a tendency to bore the pants off his audience, and to always think that he is right. In general one could say that Sulphur's first love is knowledge for its own sake, and his enjoyment of sharing his knowledge is secondary. Consequently, Sulphur is usually very well informed on his favourite subjects, and is less condescending in his delivery than the intellectual Lycopodium strutter, whose main interest is not the intellectual content of his delivery, but the admiration he can win with it.

Part of the act of the intellectual strutter is an elaborate attempt to justify or detract attention away from his failings. For example, I once knew a young man who had not worked for many years, relying on the State to pay his bills. He said that he had obtained a certificate from a doctor friend of his (the intellectual strutter is always a personal friend of his doctor) to the effect that he could not work on account of 'nervous tension'. Whilst he was something of a nervous man, he appeared perfectly capable of working, and he affirmed that this was indeed the case. However, he justified his avoidance of regular work by saying that the healing work he was engaged in required all of his time. He had attended numerous courses on alternative medicine, and had certificates all over his walls to this effect. They were in the name of 'Jonathan Earth Spirit', a name he had adopted and acquired by deed pole. He ran local meditation meetings from his home, one of which I attended. There were only four of us there, but undaunted, he announced whilst in a pseudo-trance that he had been called upon to be a centre of healing for his community. He subsequently sought treatment from me for nervous indigestion. I gave him Lycopodium 10M, after which he entered a brief but profound depression. Following this he ended his meditation meetings, reverted to his real name, and got a real job. Such is the power of the similimum to eradicate what is false (at least sometimes).

I cannot resist mentioning one more example of the remedy's ability to eradicate false pride. The middle-aged Lycopodium man I mentioned previously who had been taught to love everyone took great pride in his youthful appearance. His brilliant white smile would flash when you talked to him, endearing him instantly. He was a womaniser and a former travelling salesman, and had used his boyish charm to good effect in both these activities. However, he too had not worked for years, relying on a diagnosis of epilepsy to obtain a pension. (Despite the fact that he had no more than one fit per year.) I eventually treated him for epilepsy with Lycopodium 10M. Within a day of taking the remedy his false front tooth had fallen out, leaving an unsightly gap which he tried frantically to fill by sticking the tooth back with super-glue. It seems that the remedy caused his body to reject not only his psychological, but also his physical falsity. (He had one grand mal seizure after stopping his anti-epileptic medication and taking the remedy, followed by a period of depression and a profound reappraisal of his life. Like Jonathan Earth Spirit he too decided to go back to work, and enrolled in a training programme at the age of fifty something. Several months after treatment he had had no more seizures, and was off medication.)

### The Average Lycopodium

Most Lycopodiums are neither wimps nor strutters. They have a little of each of these types in them, as well as a degree of genuine confidence and an ability to interact without defensiveness, at least some of the time. Most Lycopodiums will admit to the homeopath that they tend to worry, especially about their work, and also about whether people like them. They will also tend to underplay their weaknesses at times, or to deny them. In this sense they sometimes pretend to be stronger than they are. Often only Lycopodium's wife has any idea of the worries in her husband's head. He may be a prominent businessman or a respected lecturer, who usually gives an impression of calm assurance, yet inside he worries that he will get it wrong. Since he has a little of the bravado of the strutter in him, he may occasionally boast a little, in a subtle way. For example, he may buy a flashy new car, and drop it into the conversation for a while. Or he may tend to use letterheads for personal use which display his professional qualifications. (He will

116

tell himself that he is just saving money by using his business stationery at home, but unlike the strutter, he will know there is more to it than that, but will allow himself this little indulgence.)

The average Lycopodium is very easy-going. He is a very 'reasonable' person, who is not given to strong moods of either elation or depression. Like the intellectual strutter, he tends to rationalise a lot, but not so defensively. Lycopodium is a mental type, in the sense that he lives more in his head than in his feelings. He usually relies on rational intellect to make sense of his world, and respects those who express themselves logically. Here he can be a little chauvinistic, gently patronising his women friends for their illogical emotionality. On the other hand, the average Lycopodium man loves women in general, and gets on with them very well. There is something of the charmer in most Lycopodiums, and a weakness for a pretty woman. His charm lies in his boyishness, which is irresistible to many women. He loves to be mothered, and those women who love to mother will flock around him, flirting with him whether they be his mother-in-law or his daughter. Because he is mild and boyish, he appears harmless, and this quality endears him to women who would never flirt with deeper or more powerful types.

### *Detachment*
Emotionally, the average Lycopodium man never really grows up. In his relations with others he is either pleasant but aloof, or dependent. In close partnership he tends to seek a mother figure, since he wants to be loved unconditionally, without having to give back very much. Most Lycopodium men were very close to their mother when children, and it may be that this closeness prevents them from getting too close to other women. They loved their mothers, but also took them for granted, and their love was gentle rather than passionate. This pattern is often repeated in adult relations with women, who are treated more like mothers than lovers.

Many Lycopodium men would rather play with the boys (or girls) than spend time being intimate (as opposed to sexual) with their partner, since they feel uncomfortable with true intimacy. True intimacy requires a certain amount of responsibility, and Lycopodium is not fond of responsibility, at least not when it involves emotional commitment. This is expressed in the older Materia Medicas as a propensity to leave wife and children suddenly without remorse. Whilst there are a great many Lycopodium men who are committed husbands and fathers, there are also a lot who avoid the commitment of marriage, who seek extramarital affairs, or who leave their family when a pretty woman comes into their life. Lycopodium is not a deeply emotional type. Emotionally Lycopodiums are 'lightweights' who enjoy the closeness of a partner without great passion or intimacy. Within a marriage Lycopodium is likely to be a good friend to his wife, sharing common interests, and helping out with the chores and the kids, yet remaining essentially separate. This detached quality is infuriating to many women, but soothing to others.

The above description may give the impression that Lycopodium is a cold type, but this is not usually the case. The average Lycopodium is warmer than the average Natrum man, (that is, he shows his affection more) and is quite fond of cuddles and kisses. He has no difficulty in saying 'I love you', and means it. It is just that his love is a gentle fondness rather than a passion. He is a mild, easy-going person, who will help anyone out who asks, but is not keen to tie himself down, and who rarely feels great depths of emotion. Such men often evoke highly emotional outbursts in their partners, who will do anything to get them to show more emotion, which they equate with love.

Another traditional rubric applied to Lycopodium is his preference for company in the next room. This is often literally true. Lycopodium will feel lonely in a house by himself, but oppressed when sharing his life too intimately with another. The preference for someone in the next room to his is a good metaphor for his emotional life as a whole. He needs the support of other people, but he also needs his space. This may often derive from his having had an overprotective mother, who leaves him dependent and yet feeling stifled at the same time.

Whilst Lycopodium's detachment can cause some difficulties in close relationships, it is a positive asset at work. Most jobs require a logical, detached mind, and this is especially true of scientific posts. Lycopodiums, like Kalis, make very good scientists. Both types have a love of logic, and an ability to follow rules and protocol. A visit to any university department of pure science or engineering will reveal a student body composed primarily of Lycopodiums, (since the type is so much more common than other highly rational types like Kali and Sulphur). These students will have many characteristics in common. For example, most will fit the traditional Lycopodium description of being 'keen intellectually but of weak muscular power', with rather thin, bony physiques, and a tendency to wrinkle the brow, either out of worry, or intellectual concentration. They will often have practical hobbies that require little physical effort, such as model making, or rebuilding engines. Socially they will tend to be conformist, rather than individualistic. This is due to the desire to fit in, and hence be popular. It is reflected in the clothes that Lycopodiums tend to wear, which are at once fashionable and conventional. Engineering students in particular are notorious for the amounts of alcohol that they consume together, and my little experience of them tends to support this. This group camaraderie is very characteristic of Lycopodiums, and is facilitated by alcohol, which loosens up characters who would otherwise be inhibited by their highly rational nature.

The average Lycopodium man is both cautious and ambitious when it comes to material advancement. As a result, he often works his way up from the bottom in the business world. Since he is a people-pleaser he is suited to big corporations, where he will steadily rise up the corporate ladder until he reaches a position which stretches him as far as he is willing to go. Although not a natural leader in the sense that Nux and Sulphur are, Lycopodium can often gradually acquire the skills and the self-confidence that is needed to exercise authority over a large number of people. By gaining steady promotion, he can grow in stature within the company gradually, without activating his fear of failure excessively. The average Lycopodium makes a pleasant boss, who is reasonable and understanding, and enjoys a certain amount of friendliness with his staff. Natrum bosses are also often like this. It is the vulnerability within these two most common constitutional types which makes them humane and approachable when in positions of authority. (Nux and Arsenicum tend to be tougher, whilst Sulphur is generous not out of vulnerability, but out of his 'largeness of spirit'.)

Lycopodium's detachment is in part a result of his rational, non-emotional nature, but also in part a front to disguise insecurity. Some Lycopodium men are very straight people, with little vanity, and no need to impress . Others develop a 'cool' image that is similar to the cool front used by so many Natrum men, an appearance of being nonchalant and unruffled whatever the circumstance. These cool Lycopodiums resemble Natrum and even Nux in the consulting room, but in personal relationships their softness and vulnerability is usually more apparent . Even the coolest of Lycopodiums tends to like to be mothered by his mate, and is more likely to be open with her about his worries than the average Natrum man. The cool Lycopodium is more easily spotted by talking to his partner in many cases, unless he is a strutter, in which case his attempts to look nonchalant are so obvious that they have "Lycopodium" stamped all over them.

### The Opportunist

To be an opportunist, one has to be both emotionally detached and flexible. Thus the more emotional types like Natrum and Sepia tend to put emotional loyalties before self-gain, and the detached but rigid types like Kali and Arsenicum tend to put both safety and principle before opportunism. The detached, flexible types include Phosphorus, Lycopodium, Argentum, Medorrhinum, Nux, Staphysagria and Tuberculinum, and all of these tend to be opportunists. In my experience, Lycopodium and Tuberculinum are the most opportunistic of all.

Tuberculinum is opportunistic because he has a great hunger for freedom, and will take whatever opportunities come his way to preserve this freedom. Lycopodium also loves freedom, but is not so courageous nor so reckless as Tuberculinum. His opportunism is in part due to a love of freedom, and in part due to his tendency to take the easy way, to make gains without either hard work or commitment. Perhaps he is still in the mother-child relationship, except now the whole world is the mother, who will provide without expecting anything in return. (Hence the disproportionate large number of Lycopodium men who do not work.) Like Phosphorus, Lycopodium expects to get away with his gambles, both because he is quick witted, and because he is charming.

One common expression of Lycopodium's opportunism is the womaniser. Romeos who flit from one woman to another, getting out when the going gets rough, are very often Lycopodiums. Many Lycopodium men are virtual gigolos, relying on their charm with women to avoid a life of emotional and professional commitment. It is not uncommon for a Lycopodium man to rely upon his lover for financial support, including being baled out of debts and other self-inflicted dangers. In return he offers sexual favours, and congenial company, and considers that his woman is getting a reasonable deal.

The crook is another variant of the Lycopodium opportunist, and many Lycopodium crooks are also womanisers. Examples of the Lycopodium crook include the shady dealer in second-hand cars, the spiv who sells anything that 'fell off the back of a lorry', and con-artists of all types. What these have in common, apart from a lack of moral conscience, is a quick, tricky mind, that jumps at any opportunity to make a penny. Petty crooks in particular are liable to be Lycopodium. To be a big time crook you need to have a lot of nerve, and a ruthless streak, and these are not qualities typical of Lycopodium. The Lycopodium crook may turn a blind eye to a great many consequences of his thievery, (Lycopodiums of all types are very good at turning a blind eye when it suits them), but he is not cold-hearted enough to sanction murder, unless perhaps he is a physical strutter, in which case he may have a lot of anger inside. Petty crooks take the easy way out wherever possible, and this is another Lycopodium tendency.

A wonderfully humorous and accurate portrait of the Lycopodium petty crook can be seen in the character of the Innkeeper, in the stage production of the musical 'Les Miserables'. The following lyrics from the show will paint the portrait more clearly (and more entertainingly) than I could myself:

'Welcome Monsieur! Sit yourself down
And meet the best Innkeeper in town
As for the rest, all of them crooks,
Rooking the guests and cooking the books.
Seldom do you see  honest men like me,
A gent of good intent who's content to be
Master of the House, doling out the charm,
Ready with a handshake and an open palm.

Tells a saucy tale, makes a little stir.
Customers appreciate a bon-viveur
Glad to do me friends a favour,
Doesn't cost me to be nice,
But nothing gets you nothing, everything has got a little price.
Master of the House, Keeper of the Zoo
Ready to relieve them of a sou or two;
Water in the wine, making up the weight,
Picking up their nicknacks when they can't see straight.
Everybody loves a landlord, everybody's bosom friend,
I do whatever pleases, Jesus don't I bleed 'em in the end!
Master of the House, quick to catch your eye.
Never wants a passer-by to pass him by.
Servant to the Poor, Butler to the Great,
Comforter, philosopher and life-long mate,
Everybody's boon-companion, everybody's chaperone,
But lock up your valises, Jesus won't I skin you to the bone!

(The Innkeeper's Wife:)
I used to dream that I would meet a prince,
But God Almighty have you seen what's happened since?
Master of the House  isn't worth me spit,
Comforter, philosopher and life-long shit,
Cunning little brain, regular Voltaire,
Thinks he's quite a lover but there's not much there.
What a cruel trick of Nature, leaving me with such a louse,
God knows how I've lasted living with this barstard in the house!

Not all Lycopodiums are without scruples, but most are opportunists to some extent. Like Sulphur some are constantly hatching grand schemes to get rich quick, which invariably amount to nought. On the other hand, many Lycopodiums have sufficient 'savvy' to set up profitable businesses of their own, taking advantage of gaps in the market, and using advertising and business connections to the full to get established. The average Lycopodium, like the average Natrum, is a bit of battler. He would like to just have an easy life, but he knows that he will have to fight for it, and whilst he doesn't relish the fight like Nux, nor assume that he will always succeed like Sulphur, he is sensible enough to know that it's worth the effort, and he has a sound enough brain and a way with people that will help him get through.

Speaking of Lycopodium businessmen, I would like to mention a common mistake that some inexperienced homeopaths fall into. Many Lycopodium business men are quite obsessed with their job, and appear in the consulting room to be no-nonsense go-getters who are brimming with confidence. This is to some extent an act, which fools the unwary homeopath into prescribing Nux Vomica, which does not act. The differentiation can be subtle and difficult, especially when the physicals are common to both remedies, as is often the case (eg dyspepsia when stressed). I usually find it helpful to enquire into the personality of the patient as a child. Very often the confident Lycopodium will admit that he worried a lot before exams, or that he underestimated his abilities as a child, even though he will admit to no weaknesses now. Also, when asked the question, 'What is your greatest fear in life?', it is surprising how many confident successful Lycopodiums reply, 'That my life will amount to nothing', or 'That my business will fail'. Such thoughts never even enter into the head of a Nux Vomica.

The average Lycopodium is not an all-out Romeo, but he will often be a bit of a sexual opportunist. This may consist of nothing more than flirting with the girls, or pinching their bottoms. On the other hand, the married Lycopodium man is more likely than most to succumb to the temptation of having an affair, once he has started taking his wife for granted. It's not that he doesn't love her. In his own, gentle and detached way he still does, but the thrill he gets from entering into a new affair may prove irresistible.

Whilst on the subject of Romeos, it would be appropriate to consider briefly Lycopodium's sexuality. Lycopodiums are particularly touchy on this subject, since it comes so close to the subject of impotence in general. Most Lycopodium men are not impotent, but many have a fear of being so, which is just another facet of the general fear of failure. The average Lycopodium is relatively highly sexed, and tends to indulge in sexual fantasy when sex is not available (and also when it is). The more physical types, like the physical strutter, and also some of the Romeos, are likely to enjoy sex every night, and may stray from their partner if they are not satisfied. More cerebral Lycopodiums are more average in their sexual appetites, but most are still on the highly sexed side of average. As with men of many other constitutional types, Lycopodium may have some difficulty in being emotionally intimate whilst he is being sexually intimate. This is just another version of liking to be in the next room—close, but not too close.

Most Lycopodium men over-value their sexual prowess to some extent, or are overly concerned with maintaining it. They may have been very highly sexed in their early years, and then, as the libido begins to settle down to a more moderate level, they may interpret this as a sign of waning virility, and worry about how far this trend will go. When they do have some difficulty with maintaining an erection, or with premature ejaculation, as most men do at some point in their lives, particularly when under stress or with a new partner, Lycopodium men are liable to over-react, and this may lead to a haunting fear of sexual failure, which itself can produce what is feared in the long run (Kent: 'Sexual passion diminished'). As a result, such men may turn to the use of alleged aphrodisiacs in a frantic attempt to prevent deterioration of sexual functioning, and may hesitantly inquire of the homeopath whether the remedy will help in this regard. I remember an old gent of about seventy years, who came to see me for homeopathic treatment. He was a widower, but had a lady friend whom he saw only occasionally. His sole complaint was that he was unable to reach climax when masturbating, which he did several times each day. He was less concerned with his lovemaking, although there too he was no longer able to reach a climax. It was interesting to see how totally unselfconscious he was about his complaint. He described it in detail with no sign of embarrassment, or of acknowledgment that this was an unusual concern in a man of his age. His appearance and the rest of the history fitted Lycopodium, and he returned after a dose of 1M to say that his problem was much improved.

Another, much younger man came to see me with the same problem. He was very skinny, and fancied himself as an expert on yoga and Eastern mysticism. He told me with great pride that he used to make love for six or eight hours at a time, but now he had a new partner and he was having difficulty maintaining an erection. It did not surprise me when he said he was having investigations to determine whether he had a vascular problem at the root of his impotence. (It somehow sounds less of a personal failing to have a vascular problem than to admit other causes which may be more closely related to personal responsibility.) His pride both in his former sexual prowess, and in his knowledge of yoga, was so obvious and exaggerated that I had no difficulty in choosing the remedy. After a dose of Lycopodium 10M he returned noticeably less 'cocksure', and also far less concerned about his problem, which had more or less gone as a result of his ending the relationship.

### The Intellectual

At the risk of confusing the reader with a profusion of subtly differing subtypes, I feel that I must distinguish what I call the Lycopodium pseudo-intellectual from the true Lycopodium intellectual. The pseudo-intellectual lies somewhere between the intellectual strutter and the true intellectual. He can be thought of as an intellectual strutter who does not have the confidence to advertise his ideas very forcefully, but to be fair to him, his ideas do tend to be a little more subtle than the strutter's. The pseudo-intellectual does not have the intellectual depth or discrimination of the true intellectual, but his analytical mind is occupied much of the time in devouring one concept after another, like a child who samples each of the desserts on the trolley. This kind of intellectual dilettantism is an attempt by some Lycopodiums to feel a greater sense of self-importance. They feel (subconsciously in most cases) that the more they know, the more significant a person they are. They are usually quieter people than the intellectual strutters, and will only try to share their knowledge with friends, who are not likely to reject or ridicule them. The pseudo-intellectual will often settle on a subject like a bee on a flower, and graze there for several weeks or months, before moving on to another topic of investigation. During this time the subject occupies much of his attention, as he reads one book after another in an attempt to become something of an authority on it. I once treated such a man, whose main complaint was a sensitive stomach. He told me that he was in the process of studying 'Chaos Theory'. He said this in a very grave manner, as if to emphasise the importance of his studies, and said that he intended to write a book on the subject, but when I asked him more about 'Chaos Theory', he gradually became more and more vague, explaining somewhat tentatively that he was interested in how 'order tends to arise out of chaos, particularly in human systems'. He worked as a computer operator, and had had no background in Chaos Theory apart from the current book he was reading. It soon became clear to me that he was attracted to the idea of studying 'Chaos Theory' because it sounded impressive, and would hopefully make him appear more interesting. He was a lonely man, with no close friends, and he had difficulty in approaching and getting to know women, since he was afraid of being rejected. He admitted these problems very reluctantly and after much questioning on my part. Like other Lycopodium pseudo-intellectuals, his main aim in life was to appear interesting enough to attract friends, a girl-friend, and a modicum of respect from other people, and it was to these ends that he collected facts, and tried to interest people in them.

I gave him Lycopodium 10M, and the next time I saw him he said he was most impressed by the effects of the remedy. At first he had felt quiet and subdued for a day or two, after which time he noticed that his indigestion had stopped bothering him, and he no longer got numb feet when sitting cross-legged to meditate. He seemed more relaxed to me, and no longer tried to impress with his learning. When I asked him how he was getting on with his investigation of 'Chaos Theory', he said that he hadn't given it much thought lately.

The true Lycopodium intellectual is less common than the pseudo-intellectual. He is genuinely fascinated with his subjects of study, and does not seek primarily to impress people. He is generally an expert on a particular field, but the field itself may be anything from quantum physics to linguistics to philosophy. To the Lycopodium intellectual his academic work is frequently the centre of his life. It absorbs him entirely for much of the day, and gives him a sense of satisfaction, and a purpose in life. He is probably the driest of the Lycopodiums, since his focus is so exclusively on intellectual matters. He is likely to be shy, having spent much of his life buried in books, and although he may lecture competently, he has none of the flamboyance of a Sulphur intellectual, nor the conviction and forceful delivery of a Nux intellectual. However, he is patient and painstaking with his audience, and thorough in his understanding of a chosen subject. The Lycopodium intellectual is the boffin in the white coat with the high receding forehead, who spends his life hidden in the laboratory pursuing some highly specific scientific matter, forever dissecting and analysing. He is less inspired than the Sulphur genius, but he is dedicated, and derives real satisfaction from his work. If he is an academic rather than a practical scientist, his ideas are likely to be learned through the usual channels of education, unlike some Sulphur intellectuals, who are highly original, and can come up with theories from seemingly unconnected observations, and incorporate information from a wide variety of disciplines.

Science teachers and professors are very often Lycopodium intellectuals. I remember my own physics teacher, and as I think back to those lessons I am sure he was a Lycopodium. His manner was thorough but relaxed (unlike a Kali or an Arsenicum, who would be thorough and regimental in all likelihood), and he was a very unassuming person, with no tendency to impose his power upon his pupils. He was a quiet man, who enjoyed sharing his knowledge, and sometimes lit up with enthusiasm when he strayed from the syllabus and taught us about exciting things like black holes and relativity, but was mostly on a very even keel. He was a little shy, and was noticeably embarrassed whenever we gently pulled his leg.

### The Hippy

In the sixties a great many young people joined the hippy movement to some extent, and no doubt they belonged to the whole range of constitutional types. I have found, however, that the majority of those people who still cling to this way of life are either Lycopodium or Natrum constitutionally. The Hippy lifestyle involves dropping out from mainstream society, and whilst this may at first seem out of keeping with Lycopodium's tendency to conform, it is very much in keeping with the type's tendency to avoid responsibility. Most present-day hippies have no regular job, and many rely on state benefits to survive. They usually justify this by saying that the system is corrupt, and hence fair game for abuse, or by saying that their lifestyle is a positive example to the community. Both of these justifications are examples of Lycopodium's ability to rationalise. The hippy lifestyle also involves 'free love', which usually means sex free from emotional commitment, and this also is very attractive to many Lycopodiums. Furthermore, the hippy community is a source of unconditional love and approval for its members, something that is very dear to the average Lycopodium.

I once treated about ten members of a community who were followers of the late Indian guru, Bhagwan Shree Rajneesh. Rajneesh had a very liberal approach, encouraging his followers to enjoy themselves above all else, and this resulted in a great deal of sexual permissiveness in their community. Every one of these patients of mine complained of dyspepsia, and every one was Lycopodium constitutionally. (It became a bit of a joke—I would have the Lycopodium ready and waiting for the next 'Sannyasin' (follower of Rajneesh). I did do my best to remain unbiased with each new case, but they did respond to the remedy.)

The hippy community of today is extremely dependent on the use of marijuana to make life pleasant, and this is perhaps an example of Lycopodium's escapist tendency. In order to avoid worrying, work and feelings of inadequacy in the face of conflict, many Lycopodiums develop a peculiar blindness to problems. This perceptive impairment is facilitated by the use of alcohol and marijuana, and enables many Lycopodiums, including the majority of the hippies, to live in a kind of fool's paradise. A more conventional example of this can be seen in the cartoon character Andy Capp. Whenever he is berated by his long suffering wife for gambling instead of paying the bills, he is apt to reply, 'Never mind pet, come and 'ave a drink'.

Within a community such as the hippy community, Lycopodium feels that he is accepted and belongs, and hence it does not matter that he is going against the grain of the rest of society, since he is still very much conforming to an acceptable norm. (Witness the extraordinary conformity of the hippy culture, with its flowery shirts, long hair, homespun jewellery, and ethos of peace and love.) The relatively secure Lycopodium is able to develop a greater degree of individuality, and this process is often initiated by a dose of Lycopodium 10M.

### Sentimentality and Soft Heartedness

Most Lycopodiums are soft hearted. Even the physical strutter is likely to send his mother flowers on Mother's Day. The majority of Lycopodiums genuinely love people, even though their love is gentle and rather impersonal. They have a soft heart, and can usually be moved by tales of sorrow and hardship. Lycopodium has often suffered from feelings of inadequacy himself, and so he is usually in favour of the underdog, since he can empathise to some extent. (Yet he also admires success in all forms, and attempts to emulate it.) The average Lycopodium man makes a reasonable and also considerate partner, and an indulgent parent. He is particularly likely to be indulgent with daughters, and may be a little hard on his son, seeking to live out through him some of his own unfulfilled dreams. The Lycopodium family man uses his easy-going friendliness and charm to good effect at home, and since he is still a bit of a kid, he tends to enjoy playing with his children, and often seems more like a mate to them than a father. He is likely to be very proud of his children, and to relish doing manly things with his boy, like fishing and playing football. (Simpson's addicts will recognise Homer Simpson here. The father of the world famous cartoon character Bart Simpson is a wonderful caricature of an 'average' Lycopodium family man. He is a coward who dreams of greatness, ignores his family half of the time because he is too busy playing with his mates, and sentimentally indulges them the other half of the time. Although his family have many complaints about him, they never really doubt that he loves them, and they know that they can rely on him when the chips are down. The rest of the time they play it by ear.)

Because Lycopodium seeks to be accepted (and hence feels subconsciously that he is not accepted), many exhibit a characteristic kind of sentimentality—a tendency to weep when warmly welcomed or appreciated (Kent: 'Weeps when thanked'). Like the Prodigal Son returned from exile, they are often overcome with emotion when offered an unequivocal show of love. In general Lycopodium men can cry far more easily than Natrums, and are not so reluctant to do so publicly. Although some abuse their partners and sons, most Lycopodium men are very aware of how much their happiness depends upon their loved ones, and they can become quite emotional during farewells, reunions, and occasions like wedding anniversaries, when they are asked to make a speech, and genuinely cry with gratitude for the love of their wife and children.

### Depression and Despair

One does not normally think of Lycopodium as a depressive type, and the majority of depressed patients will need other remedies, yet any constitutional type can become depressed under adverse circumstances, and Lycopodium is no exception. The depression of a Lycopodium person will respond to the remedy, unless it is due to grief, in which case Natrum Muriaticum or Ignatia may be needed.

I have not seen many depressed Lycopodiums, and hence my remarks will be brief. Those that I have seen had had difficult lives, with little parental approval or love during childhood. Their depressive state was similar to that of Natrum Muriaticum, with some typical Lycopodium features 'added on'. Thus they tended to withdraw from company when depressed, and yet preferred to have company available. They tended to sit and brood about their troubles, and about the past, and had very little self-respect. This state of depression is hard to differentiate from a Sepia or a Natrum depression, and the pre-morbid personality should be used as a pointer. There will usually be some typical Lycopodium features in the depressed Lycopodium patient, such as anticipatory anxiety and unrealistic fear of failure. Indeed, these anxious tendencies are likely to be heightened during a depressive period. My depressed Lycopodium patients exhibited quite a lot of despair, as if they were on the verge of giving up on life. Suicidal thoughts were a feature in some, and were intensified during the initial aggravation from the remedy (although I have never come across a depressed patient who committed suicide during a homeopathic aggravation). Kent says of the depressed Lycopodium patient, 'does not want to be talked to, or forced to do anything, does not want to make any exertion, yet at times when forced to do so she is relieved'. Unfortunately, such remarks tend to apply to most depressed patients. When considering Lycopodium in cases of depression, one must take the totality of the patient's history into account. One useful feature of Lycopodium is that depression is liable to be at its worst upon waking, and tends to improve as the day goes on (Kent: 'Suicidal on waking'). The depressed Natrum is also often worse upon waking, but does not tend to improve so much later in the day.

### Senility and Dementia

Lycopodium is a little like Baryta, in that there is a certain immaturity to the type, which becomes exaggerated in cases of senility. (The same can be said of Sulphur.) The principal features of the demented or senile Lycopodium individual are exaggerations of characteristics commonly seen in younger Lycopodiums.

Forgetfulness is common to all cases of senility, but there is a characteristic Lycopodium form of forgetfulness that is seen even in non-senile people, which becomes more apparent with advancing years and failing mental powers. This is the tendency of Lycopodium to forget proper names. On meeting an acquaintance, Lycopodium can suffer a paroxysm of anxiety and embarrassment trying to remember their name, even though they have met many times before (Kent: 'Memory poor-proper names'). The senile Lycopodium gent has a habit of substituting 'Wos is name' for virtually everybody, even his own family.

With advancing age Lycopodium tends to become less acquiescent and more cantankerous. (Kent: 'Taciturn', 'Quarrelsome', 'Rudeness'.) The elderly Lycopodium man is often something of a little Hitler, ordering people about as if they were servants (Kent: 'Haughty'). It is as if he were finally courageous enough to fight the battles he had always avoided, but finding himself removed from the battle-field, he vents his fire on his attendants instead. Demented Lycopodium men in nursing homes have a habit of attacking their nurses when being undressed or put into the bath, at which times they will swear obscenities and kick and bite. They will also flirt openly with the nurses, and offer their sexual favours, in comical imitation of the younger Lycopodium Romeo.

The chronic fearfulness of many Lycopodiums may translate into suspiciousness in old-age (Kent: 'Distrustful, suspicious and fault-finding). In true Lycopodium style, the demented Lycopodium will dissect a sentence, look for any signs of aggression in it, and then proceed to take exception to one point after another (including many points which were imagined), pontificating like an ultimate authority of the truth. This verbal fencing is an exaggeration of the intellectual strutter's tendency to preach and to contradict. (The dementia of Sulphur has many similarities, differing mainly in the tendency of Sulphur to project himself as even more important than the demented Lycopodium—the classical Sulphur delusions of grandeur. Also, Sulphur will tend to ramble on endlessly about factually correct information that he gathered during his life which fascinated him.)

### The Lycopodium Woman

I have not left the subject of the Lycopodium woman till last out of chauvinism, but rather because much of what has been written so far applies to Lycopodiums of both sexes. In my experience about one in ten Lycopodiums are female. In view of the high proportion of the population that resonate to the remedy, this means that Lycopodium women are relatively common, and I see them about as frequently as Sepia women, and more frequently than Pulsatilla or Silica.

Lycopodium women are generally more straightforward than the men, because they don't try to hide their insecurity behind a screen of bravado or intellectual rationalisation. All the Lycopodium women that I have treated were very open about their anxiety, which was considerable in most cases, and quite crippling in some. There is the same fear of failure that we see in the Lycopodium man. In women this often translates into a fear of being an inadequate wife or mother. Those women who go out to work generally have a lot of anxiety about their performance at work, especially if they have to speak to groups of people. One Lycopodium woman came to see me for treatment of nervous diarrhoea. She had quite a high powered executive job, which involved giving presentations from time to time. Her anticipatory anxiety had gradually increased to the point where she had to rush to the toilet just before every meeting, and also in the middle of the meeting, before her turn to speak. This kind of anxiety is not seen very often in Lycopodium men to such an extreme degree, since they have more effective mechanisms for avoiding anxiety by boosting their ego. The lady's nervous diarrhoea gradually faded into the background along with her anticipatory anxiety after a few doses of Lycopodium 10M.

The one kind of ego boosting that I have seen Lycopodium women go for is physical fitness, particularly gym work and body-building. Many of the female gym instructors I have gotten to know have been Lycopodiums. (Having said that, there are many female fitness enthusiasts who are either Natrum or Tuberculinum.)

As well as being more obviously nervous than the men, Lycopodium women as a whole try even harder to please people. They are generally rather acquiescent and timid, and quick to offer praise and assistance to other people. I remember one Lycopodium woman of about twenty years, who appeared to be much younger, on account of her timidity. She told me that as a girl at high school she was asked to 'go behind the shed' with a couple of the more forward boys. She had for months listened with a mixture of horror and fascination to the tales of the precocious girls who regularly went behind the shed with the boys, and had come to think that there was something wrong with her because she had not been asked. When she was finally asked she was paralysed with indecision, torn between her desire to be popular, and her fear of the boys. She had never quite gotten over this experience, and replayed it in various guises again and again. This characteristic of trying hard to please is seen just as frequently in Natrum, Pulsatilla and Staphysagria women, and the homeopath would do well to remember all four of these when considering the case of an acquiescent woman.

All the Lycopodium women I have seen seemed to fit the term 'girl' better than woman. This cannot be simply on account of their fear or their willingness to please, since I have treated Natrum women who were equally fearful and keen to please, who seemed more like women than girls. Similarly, many Lycopodium men seem somehow boyish in comparison with their Natrum peers. I suspect this youthful impression has more to do with Lycopodium's lack of emotional depth, and tendency to avoid responsibility, although the characteristic lack of self-confidence doubtless compounds the effect.

The girlish impression of the Lycopodium woman is not only objective, but also subjective. I have heard Lycopodium women say that they do not feel fully confident of their 'womanhood', just as many of the men doubt their 'manhood'. I believe that in both cases this is a result of an inner sense of impotence. A woman's sense of womanhood is just as much a sense of personal power as a man's sense of manhood, and it is this that Lycopodium tends to lack. It is often compounded in the woman by her physique, which is often bony, flat-chested and hence rather androgynous.

Like the Lycopodium man, the woman usually has a good ability to reason analytically, (when she is not overcome by anxiety). She also has something of the mellow detachment of the male, which makes her seem far less emotionally intense than the average Natrum woman. When she is not worried, she appears light and often playful, almost like Phosphorus, though a little less brilliant. Although not without her sexual charm, the Lycopodium woman has to me a sisterly quality to her, which is light and 'pally', a good sport who likes to play, and also to chat, once she has overcome her initial shyness.

The Lycopodium mother and wife has a lot in common with her Sepia sisters. Both have a certain detachment from their loved ones, despite the fact that they worry unduly about them. This is usually healthy, in that it combines love with a relative lack of attachment, which allows the woman to retain a sense of independence and identity separate from her family (something Natrum, Staphysagria and Pulsatilla women often fail to do). This detachment is usually less than that seen in the male Lycopodium, but occasionally it can be strong enough to be a problem, when the Lycopodium woman, like some Sepia women, fails to feel much of a bond with her family (Kent: 'Indifferent to her children). In the majority of cases, however, the female Lycopodium is even more soft-hearted than her male counterpart, and loves with a gentle but steady flame in her heart.

## Physical Appearance
The classic Lycopodium physique is medium-tall and very skinny. The 'whimp' has a puny under-developed physique, and is typically stoop-shouldered. The chest is quite often sunken to some degree. Many less 'whimpish' Lycopodiums also have a small frame.

The Lycopodium face tends to be angular, in keeping with his clear rationality. The brow is frequently wrinkled, as a result of chronic anxiety, and the hair is usually dark, straight and thin. A great many Lycopodium men go bald at a young age, and this is frequently a cause of concern for them, since they tend to associate it with a lack of virility. Even Lycopodium women tend to have hair that is sparse, and falls out easily when brushed.

The wearing of beards is a characteristic adopted by a great many Lycopodium men. Especially characteristic is the 'goatee' beard, which is almost specific to Lycopodium. Moustaches are also worn more often by Lycopodium men than by any other type, and I suspect they are worn principally to produce a more masculine, virile appearance. (Just as moustaches are more common in the police forces of many countries.)

In keeping with the theme of virility, or the lack of it, a great many Lycopodium men have very little bodily hair, and ironically they often take a very long time to grow a beard or moustache.

The more puny looking Lycopodiums (who are usually 'wimps' psychologically) often have wizened features, which have been likened to dried prunes. As babies they usually look like little old men, and as they grow older their small faces and close-set eyes sometimes take on a ferret-like appearance.

There is a variant of Lycopodium who has a broad squarish face, and often a broad muscular body as well. This type is generally the most vain, and has the most tendency to womanise. He is either one of the genuinely confident Lycopodiums, or a strutter who gives an appearance of confidence.

Most Lycopodiums preserve a youthful appearance as they get older, and often look 'boyish', which is a consequence of their emotional detachment.

Lycopodium women share with the men a thin physique, and angular facial features, including the wrinkled brow. They usually have small chests, and generally have a 'girlish' appearance.

Although Lycopodiums are constitutionally thin, quite a few become obese as a result of either drinking alcohol or eating a lot of sweets. In these cases the hips and legs are characteristically thin in comparison to the enlarged abdomen.

# *Medorrhinum*

*Keynote:* The passionate adventurer

Medorrhinum is a fascinating and often missed constitutional type. The mentals are very poorly represented in the older Materia Medicas. Furthermore, the very breadth of character of Medorrhinum can lead the homeopath to mistake it for many other types. It spans extremes of temperament, from introverted to extroverted, from kind to cruel, from intellectual and detached to highly emotional and intuitive.

In order to make some sense of this variety and diversity of expression of the Medorrhinum psyche, it helps if one remembers that the Medorrhinum individual has an enormous appetite for life, and for experiences of all kinds. As a result, he may be tempted to embrace all manner of experiences, both socially acceptable and otherwise, just to see what they are like. The origin of the remedy is itself a reminder. The gonorrhoeal taint was usually acquired by indulging the appetite for exciting sensual experience. (Whilst the acquisition of gonorrhoea can superimpose a Medorrhinum state upon another constitution, the majority of Medorrhinum individuals inherited the constitution, presumably as a result of gonorrhoeal infection of forebears.)

Medorrhinums are adventurers. Some explore the physical world, fearlessly drinking in the nectar of new experiences as they travel the globe. Some explore the world of emotion, forming one intense relationship after another, often with widely differing personalities. Others explore the vast vistas of intellectual ideas, devouring philosophies as eagerly as they devour scientific theories and developments. And some take heady excursions into the realms of imagination and mystical insight. Most Medorrhinums are enthusiastic adventurers in all of these aspects of life, willing to learn from the unknown, and optimistic that they will survive its perils.

When I was travelling in California I came across Medorrhinum individuals far more often than I had done whilst practising in England. The early North American settlers spread across the continent from East to West, separating out into communities that were distinguished by their degree of adventurousness, rather like an electrophoretic strip that separates proteins according to their molecular weight, the lightest travelling the farthest. Those pioneers that made it to the West Coast were adventurers and opportunists, hungry for more of everything in life, both emotional and physical. Many of them must have been Medorrhinums, who along with idealistic

Sulphur and determined Nux Vomica sought a new life of freedom and bounty, uninhibited by the restrictions of the past.

## The Medorrhinum Child

All children are adventurers, expanding their horizons with every new experience. The Medorrhinum child is particularly adventurous, constantly seeking more information about the world around him. He is liable to reach his developmental milestones relatively early, since he is in a hurry to explore more and more of his surroundings. Almost every Medorrhinum child I have seen has been precocious in some way. Most are particularly good at verbal skills, not only in terms of vocabulary and pronunciation (I once cycled around the Nepalese capital with a gorgeous three year old Medorrhinum child on my back. She was Danish, and appeared to understand nothing of what I said. I chatted to her anyway, to be friendly and to put her at ease. As I paused at the end of a sentence, she caught me by surprise by uttering a perfectly articulated "Kathmandu!"), but also in terms of the maturity of their social interchange. I once commented to a five year old Medorrhinum boy that I was tired because I hadn't slept well, and he replied casually, "Yeah, sometimes that happens."

Medorrhinum children are amongst the most fearless of all youngsters. They are not shy, and they usually love to talk to complete strangers, providing the latter appear to be nice. Needless to say, this fearlessness causes their parents a few headaches. The Medorrhinum child is extremely inquisitive, asking a constant stream of "Whys?," and exploring the immediate environment with untiring zeal. He is likely to resent restriction, and ignore his parents strictures when it suits him. At such times he will most probably come up with some clever justification for his disobedience, or alternatively charm his way back into favour by raving excitedly about his latest discoveries. Such children are a delight for the most part, but their boundless energy, combined with the insistence of their questioning and exploring, can be a little wearing. One such three year old would constantly scream with delight as he roamed around a vegetable patch I was digging. His speech was intelligent but very loud, delivered with both enthusiasm and a determination to be heard. He was the son of a friend of mine, and I had long suspected that he was a Medorrhinum. After several days of having my ear bent by his vocal cords, I offered to treat him homeopathically, and his parents soon confirmed my suspicion. Within a few days of him taking Medorrhinum 10M he was back in the vegetable patch, but this time his voice had lost its insistent quality, and though he was still boisterous, he no longer threw tantrums when denied his demands. (Such miraculous transformations in a child's character are by no means rare as a result of homeopathic treatment, but they are often transient, and require repetition of high potencies from time to time to maintain them.)

Medorrhinum has something of a reputation for cruelty, but in my experience this is only true of the young Medorrhinum child. Very often Medorrhinum patients will confirm when asked that they enjoyed tormenting insects when they were young, or using a magnifying glass to fry them in the sun's rays. Some go as far as tormenting dogs or cats, by throwing them into the bath, or whirling them round by the tail. Generally though this cruel streak does not extend to hurting people, except perhaps when the Medorrhinum toddler punches his playmate in order to steal his toy, and it has usually disappeared before the child reaches his teens. The reason for this cruelty to animals is not clear, in view of the sensitivity of the older Medorrhinum. It is presumably a means by which the young Medorrhinum flexes his muscles, in order to gain a sense of power. By the time he reaches adolescence he generally has sufficient confidence to dispense with such methods.

Sexuality is an area in which the Medorrhinum child is especially likely to be precocious. The remedy is made from a sexually transmitted bacterium, and this is reflected in the predominance of sexuality in the lives of most Medorrhinum people. Freud revealed that children usually have a strong sexual interest, particularly between the ages of three and five, which subsides during the 'latent period' (aged six to ten), and then resurfaces at adolescence. This 'prelatent' libido is particularly strong in Medorrhinum children. It is not unusual for Medorrhinum babies to masturbate aggressively, and Medorrhinum toddlers are generally fascinated both by their own genitals and by those of other children. They are more likely than other children to engage in sexual games, which are harmless so long as the parents do not object and inject guilt into the child.

The precocity of the young Medorrhinum girl has a quality that to me is unique to the type. I have found that many Medorrhinum girls have a charm that is vivacious and sensual, even at the age of three or four. These very young Medorrhinum girls flirt with men that they like in a manner that is neither shy nor coy like Pulsatilla, nor overt like Platina, but rather in a confident, natural way, much like a mature woman who is enjoying the interchange, without being insistent or devious. Most Medorrhinum people are fortunate in the way they maintain a natural, childlike enjoyment of their senses, and of being themselves, long after most other types have lost their spontaneity. This natural enjoyment of simply being themselves is reminiscent of Phosphorus, but whereas the latter often loses his own identity in a wave of emotion or ecstasy, Medorrhinum is more 'grounded' in the body, remaining 'present' in the midst of his pleasure. In this sense Medorrhinum tends to appear more mature than Phosphorus.

At puberty the Medorrhinum adolescent develops a very powerful sex drive, which usually results in both romantic and sexual experiences at a relatively young age. The Medorrhinum teenager falls in love and in lust equally passionately, and usually together. Some find sufficiently stimulating and compatible partners early on and stay with them, but many young Medorrhinums have a long string of sexual partners before they settle down.

With the upsurge in libido comes vanity, which can be strong in the Medorrhinum teenager, who misses no opportunity to look in a mirror, or in his reflection in shop windows. This vanity can be so excessive that it exasperates parents, particularly fathers, who find their son's constant hair-combing unmanly. Medorrhinum is a very sexual type, and is usually both attracted to, and attractive to the opposite sex. Medorrhinums of both sexes appear vivacious and passionate, and tend to have no trouble attracting a partner.

### The (Wo)Man of the World

The average Medorrhinum individual is as down to earth and objective as he is passionate and adventurous. There is a detached, intellectual aspect of the Medorrhinum character that enables him to learn a great deal from his diverse experiences. The early American pioneer would have had to have learned a great deal of practical wisdom fast as he blazed a trail across the continent. If he were simply a dreamer he would as like as not end up at the bottom of a river, or dying of thirst. I have found Medorrhinum people to be accomplished 'all-rounders' more than any other type. Nux may excel at everything he does, but he does not have the emotional sensitivity of Medorrhinum, nor the intuitive and mystical insight. Sulphur likewise tends to be less sensitive, and also more obsessive than Medorrhinum. The more emotionally healthy members of the Lachesis and Ignatia tribes are usually good all-rounders, and can be hard at first to distinguish from Medorrhinum. The main difference is that the latter is equally objective and passionate, whereas the former two types are more passionate than objective. Medorrhinum wants to experience everything in life, and to understand it, and is generally well equipped to this end, intellectually, emotionally and physically.

As one would expect, Medorrhinum tends to be more reckless during adolescence, and then matures surprisingly rapidly. Like other confident types he may be a hell-raiser in his youth, plunging apparently blindly into sensual indulgence, in the form of alcohol, sex and other stimulants. Even at such times, however, he is more in control than he appears. That cool intellect is watching, a dispassionate observer of his passionate antics. One Medorrhinum man commented to me that he used to marvel as a youth at the clarity of his intellect when he was drunk. His mind would watch himself reeling about, totally lucid, and faintly amused at his uncoordinated body.

This tendency of Medorrhinum to maintain perspective despite his sensual indulgence is beautifully displayed by the character of Prince Hal in Shakespeare's Henry IV Part 1. Hal is a profligate prince who shames his father the King by spending his time revelling in the tavern with thieves and whores. And yet in the midst of this debauchery he turns to the audience and delivers a sober soliloquy, which begins with the words, "I know you all, and will awhile uphold the unyoked humour of your idleness," and ends, "I'll so offend to make offence a skill, redeeming time when men least think I will." When his country calls him, Hal suddenly turns into a brave and shrewd captain of fighting men (in Henry IV Part 2), and eventually into a sober, respected King (in Henry V). Throughout his years of revelry he had never lost sight of himself. He indulged his appetite for fun and adventure without losing either self-respect or sharpness of mind, and rapidly dropped his games when the time came for more serious endeavours.

In the consulting room the homeopath may have difficulty in identifying Medorrhinum from the mentals, simply because he is such an all-rounder. We usually rely on the relative excesses and deficiencies of character to help us identify the constitutional type, and these may be very few in Medorrhinum. It is true that Medorrhinum is sometimes given to excess, particularly sensual excess, but this hedonistic tendency is usually modified by common-sense in the Medorrhinum adult, and may only reveal itself as a love of good food, good music, and of making love.

The Medorrhinum patient is generally open and friendly in the consulting room. He usually interacts enthusiastically, but maintains a certain self-possession and objectivity - the man of the world, who has experienced a lot in life, who loves the world and life itself, but is able to take it in his stride. He will not display the unrestrained idealism or egotism of Sulphur, or the lack of personal boundaries of Phosphorus. Yet he will not hold back from personal interaction like Natrum either. In this sense he resembles the confident Lycopodium, who is both objective and friendly. However, Medorrhinum is certainly less detached from emotion, and more intuitive than Lycopodium.

Because of this broad spectrum of psychological development, there is a certain androgynous quality to Medorrhinum. The women are generally confident and intellectually objective, without surrendering any of their femininity (unlike many Natrums and Ignatias). The men are passionate and emotionally sensitive, without appearing weak or effeminate. This all-roundedness, together with Medorrhinum's high sex drive and hunger for different experiences, leads quite a few into experimenting with homosexuality, or more commonly, bisexuality. Many Medorrhinum people have had homosexual encounters in their youth, but the majority settle down into hetero-sexuality as they mature, having lost the hunger for 'different' experiences.

### Independence, Sociability and Flexibility

Medorrhinum is one of the more individualistic types, along with Argentum, Mercurius, Nux, Silica, Sulphur, and Tuberculinum. Each of these types has a strong intellect in most cases, which is likely to favour its independence, and resist adherence to 'isms'. Unlike most of the above types, Medorrhinum is not really a stubborn person. He tends to do 'his own thing,' but not wil-fully. This is probably because he is less attached to his desires than all of the above except Argentum. Medorrhinum, Mercurius, and Argentum have a truly detached quality that makes them not only independent, but also flex-ible. Lycopodium is also detached, but is not so independent or individual-istic, since he needs to please other people. Phosphorus is flexible, and also detached in some cases, but is not usually very independent, since like Ly-copodium he needs people. Only Medorrhinum, Mercurius, and Argentum tend to combine these four qualities of independence, individuality, flexibil-ity and detachment, and Medorrhinum is usually more of an all-rounder than Argentum, because the latter is usually restricted by anxiety.

Although most Medorrhinums are free-thinkers, they are seldom loners. They enjoy stimulating company too much for that. Being all-rounders, they usually have an ability to get on with all types of people (like Prince Hal, who was equally at home in Palace and tavern). One Medorrhinum friend of mine uses this ability in her work, which involves mediating between colleagues when disputes and personality clashes arise in a large company. Like her daughter, her Medorrhinum mother is also a psychologist, but applies her social skills to the counselling of difficult children, and their parents. Medorrhinum is ideally suited to be a mediator, since she can see all sides to a problem, and is emotionally sensitive enough to be tactful about her insights.

In relationships, Medorrhinum is warm, without being possessive. She likes to keep in touch with a wide range of people, and is likely to understand if her partner does the same. Despite their many positive qualities, most Medorrhinums are not very proud, and have little time for people who are. They seldom make less confident acquaintances feel uneasy. As one would expect, the Medorrhinum man is a little more self-satisfied than the woman, but this is usually subtle, and is likely to be expressed more as tongue-in-cheek self-praise than genuine boasting.

### Clairvoyance, Anxiety and 'Spaciness'

Thus far our analysis of the Medorrhinum psyche bears little resemblance to the brief sketches contained in classical Materia Medicas. This is because the latter concentrate almost exclusively on extreme negative characteristics, and hence give little idea of the whole personality. It is when we consider Medorrhinum's clairvoyant faculty, and the fears associated with it, that the classical student will be on more familiar ground.

Medorrhinum, like Phosphorus, Lachesis, Ignatia and China, is intuitive, imaginative, and prone to genuine clairvoyant insights (predictions of the future, telepathy, precognitive dreams). Any thorough understanding of the human psyche reveals that these abilities do exist, and to those who doubt it, I can only quote that master of human understanding, William Shakespeare, "There are more things in Heaven and Earth than are dreamt of in your philosophy."

The more prosaic expression of Medorrhinum's imaginative faculty is daydreaming. Some of the more lazy Medorrhinums I have treated, and also some of the unhappier ones, tended to indulge a lot in daydreams. One young man whom I treated for severe eczema was unhappy because his father was very strict and fought with his mother. He was about seventeen years old. He told me that he spent much of his time watching fantastic battles in his mind between sorcerers, dragons and warriors equipped with magic weapons. These day-dreams were entirely under his control, unlike the more scary visions of Stramonium. Others slip into a kind of fugue state, in which they feel far away from everything (Kent: 'Everything seems unreal'). This is a very commonly reported by the Medorrhinum patient, and may be his principal complaint. It is described in various ways. Some say that their head feels 'woolly,' whilst others describe it as a feeling of being separated or far away from everything, as if they are witnessing ordinary events from somewhere else, from another dimension. Yet others say they feel 'spacey,' meaning that their mind seems to be expanded. This sense of detachment and expansion is very characteristic of Medorrhinum, especially during times of stress. Similar states are described in Alumina cases, but these are generally more severe and more lasting. The Alumina patient feels as if she is not really there, rather than just witnessing the world from a distance. Cannabis Indica cases can be harder to differentiate from Medorrhinum, since they describe a very similar state of detachment and expansion. However, the mentality of a person needing Cannabis Indica is usually more generally disturbed, resembling a state of chronic intoxication and excitation, with hallucinations and delusions, such as one sees in actual cannabis poisoning.

Medorrhinum's tendency to 'space out' gives rise to a very characteristic fear, that of going insane. I have never come across a Medorrhinum person who went insane, but many have this fear. One Medorrhinum friend of mine told me that she would know when she had gone over the edge, when she picked up the milk bottles on the doorstep and then dropped them, watching the milk and glass fly. She was perfectly sane, and showed no outward sign of mental instability. She often experienced one of the more common forms of intuition, that of knowing just before a good friend would ring her on the telephone.

Associated with this fear of madness (Kent: 'Fears loss of reason') is a sense of 'wildness' in the head. This is exactly how Medorrhinum usually describes it. It is particularly likely to occur during times of stress, but may occur at any time. This sense of wildness seems somehow in keeping with the adventurous nature of the type, and also with the origins of the remedy. It is as though the mind is becoming overloaded with diverse experiences, and slips into a more expanded but chaotic realm. Such experiences are common in any constitutional type as a result of taking hallucinogenic drugs, but Medorrhinum needs no drugs to have them. Not surprisingly, Medorrhinum individuals are very sensitive to drugs and will get 'high' very quickly from both alcohol and other disinhibiting substances.

One characteristic of Medorrhinum that is pure gold diagnostically when volunteered, but virtually worthless when specifically elicited, is the feeling that someone is behind them in the dark. This feeling is extremely common amongst Medorrhinum individuals, and sometimes is so strong that it prevents them from going out alone at night. Another related sensation is the tendency to see faces in the dark which are not there. This is seldom a vivid hallucination of the kind that Stramonium or Hyoscyamus may have, but more a result of a vivid imagination misreading the shadows, in much the same way as Phosphorus might. It is the kind of experience that tends to confirm Medorrhinum's fear of madness, and hence heightens the wild feeling inside. These unusual perceptions appear to be more common in Medorrhinum women than men, as is the general level of anxiety that often accompanies them. Most Medorrhinum men are more or less fearless, like Sulphur and Nux. Many of the women, however, do suffer from some anxiety, usually of an irrational kind which is free-floating and unrelated to any real dangers. It is in this sense that Medorrhinum suffers from anticipatory anxiety. Whereas Lycopodium, Argentum and Silica will worry before a performance of some kind, Medorrhinum will feel anxious before some major life-event, such as getting married or moving house. This is not a fear of failure, but rather a sense of losing control, which may result in an irrational fear that something awful will happen (Kent: 'Frightened sensation on waking, as if something dreadful had happened'). This fear of losing control is also seen in Phosphorus, and it has the same origin in both cases, an oversensitive mind that is more open than most to what Carl Jung called 'the collective unconscious'. The latter is often symbolised by the ocean, and I have come across several Medorrhinum women who had a fear of deep water, although they could swim.

It is well known that Medorrhinum feels better after sunset. This is true not only physically, but also emotionally. More specifically, Medorrhinum switches at sunset from the rational, objective mode of being to the more spontaneous, lyrical and romantic mode. In such a state he sees the world more from the viewpoint of the poet or the artist, and is disinclined to pursue logical trains of thought (Kent: 'Aversion to mental work,' 'Exhilaration in the evening'). He may be quite happy keeping down an office-job from nine to five, so long as he can switch off in the evening and enjoy the beauty of life.

This expanded, non-rational part of Medorrhinum's experience tends to be very enjoyable (when it is not generating anxiety), and results in Medorrhinum being an optimist in most cases. This optimism is generally well-founded, since being an all-rounder with a good degree of common-sense, Medorrhinum can usually attract good times, and avoid the pitfalls of the more impressionable Phosphorus individual.

One weakness of Medorrhinum that is related to the tendency to become absent or 'spaced-out' is a tendency to forget words, particularly nouns (Kent: 'Forgetful of his own name'). Like Phosphorus, Medorrhinum lives either in the present or in the future, and this gives rise to a very peculiar forgetfulness; the inability to remember what has just been said, what he was about to say, what has just been done, or what he did yesterday. He may be able to retain all the facts he needs to sit an important examination, but be quite unable to tell you what he had for breakfast. Or he may run to the top of the stairs, and then be unable to remember what he had gone upstairs for. In this sense, Medorrhinum is sometimes scatterbrained and unfocussed. This lack of focus is usually mild, but can become extreme as a result of stress, and also from abusing drugs, and drive the patient to seek help from a homeopath. Whenever a patient appears vague, or scattered in the mind, Medorrhinum should be considered, along with Alumina, Argentum and Cannabis Indica.

Yet another Medorrhinum characteristic associated with the tendency to space-out, and with the mental 'wildness' inside, is hurriedness (Kent: 'Propensity to hurry'). The sense of being out of control mentally leads to a kind of panic, which in turns leads to hurriedness, of both thought and action. Exactly the same thing happens to some Lachesis and Alumina people. The average Medorrhinum individual may at times be in a hurry to indulge his strongest appetites, but in general it is the anxious Medorrhinum who fears insanity who hurries excessively.

### *Physical Appearance*
Medorrhinum's rounded personality is expressed in the facial features (which are not rounded, but angular). The face is broad, reflecting an open temperament, with a pear-shaped, angular outline, and a straight nose, re-

flecting a strong intellect. The lips are full and sensuous, and the eyelashes are long in both sexes, reflecting both sensitivity and sensuality. The complexion is usually dark, but may also be reddish or blonde. The body is usually well-proportioned, and relatively hairy, in both men and women. The hair is generally very thick, cascading in a mass of gentle curls.

Some Medorrhinums have a dreamy look in their eyes, which is an outward expression of the tendency to day-dream, and also the ability to feel ecstasy.

Examples of famous men who have the appearance of Medorrhinum include Freddy Mercury, the sensual lead singer of the rock group 'Queen', Tim Curry, who played the equally sensual 'Frank N. Furter' in the cult film 'The Rocky Horror Picture Show', and Mick Jagger of the 'Rolling Stones'.

The screen actress Helen Bonham Carter is a good example of a Medorrhinum woman.

I have found Medorrhinum to be equally common amongst men and women.

# Mercurius

*Keynote:* The medium

**M**ercurius is a fascinating type. It is probably harder to 'get a handle' on the Mercurius personality than on that of any other constitutional type. How do you get a handle on something so multifaceted, so changeable and so contradictory? I suggest we start by considering the curious relationship between the Mercurius personality and the image of the Roman god Mercury, and particularly his Greek predecessor, Hermes.

Mercury is the messenger of the Gods. He is fleet-footed, possessing winged sandals, and also quick witted, as can be seen by the wings on his helmet. His father is Zeus himself, the ruler of Heaven, and his mother is a lowly earth nymph who was ravished by Zeus. Thus Mercury is semi-divine, semi-earthling, and hence a perfect candidate for messenger between the Olympian gods and the mortals below. Mercurius individuals generally have one foot in the world of dreams, and the other in 'the real world'. They alternate between cold logic and surprisingly astute intuition, between pragmatism and mysticism, between austerity and sheer hedonism. This tendency of Mercurius to occillate between two extreme modes of being is highly characteristic of the type, and is unique to Mercurius. Anacardium will alternate between a normal (or a sublime) and a demonic personality, each one stable and complex. Mercurius will ossillate between the poles of any number of different qualities, including introvert/extrovert, optimist/pessimist, pragmatist/idealist, moralist/opportunist and so on.

The reason that Mercurius is able to be so flexible has to do with his inherent neutrality. He is the messenger, the medium. He has no fixed personality of his own. He merely relays whatever comes through him. This neutrality can be very confusing to Mercurius himself. At times he does not know who he is, or what he thinks. One day he is a moralist, having been inspired by the purity of a religious figure's speech, and the next day he is a sensualist, idealising the path of hedonism, having watched a film like 'Emanuel'. Mercurius' neutrality can feel like emptiness. At times there is nothing flowing through his highly receptive brain, and then he is sitting in a void. At such times he may feel very alone, as if he were sitting in a huge wasteland, or just bored, or else terrified of his own anihilation.

The inherent neutrality of Mercurius means that he is very impressionable. He picks up influences from the environment and becomes them for a while. I once treated a young woman who said that she had a 'medial personality'.

I did not know what this was, so she explained that a medial personality is so influenced by her environment that she cannot hold onto her own identity. She complained of alternating moods of depression, despair, anxiety and restlessness. The remarkable thing about these moods was how transient they were. She would enter a profound depression, but it would only last a day, before some other mood would take over. This lady appeared quite androgenous, like a youth who could be taken for either sex. Many Mercurius individuals appear androgenous, since they are so neutral.

She spoke hesitantly, because she found it very hard to describe her own mental state, which was so complex. It was acutely important to her that I understand, and she was obviously highly articulate and intelligent, and so she very slowly and very deliberately explored her own mental landscape with her words, gradually painting a strange picture of mental splitting and virtual disintegration, and the battle to hold the pieces of her mind together. It can be fascinating to have such a flexible mind, but Mercurius often pays the price of instability, and even mental disintegration. The picture of mental sharpness and depth, combined with androgenous qualities, and mental scattering, led me to the prescription of Mercurius 10M. This produced a rapid integration of my patient's experience, leading her to say that for a few days after taking the remedy she was ecstatic, since she was experiencing a degree of integration of her mind that she had not dared to hope for. Although this dramatic improvement was only temporary, it was followed by a steady increase in her sense of 'centredness' on a regular daily dose of Mercurius Vivus LM6.

The scope of the Mercurius personality is truly vast. On the one hand there are immature Mercurius youths who are extremely impressionable, flighty and unreliable, and on the other hand mature individuals who have a lot of wisdom and a lot of personal power. The former resemble young foals whose energy is intense but clumsy. I remember one such case, a youth of about eighteen years who came to see me for treatment of Attention Deficit Disorder. He was bright and exciteable, and very forthcoming. He was excited because he had just self-diagnosed himself , having read a book on ADD, and was eagerly looking forward to some relief. He gave the typical ADD history of mental scattering, with poor concentration and easy distractability, together with impulsiveness and lack of self-esteem. This in itself was enough to suggest Mercurius, but there were many confirmatory characteristics. His openess was one. Such bright and eager openess suggests Phosphorus, Mercurius and Argentum Nitricum. Although his speech was somewhat erratic, in the sense of tripping over his words on account of his impulsive enthusiasm, he said that communication was his strong point. He told me that he loved to teach others what he knew, and was good at it. I believed him in spite of his erratic delivery, because I could already see the mental brightness and curiosity that is so often characteristic of the Mercurius individual. Although Mercurius is open and impressionable like Phosphorus, he is far more mental, as opposed to emotional, than the latter. Only Argentum comes close, being another erratic but sharp mental type. Curiously, for all his impulsiveness and his contradictory extremes, Mercurius does not appear eccentric like Argentum. He is flighty and unpredictable, but his intellect is somehow so spot-on when it focusses that it gives an impression of directness rather than eccentricity, which invloves a certain skewing of perception.

My young patient said that he had few friends, because people found him opinionated. It is true that Mercurius tends to say what he thinks, and the young Mercurius in particular is liable to be cock-sure in his delivery, since he has not learned the subtleties of social interaction, and also because his genuinely acute perception can give him a sense of superiority. I gave him Mercurius Vivus 10M followed by LM6, and he soon reported an improvement in his concentration. He had got himself a job as a vacuum cleaner salesman, and he proudly explained to me the superior qualities of his product. He also looked proud when he told me that he had just won a prize for reassembling the parts of a new vacuum cleaner in record time. Mercurius is very quick. He is also very adaptable. His mind will effortlessly embrace any experience and any concept, because it has no fixed reference point. This gives him great breadth and flexibility, but also great instability. It is only the more mature Mercurius individual who manages to discipline himself sufficiently to make full use of his talents by ignoring distractions and by prioritising.

Mercurius individuals tend to be intuitive. They live on the borderline between rational intellect and intuitive insight, and often oscillate between the two. This is in itself something of a contradiction. On the one hand Mercurius discriminates, classifies and compartmentalises the world more than most other types. For example, he will make instant judgements about a person's character, and thenceforth either befriend them or shun them. He will be surprisingly black and white about his opinions and his preferences, often without a great deal of objective knowledge about them. He may sound opinionated and didactic about a point which he has never given a great deal of thought. The Mercurial mind takes snapshots of the world before it, and instantaneously classifies the contents of the picture, and then files it away. This can lead to hasty judgements and even prejudice, but having said that, the perception of the Mercurial mind is often so quick that it arrives at accurate conclusions in apparently impossibly short bites of time. (The term bite here seems appropriate, given Mercurius' affinity with computers. Like the latter, the Mercurial mind is very fast, and often eerily detached).

On the other hand, many Mercurius individuals are capable of suspending logical thought and opening up their minds to subconscious and 'superconscious' sources of information. This is often done involuntarily, when intuitive insights suddenly pop up and reveal themselves 'out of the blue'. Many Mercurius people learn to take notice of this intuitive gift. Mercurius may also deliberately seek out this connection with deeper realms of the mind. In my experience Mercurius frequently has a facility for meditation, which at face value may appear surprising, given the often scattered and incessantly busy nature of many Mercurial minds. It is true that Mercurius may be driven to distraction by excessive thinking, but it is equally true that he has a choice, and when he seeks to turn his attention inwards beyond the rational intellect, he finds it surprisingly easy to still the chatter of the every-day mental processes, and open himself to the insights of the non-rational mind. Here we see why Mercurius is so closely identified with Hermes. The latter may be a mischievous gadabout who can't keep still, but he is the apointed conduit between the world of the gods and the world of men. He is an amphibious creature, equally at home in the waters of the underworld, and on dry (rational) land. Unlike China, who may become totally immersed in inner worlds and lose touch with this world, Mercurius is generally very much here most of the time, but able to slip down into the depths (or soar to the heights) for a quick trip to never never land, to the land of dreams, or to deeper, more transcendental realms. This is what gives the Mercurial poet his depth. It can also be a kind of possession, an unwanted intrusion into the Mercurial mind of irrational or symbolic contents which he would rather avoid. The following poem by a young Mercurius poet illustrates this:

its amazing how many unconscious symbols you can find in a
kitchen
theyre alive and well
just in a comic state of unreality
i must admit
i turn off when i read the signs
i really fight them intruding into my space
Jung's gremlins
Faust's demons
roleplaying elementals from the deepest recesses
of god knows whose minds
i dont give a damn
so long as they let me do something else
cept feeding these monsters,
think ill scrub that pot one more time

(this poet prefers to write without punctuation, which presumably appears like an obstacle to the free flow of Mercurial consciousness. He also likes to arrange his words in patterns which are visually striking. This combination of verbal and visual creativity is quite commonly seen in Mercurius artists).

The poet who wrote the above poem is very young, and looks even younger. He has the typical Mercurial appearance of tall 'lanky' limbs, and elfin features. In conversation he is quirky and unpredictable, one moment profound, the next childishly silly. He told me a story which dramatically illustrates both the psychic openess of Mercurius, and its inherent neutrality, its potential to be open to either god or devil. (I have just tried to type 'good and evil', but some gremlin in the machine wrote 'god or evil', which became 'god or devil'. This is how Mercury works, tripping up our minds with meaningful plays on words). He told me that he was once sitting meditating when he felt a presence enter him. It was a very strange experience, since he was not used to being possessed. The presence felt powerful and evil. It took control of both his thoughts and his body, leaving him a helpless witness. He found this presence viewing this world with fascination, and a gleeful anticipation at the thought of using and subduing it. His body walked out of the house and viewed the street outside. He could feel the presence relishing the thought of manipulating this new world before it. Then he/they walked back into the house, and said to the poet's girlfriend 'He's not coming back'. She was alarmed, having seen the evil look in her partner's eye, but she had the presence to demand, 'But I want him back!'. Surprisingly the spirit said 'O.K.', went back to the bedroom, sat down and departed, leaving the poet back in charge of his body and mind and sitting where he had been crossed legged on the bed. Now this would have been extraordinary enough, but what followed completes the picture of mercurial possession more perfectly than if I had made it up myself. No sooner had our young poet found himself free of the malefic power, than another being entered him. This one was quite different from the first. It felt wholly good and wise. It stayed for a few minutes, and during that time taught the poet a great many things. The latter found that he was free to communicate with his new arrival mentally, and that any question he asked would be instantly answered by the spirit. The form of the answers is interesting. They appeared written on a mental screen, like that of a TV or computer. He asked what would happen if he chose such and such a course of action, and instantly the consequences appeared, consequences both immediate and distant. He then asked what would happen if he took a subtley different course of action, and a whole new set of consequences appeared. Deep philosophical questions about the nature of life were answered in an instant. There was nothing that this presence did not appear to know. It left as suddenly as it came, leaving the poet to marvel at what had happened. I am sure what he told me was true, both because I know the man, and because his girlfriend was there at the time, and she shuddered at the thought of what had happened.

I can think of no clearer illustration of the ambiguous nature of Mercurius' psychic receptivity. When the Mercurius ego is inflated, it can abuse the insights it gains, seeking personal power. This is the shadow side of Mercurius, The Magician. Stage hypnotists who make their audience do ridiculous things are liable to be this type of Mercurius. So are certain individuals who deliberately play with magic (real magic, not conjuring) to gain power over others. This type of character is portrayed beautifully clearly in the film 'Warlock', about a Medieval sorcerer who transports himself to the twentieth century in order to dig up scrolls which will give him enormous power. The warlock is very clever, extremely charming, and utterly ruthless. He is quite unperturbed by the strange setting of the world five hundred years ahead of his own time. He knows exactly how to manipulate twentieth century people to serve his own ends, and in the process leaves a trail of destruction. I find it fascinating how well Hollywood casting directors choose their actors. Actors in films these days nearly always play their own constitutional types. Naturally, this is why they are so convincing. Casting Jack Nicholson as the self-indulgent magician in the film 'The Witches of Eastwick' is a case in point. Nicholson always appears evil, and usually appears playful and mischievous as well. Indeed playful is one step from mischievous, which is one step from evil. Mercurius is generally at least two of these three. Nicholson's characters have the power of a Nux Vomica, but his power is of a different kind. It is charming, mesmerising, and utterly self-serving in most parts. Nux is more simple in his earnest, undisguised use of (predominantly physical) power. The Mercurial Nicholson is powerful in a deeper way, which is more slippery and hence more frightening. Nux is intimidating because he is ruthless. Mercurius can be frightening because he is evil (Kent:'Deep evils of the will'). Because of his relatively easy access to transpersonal realms of both power and information, Mercurius must choose between being a demon or an angel. Many are in the process of transition, and express both qualities alternately. It could be said that most people express both good and evil at different times, but the polarity is more starkly expressed in Mercurius (as is every other polarity), because of his more direct access to transpersonal inspiration.

### The Word Made Flesh

In Greek mythology the child Hermes studied with the Muses, those mysterious spirits who inspire poets and writers with original insights. Under the spell of the Muses the poet writes his best work effortlessly, because he is only a channel for the creative current flowing through him. Mercurius embodies all of the characteristics attributed to Hermes. He is messenger of the gods because he is transparent enough to be used by them as their voice. Many Mercurius individuals are gifted writers or speakers. Some can only create when the Muse is there, and the rest of the time they are barren. Others can tap into this creative current at will. (e.g. Paul McCartney, the Mercurial ex-Beatle). I am reminded of the gifted writer Russell Hoban's book 'Klienziet'. In it the hero Kleinziet gets sacked from his job as an advertising copy writer for writing a nonsensical advert, which had somehow been inserted into his brain and masqueraded as inspiration. He then goes through terrible trials in hospital as one organ after another decides to give up. However, Hoban manages to make a brilliant comedy out of this. Instead of medical terms, he uses musical and geometrical terminology. Thus his diapason becomes splayed, his pain shoots from A to B, and his asymptotes are skewed. (This is a good example of Mercurial cleverness with words. Mercurius loves a play on words. They are his element, and he is both reverent and playful with them). Whilst in hospital he converses with Hospital, Death, and even God, and none of them sound very reassuring (an example of the gods speaking to rather than through their messenger?). Eventually through the love of the ward sister he escapes from the hospital ward (where nobody has ever gotten out) and sets himself up in a plain empty room with only a typewriter and a few sheets of paper. He waits, and then all of a sudden he is overtaken by Word, who injects his seed into Klienziet. From then on Kleinziet grapples with the paper like a passionate lover-cum-adversary, forcing words onto it, enticing it with little ditties, and then ravaging it with full- blown stanzas. At the end of the book Klienziet makes friends with Death, who has the form of a huge hairy chimpanzee, and lives happily ever after. This wierd but brilliant little story is full of Mercurial images, and I have no doubt that Hoban is himself Mercurius constitutionally. First of all there is the advertising agency. Nobody writes advertising copy better than Mercurius. He is a wizard with words, manipulating them into any form, for any purpose. Mercurius is generally amoral, and this is useful in the advertising world. He is the ultimate performer when it comes to quick, catchy, clever phraseology, the quickest and most ingenious of word-smiths. Then there is the peculiar obsession he develops with a few rhyming nonsensical phrases, which not only cost him his job, but also lead him eventualy toward greater creativity. The Mercurius mind is sufficiently open and maleable to be prone to both sudden inspiration, and to maddening distraction by trivial thoughts, and not only that, but also possession by nonsensical thoughts which won't go away.

Klienziet's conversations with absolutes like Sky, Hospital and God are those of chats with equals, not grovelling deference to a god. This is reminiscent of Hermes who is himself semi-divine, and who not only serves the gods, but is also on first-name terms with them. After all, his father is Zeus himself. The Mercurius individual often displays a strange detachment from other people, and gives the sense that he is above this world. His detachment may be distinctly arrogant, but in the case of more integrated mature Mercurius individuals, it is not arrogance, but a sense of his own depth and stillness which keeps him apart. The healthy Mercurius has overcome his fascination with himself, and interacts with the world in a helpful but still detached way, like a wise observer. This deeper side of Mercurius is easily missed, for several reasons. First of all, the wiser Mercurius individual tends to be quiet until he finds a suitable outlet for his wisdom. Secondly, his immature Mercurius brothers are far more visible and noticeable, and hence get Mercurius a bad name, and thirdly, it takes wisdom on the part of a homeopath to recognise wisdom in his patients.

Even the mature Mercurius tends to have a weak connection to his body and the Earth. Mercurius is not very grounded. He tends to live in his head. This is another reason why he is so detached, and also why his mind may be taken over by impulses from beyond, be they inspirational or demonic (Kent:'Impulsive insanity'). Klienziet finds that all of his organs desert him one by one. He cannot rely on any of them. This is reminiscent of Mercurius' poor relationship to his body. Very often he ignores his body's needs, but follows his desires instead. Thus he may live off junk food, stay up late watching videos, and take no exercise. It is an effort for him to connect with his body, unless it is sufficiently fun to do so, such as when playing certain games. Because he gives his body so little thought, he will often pay the price in the end, in the form of exhaustion, recurrent or chronic infections, or deeper illnesses like heart disease.

The cleverness of Mercurius may be very banal. His mind tends to be constantly on the go, making connections between apparently disconnected items. This kind of thinking is brilliantly portrayed in Tom Stoppard's play 'Rosencrantz and Gilderstern are Dead'. The two principal characters are wise idiots, rather like the fool who is so often called upon by Shakespeare to amuse and to inform. They banter back and forth in a constant play on words which is both clever and exhausting, since it seldom leads anywhere. Rosencrantz and Gilderstern are actually characters out of Shakespeare's Hamlet. It is apt that such Mercurial fare be made out of one of the Bard's plays, since they are so steeped in Mercury's wit to begin with. Although he scripted his plays in advance, Shakespeare's 'word-fencing' sounds both spontaneous and brilliant in its pace. Here is a brief example from 'All's Well That Ends Well':

> Monsieur Parolles, you were born under a charitable star.
> Under Mars, I
> I especially think under Mars
> Why under Mars?

The wars have so kept you under, that you must needs have been
born under Mars.
When he was predominant.
When he was retrograde, I think, rather.
Why think you so?
You go so much backward when you fight.

And so on. This is an example of the Mercurial trickster's wit. People who
can perform like this without a script are often Mercurius constitutionally.
It takes great speed and mental agility to do so, since the rejoinders must
straddle two separate streams of logic simultaneously. This kind of banter
sounds crazy, but like Hamlet himself, there is method in Mercurius' madness. Indeed, he is even quick enough to make a jest of it himself. Hamlet:
'…but my uncle-father and aunt-mother are deceived…I am but mad north
north west: when the wind is southerly, I know a hawk from a handsaw.' It is
highly likely that the great Bard himself was Mercurius. For years I wondered
which constitutional type Shakespeare could have been, and then I discovered Mercurius, and everything took its place. Shakespeare was a formidable
word-smith, not only in the breadth of his characterisation, but also in the
agility of his jou de mots, and the depth of his perception. He was equally at
home in the sombre dignity of the palace, or the bawdy humour of the tavern. He had a special love of paradox, and its sister, illusion. Thus he fitted
kings out in beggars clothes, swapped twins at birth (twins are fascinating to
dual-natured Mercurius), and revealed the most pious to be rogues, whilst
the lowliest were found to be angels. His understanding of human character was awesome, and yet he remained light hearted, and somehow detached
('The world is but a stage, and we are but players upon it'). His love of symbolism and esoteric reference reveals a man who is equally at home in the
realms of rational logic and irrational wisdom, and his fondness for the fool
is reminiscent of Mercurius, a paradox himself, whose mind is so empty that
it can speak wisdom.

Like Shakespeare, a great many Mercurius people have a fascination with
the esoteric, and in particular with divination (the prediction of the future).
Several of my Mercurius patients were addicted to consulting fortune-tell-
ers, or to using tarot cards or the I Ching themselves to determine which
course of action to follow. This is hardly surprising when one remembers how
confusing life can be for poor Mercurius, who generally has a thousand
different options open to him. Pamela Tyler has written a brilliant book on
the astrological characteristics of the planet Mercury (entitled simply 'Mercury') which reveals the eery correspondance between the astrological
Mercury and the constitutional Mercurius personality. I was struck by the
following line in her book: ' Mercury is THE consumer in the occult super-
market'. Mercurius loves stimulation, and hence anything out of the ordi-

nary, and he feels an instinctual connection to matters psychic and occult, even when he has had no direct experience of them.

### *The Puer Aeternis*

Thus far we have considered Mercurius' impressionability, his flexibility, and his skill with words. We must now consider a far less likeable side of him; his childish self-indulgence, which can be summoned up by the term 'Narcissism'. The great psychologist Carl Jung coined the term Puer Aeternis, or eternal child, to describe a certain kind of person who never really grows up, and yet is generally charming, self-obsessed and often manipulative. His description is a very accurate description of the more immature Mercurius person, and even more mature members of the Mercurius tribe retain certain characteristics of the Puer (or Puella if she happens to be female).

The Puer feels that he is special, generally because his mother adores and spoils him, and thus helps to keep him emotionally infantile and dependent upon her. Many Mercurius people are so bright and mentally agile as children that they are seen as special by their parents. Furthermore, Mercurius is inherently good at manipulating people to get his own way, both through charm and less attractive methods, such as tantrums. Thus the Mercurius child is often spoilt, and the more he is spoilt, the more he will resemble the Puer. A good example of this is the late Peter Sellers. I was attracted to a biography of Sellers by a review of it in a newspaper. It said that 'Sellers could take on the personality of anyone, since he had no personality of his own'. This intrigued me, since it sounded so Mercurial, and so I read the book ('The Life and Death of Peter Sellers' by Roger Lewis) and found that Sellers was one of the clearest examples I have come across of a Mercurius Puer. Lewis started out as a great fan of Sellers, but the further he probed into his hero's personality, the darker it became. Sellers' own uncle remarked about the young Sellers, 'He was a horror, a monster of a child. We would gladly have cut his throat.' He was totally spoiled by his histrionic mother, and was allowed to do whatever he chose. He once pushed a visitor into the fire, burning her badly. He would spit into people's hats, dismember his toys, and squash the cat in a sofa-bed. If his mother left the room he would scream until she returned. This manipulative behaviour continued throughout Sellers' life. He would always get what he wanted, whatever the cost to other people.

Sellers had an uncanny ability to mimic the voice and mannerisms of another person after the briefest exposure to them. His daughter said that he had a psychic ability to understand other people, which he used in his impersonation act. Aquintainces said that he was always playing somebody else, never himself. Sellers himself said once, "I gave up looking for my personality years ago". He was only truly happy in front of the screen, doing what he did best, putting on another mask (One of Sellers' earlier biographies was entitled 'The Mask Behind the Mask'). He said that life was only worth living when he was filming. The rest of the time his life had no meaning. Sellers was extraordinarily gifted as a mercurial 'parrot', but he never succeeded in developing mature relationships with anyone. Lewis wrote of Sellers, "He was incapable of forming a secure friendship, with the give and take that demands". Instead, he used people. For example, he would pay his family no attention for weeks, and then drag them up on stage after the show so that he could be photographed as the family man. The Puer is very clever at getting what he wants. When Sellers caused the BBC major headaches by refusing to stick to the script (it cramped his spontaneity) his agent would receive letters from his employers compaining about his breach of contract. Sellers would reply himself in the following manner. He would begin by being reasonable and friendly, but unrepentant, and then he would start to complain himself about the way he was being treated, dropping in a few untruths to strengthen his case, until he was in full flow in a tirade of indignation towards his employer. He was so skillful at this, and his talents were so much in demand, that he would invariably receive a letter of apology from the very people he was abusing. This is the stuff of dictators, and the Mercurial Puer can easily become a dictator if he aquires sufficient power.

The Mercurial Puer is intolerant of any discomfort. I once treated a young teenage girl for attention deficit disorder. She was bright and quick, and almost unnerving in her detached cleverness. She was a computer wizzard, who had no problem concentrating with her computer, but at school she was restless and moody. (This is reminiscent of Mercurius, who is attracted to electronic gadgets, and gets bored with people). Her father told me that she had a very strong will, and would throw tantrums when she couldn't get her own way. He also said she had a powerful sixth sense. He described how she could will the dice to fall on particular numbers when playing games, and she confirmed this. Her sharp impersonal intellect, her distractability, her love of computers, and her psychic proficiency all put me in mind of Mercurius. When she had to have an injection she complained and made more of a fuss than a three year old, both before and afterwards. If she had a scratch it was the end of the world. This extreme sensitivity to discomfort comfirmed Mercurius, which had a stabilising effect upon her behaviour.

Homeopaths know Mercurius to be intolerant of both heat and cold. It is described in the materia medica as the 'human barometer'. Of course, the metal mercury itself is highly responsive to small changes in temperature, which is why it is used in thermometers. I have a Mercurius friend who sneezes whenever the temperature falls slightly. In the car he is constantly fiddling with the air-vents, the heater or the air conditioner to get the temperature on his body just right. When the car moves from sun to shade he will immediately adapt the air flow to raise the temperature, and will adjust it every half-minute if necessary. When he eats, this man is extraordinarily fussy. In a restaurant he will pick holes in the menu, and ask for all sorts of special modifications to the set meals, not because he has any particular food sensitivities, but because he has to have it exactly as he likes it. If the food arrives slightly too cool (i.e. at normal temperature to everyone else) he sends it straight back. He says that his stomach is very sensitive, not to any particular food, but to the balance of food it receives. Thus after bitter food he must have sweet food to balance it. If the food is not tasty enough he will add salt, and then it is too salty, so he must have a drink, and so on. (I am reminded of an hilarious restaurant scene in Steve Martin's film 'L.A. Story' where a group of trendy socialites are ordering coffee. The orders start fairly conventionally with cappocino, machiata, short white, and gradually get more and more finicky with orders such as half-caf, skinny decaf, skinny half-caf with cream, and finally, skinny decaf with cream, and a slice of lemon). For some Mercurius individuals, achieving a balance is almost impossible. Like a blob of mercury their sensitivities are so easily upset, and stability is so elusive. This applies to their moods, their body, and even their opinions. Mercurius is forever oscillating between one extreme and another. Rigid discipline is often either impossible, or actually damaging to Mercurius. Sellers dieted strictly in order to appear lithe and attractive to his prospective leading lady, Sophia Loren. He succeeded in losing several stone in weight, but the shock nearly killed him. At the end of his diet he had the first of many heart attacks. One of my Mercurius patients told me a similar story. He had always eaten too much, and was thus soft and flabby. At one time he resolved to diet and work out every other day. Although his work-out was not a severe one, he succeed in turning his spare tyre into firm muscle, but no sooner had he acheived his goal than he collapsed with a mystery illness that completely sapped his strength. After that he went back to eating too much and doing no exercise. It seems that for some Mercurius individuals, the forced imposition of structure upon their undisciplined lifestyle can be catastrophic.

The clearest popular example I can think of of the Mercurius Puer is the overgrown child Arthur, in the film of the same name, played by Dudley Moore, himself almost certainly a Mercurius. Arthur is totally dependent upon servants to look after him, and though he is lovable because he is charming, he is selfish and quite incapable of taking responsibility for himself, let alone anyone else. It is a great struggle for Arthur to overcome his self-indulgent neediness, and many Mercurius individuals go through this same struggle. When they have to resist a pretty woman when married, for example, they may have absolutely no will power at all, so they don't bother trying to resist. The same can be said for food, thrills, or whatever it is they desire (Clarke: 'Willpower lost'). Sellers chased after Sophia Loren whilst married, and then after Britt Eckland, whom he eventually married. Mercurius is totally impulsive in his whims, like a small child. He is also impulsive in his inspiration, and so like Sulphur he is tolerated and loved because he is charming and brilliant. (A good example of Mercurial brilliance is Dudley Moore's improvisation on the piano. He will start by skillfully playing a piece of heavy classical music, and very gradually will change the melody to something banal like the tune to 'Happy Birthday to You'.) He is also loved by women because he has a boyish vulnerability. Mercurius can be totally open with another about himself, especially with one of the opposite sex, and this in itself can be very attractive. It can also be overwhelming . He is apt to fall instantly in love, propose, and then fall instantly out of love once hitched. This happened to Sellers on several occasions, hence his numerous marriages. However, he must have had some self-knowledge from the start. According to Lewis' biography of Sellers, the latter proposed thus to his first wife, 'Anne, will you be my first wife?' The poor woman said 'Yes' all the same.

The Mercurius Puer is boyish (or girlish) in many ways. He tends to be cheeky, irreverent, irresponsible, and addicted to pleasure. I have seen this addictive tendency in several of my Mercurius patients. One young man (who looked even younger) came to see me to help him give up recreational drugs. He was a top hairdresser, and he loved his work, but he worked with typical Mercurious speed, and at the weekend he wanted to switch off and have a good time. So he took drugs. Lots of drugs. Mercurius tends to take things to extremes, and this man's drug intake was enormous. Despite his huge drug intake, he prided himself on not being an addict. He told himself that if his habit did not interfere with his work, he was not addicted, and it did not. However, it was taking its toll on his body and his relationships, and so he had come for help in giving up his weekend habit. Some of the words he used to describe himself made me smile, since they were so pure in their Mercurial essence. He said that when he took drugs, he didn't just lie around like a zombie. He had a lot of fun with a whole group of others, who relied on him to create 'the action'. Mercurius is forever on the move, hence my patient's indifference to passive 'spacing out'. He said he 'played the pied piper' for his friends, who willingly followed. The Pied Piper is an entirely Mercurial figure, a young man who trips lightly through the town bewitching first rats, and later children with his pipe. He performs the first act for a fee (the Puer is self-serving even in his playfulness), and when he does not get paid, he lures an entire town of children to oblivion. This is the dark side of the playful Puer. Cross him and he becomes a heartless demon. Even his attire is mercurial, being a mixture of opposites. My hairdressing patient gave international seminars on his trade, which was quite impressive given his youth. He said that as a child he used to stand on a soap box in his back garden and give impromptu speeches to an imaginary audience. In these speeches he would describe how great and successful he was. Here we see the Mercurius facility with words combined with the Puer's narcissism. I gave him Mercurius Vivus 10M and three weeks later he said that he had been a lot calmer, and had had no difficulty refraining from using drugs. He had entered a new relationship, and was determined that it would not be threatened by his previous extreme lifestyle. After a single dose of the similimum the Puer will start to grow up.

The Puer figure has a peculiar mixture of vulnerability and arrogant insensitivity. He thinks he is the best, but he needs approval. He spouts off his mouth without thinking of the consequences, yet he is profoundly hurt when someone delivers a criticism that rings true. He is liable to cling to a new love and base his world around her, until he gets used to her, and then he will take her completely for granted. The Puer is actually very insecure, since he bases his sense of security and invulnerability upon his mother's undying affection. When he is deprived of this, he expects the world to dote upon him like his mother did, and when it refuses, the Puer gets a nasty shock. The young vacuum salesman with attention deficit disorder looked sad and vulnerable when he said that he found it hard to make friends, and admitted that other people found him opinionated. He then confirmed that he was still in the Puer stage by justifying his attitude, saying that he wasn't really opinionated, it was just that other people couldn't take the truth he dished out. The Puer is constantly self-reflecting, yet all he sees is his superficial brilliance. He finds it very hard to see that he is selfish and unable to sustain intimacy. (How can you be intimate with another when you are in love with yourself?) The Mercurius Puer may feel like he has totally merged with another person, and this can be ecstatic for him, but he has really lost himself in the other. True intimacy involves remaining oneself and meeting the other.

An excellent example of the vulnerable, brilliant Mercurius Puer is the singer Michael Jackson. Jackson is one of the most contradictory and evanescent characters on the public stage. He is a Peter Pan who has never grown up. He lives in Never Never Land, complete with his own personal fairground, cinema and zoo. His appearance is extraordinarily Mercurial. Not only is it beautiful, lithe and very youthful, it actually changes from week to week. He is so obsessed with his appearance that he has molded his face into a reflection of his sister's. Moreover, in true Mercurius style, he appears half white and half black, half man and half woman, half human and half elf. On stage Jackson is electric in his agility. He mesmerises audiences with his moonwalk, appearing to walk backwards and forwards simoultaneously. With the aid of computer special effects he completes the illusion by turning into a panther before our very eyes. When Jackson appeared on television in 1994 to answer criticisms from the press, who had painted him as a freak, he did little to amend this image. He appeared as a frail and ghostly figure with a soft girl's voice, who felt misunderstood and wanted to love and be loved by everybody. He claimed that he plastered make-up on his face at all times because his face was turning white in patches. It is true that some Mercurius individuals have physical signs of their dual or multiple nature. For example, one of my Mercurius patients has pupils of completely different sizes. For all his strangeness and his reluctant isolation, Jackson is a brilliant creative performer. He may have been right when he said so innocently and earnestly that God gave him his gifts so that he could bring joy to Mankind.

## *The Fool*

As I write this chapter I cannot help marvelling at the way Mercurius embodies not one but three or more of the archetypal figures in the Tarot pack. He is the Fool, who is an aspect of the Puer, and also the Magician, the Heirophant and the Emperor. This has, no doubt, something to do with alchemy, where Mercurius was the spirit in the vessel to be transformed from one stage of refinement to a higher one, just as the Magician is said to be a 'higher octave' of the Fool. Since Mercury is also the messenger of the gods, the link between the unconscious mind and the rational mind, who was taught divination by the Muses, it seems only proper that he should feature so prominently in the Tarot deck, which is, after all, a symbolic representation of the stages the psyche goes through in its quest for wisdom. Ahem, I get carried away.

The Fool is a fascinating archetype, since it combines the contradictory aspects of idiocy, wisdom, innocence and the Trickster. It is thus a highly Mercurial figure. In the Tarot deck the Fool is pictured as a young man wandering carefree with a sack on his back, about to blithely step over a precipice, with a dog barking at his heels. It expresses the sanguine, unthinking innocence of the Mercurius Puer. One classic example of the Fool is the one who pops up in so many of Shakespeare's plays. (In 'Two Gentlemen of Verona' he is called 'Speed', a highly appropriate name for a mercurial figure. Shakespeare says of one of his fools, 'This fellow is wise enough to play the fool, and to do that craves a kind of wit. He must observe their mood on whom he jests, the quality of persons, and the time. This is a practice as full of labour as a wise man's art'.) Shakespeare's Fools are treated as idiots by the other players, and they usually 'play the fool' most of the time, yet their foolishness hides wisdom which derives from their detached, non-aligned status. It is the fool who will tell the King the truth about himself when none other dares or can see it. The Fool sees all, but says nothing, until he is asked. He then reveals his remarkably astute powers of observation, not with a proud flourish, nor with gravity, but with the lightness of an imp, or an impersonal alien. It is Mercurius' impersonality which causes him to appear foolish. He will often have nothing to say in conversation, since the talk centres around personal opinions or likes and dislikes, which he has no interest in. One of my Mercurius patients, a teenager who suffered from rhinitis, said that at school he was silent most of the time, because he knew nothing about the fashionable music that his peers raved on about, and he could not relate to the emotional and essentially childish way in which they mocked certain things and heaped adulation on others. He had no personal opinion about Mandy's flirting with Steven, and he hadn't learned the in-jokes about the teacher. In a sense, he appeared a fool because of his detachment, yet his detachment was not deliberate. He desperately wanted to make friends and was even willing to try to learn their language, but he was not good at appearing interested in things he considered trivial. He was very knowledgeable for his age about science, politics and history, but he was socially an outcast. Like the Mercurius Fool he would talk with anyone, yet they found him strange to talk to, since he did not seem like one of them. He was smarter, and yet appeared completely ignorant of the matters they considered important.

The Mercurius fool is not a proud type. He will talk to anyone. The question is, will anyone listen? Generally it is only those people who are both willing to be honest about themselves and who are able to look beyond personal preferences that will take the time to listen to the Fool. The Tarot Fool is the first of the major arcana cards. Yet he is not representaive of the first stages of human evolution, but rather the first stage of conscious development beyond 'mass-consciousness', namely that of opening to the realisation of our own ignorance. He represents a willingness to step into the unknown, unprepared and trusting to Fate, and this innocent adventurous trust is often seen in Mercurius.

The Mercurius Fool is a playful type. Some are self-indulgent Puers who need to play, and who become morose, irritable and demanding when they have to work. Others are more selfless, and these most closely resemble Shakespeare's Fool. They are mischievous and sharp, but not malicious. The young Mercurius Poet I treated was one such 'fool'. He would play the fool with relish, joking about like a child and sparring with clever word-games. Like many Mercurius individuals he projected two opposite characteristics simultaneously. He appeared very young, open and somewhat 'green' and gawky, and he often spluttered over his words like a fool, and yet his words (particularly his poetry) held profound wisdom. Frequently he played the fool socially, since it won him more approval than being profound, and left him feeling less vulnerable.

After I 'discovered' Mercurius as a constitutional type, it gradually dawned on me that the majority of stand-up comedians belong to this type. The stand-up comedian has to have a very quick wit, and especially a plastic persona that can imitate different characters. Moreover, those that write their own material need to be sharp observers of human nature. The best humour often depends upon the unmasking of behaviour and attitudes that we have all seen a million times but never really thought about. The comedian must be able to isolate these automatic attitudes in order to exploit them. This is where Mercurius' 'all seeing eye' comes in. Performers like Ben Elton, Robin Williams and Jim Carrey are highly Mercurial. They are 'motor-mouths' who can speak extraordinarily quickly in a wide variety of accents. They are generally quite ruthless in their unmasking of unconscious attitudes, yet they do so without appearing angry or malicious. Like a good courtroom attorney they will home in on an unconscious gesture without mercy, and yet without malice either. Mercurius is good at stating both profound and disturbing truths without being affected emotionally. It works well in comedy, and in the courtroom, but socially Mercurius can lose friends quickly unless he learns to soften the blow of his acute observations. Like the young vacuum salesman, he may offend others with his uncompromising observations, and then wonder why he is lonely. Nux Vomica is also highly outspoken, but there is a difference. Nux deliberately 'bursts people's balloons', and almost relishes their discomfort. Generally Mercurius is less aggressive. He says what he sees, and does not stop to think how it might hurt the receiver, or else he rationalises that it will do them good, but he does not speak out of anger in most cases. Mercurius is far more neutral and detached than Nux, though his sharp, forthright manner can remind the homeopath of the latter.

The Puer has aspects of foolishness because he does not think before he speaks or acts. He is so spontaneous that he is able to take advantage of any circumstance that Fate delivers. And since he is also very 'plastic', he is able to go with the flow and adapt, which can make him appear very lucky. On the other hand, he can get himself into all sorts of sticky situations because he does not look before he leaps. A good example is the Mercurius Puer's tendency to jump into relationships impulsively. Several of my Mercurius patients have reported this. They go for the excitement of the new liason, without stopping to think where it may lead. Sometimes it works out, other times it has disastrous results. The Mercurius fool tends to be very absent minded. One reason is that he lives entirely in the present. This means that he does not learn from past mistakes. It also means that he does not plan. For example, the wife of one of my Mercurius patients told me that when they go away for the weekend she has to plan the route, otherwise he will just guess it, and get hopelessly lost as often as not. He has supreme confidence that he can 'wing it', and often he falls flat on his face. Similarly, the Mercurius fool is liable to leave home without his keys. He just didn't think. He may be able to connect abstruse pieces of scientific or esoteric information, but he cannot remember to take his keys. This is an example of the tricky, unreliable nature of the Fool. If, through negligence, he fails to perform some entrusted task, he will use his quick wits to excuse himself. Or else his mind will be a blank, and he will give no excuse. Mercurius is apt to be empty or blank mentally some of the time (as with everything mercurial, it is a case of all or nothing). It is this very emptiness which allows him to observe so objectively, and also to be open to inner wisdom. However, it can also leave him stupified, with nothing to say. Peter Sellers' headmaster said of his former pupil, "Sellers made no impression whatever. He merged into the woodwork. He had little in common with any of us." This same Sellers made an enormous impression as an impressionist since he did not have to play himself! Mercurius can appear foolish both because he is hasty with words (Kent:' A marked feature running all through is hastiness'), and also because he says nothing at all. Peter Sellers played such a blank fool in the film 'Being There'. (There have been a series of movies made in recent years about fools, and all of them have starred actors who appear to be Mercurius constitutionally. I am thinking of 'Being There' by Peter Sellers, 'The Jerk' by Steve Martin, 'National Lampoon's Vacation' with Chevy Chase, 'Rainman' by Dustin Hoffman, 'Forrest Gump' by Tom Hanks, 'Hudsucker Proxy' with Tim Robbins and 'Dumb and Dumber' with Jim Carrey. Also Bill Murray in various films. Each of these actors has certain Mercurial features in common. They appear youthful, innocent, detached, 'bright and sparky'. Their facial features and physiques are also highly consistent with Mercurius. These Mercurius actors have been chosen to play humerous idiots because they are naturally able to portray the curious combination of mental blankness and bright spontaneity which is so often seen in Mercurius).

## The Trickster

Carl Jung used the term Trickster to describe that aspect of the unconscious mind which trips us up. It makes us fall over our words, make Freudian slips, and even lie when we expected to tell the truth. The Trickster is out to get us. He will fool us into choosing the wrong path, saying the wrong thing, buying the worst possible dress. He is the gremlin, the demon, the leprechaun, the little one who is always up to his tricks. Some Mercurius people personify the Trickster, who is yet another alter-ego of Mercury. In Greek Mythology Hermes was up to his tricks as soon as he was born. He decided to steal his brother Apollo's cattle, and so he tied large sandals backwards onto the animals' hooves, so that when he led them away, their prints appeared to travel in the opposite direction. This enabled him to evade detection. When Apollo discovered what had happened he was furious, and hauled his half-brother up before their father Zeus. Zeus admonished Hermes, but he was so amused by his son's ingenuity that he let him off lightly. The Mercurius Trickster has such 'chutzpah' that he tends to get away with his tricks. These tricks may be nothing more than playful practical jokes. Peter Sellers had a great love for them. For example, in the middle of a stage act he went into the wings, put on a fireman's uniform, came out and shouted "Fire! Fire!", which nearly cleared the auditorium. On another occasion he insisted on retake after retake of a brief television interview, which ended up taking three hours to film five minutes of interview. It happened to be April Fool's Day. The Mercurial trickster can be cunning in a self-serving, deceitful way. He can weave and manipulate in order to get exactly what he wants. Sellers in his early days pretented to be a distant relative of anyone he could find with the same surname who was rich. He actually wrote letters to each wealthy Sellers pretending to be a long lost cousin, and appealing for funds to get his career started. For once he did not succeed. Lewis wrote of Sellers, 'He had no moral sense, no judgement, and he was never sure how to behave, or he would see what he could get away with'. This line gives us a clue as to why Mercurius can behave so cunningly. He is not sure how to behave, both because he is isolated from other people, and also because he must work out quickly how to cover up his tracks. The utterly self-serving kind of Mercurius is generally slippery rather than aggressive in getting his own way. He will constantly weave and dodge to evade being found out. There is generally a deep fear in this kind of Mercurius of being caught. Sellers once said, 'I have no friends, and I suspect everybody'. He spent much of his later years living in the Dorchester hotel in London, having left his long-suffering family. At least in the hotel he need not worry about behaving decently. There he had no obligations to anyone.

Not all Mercurius individuals are as selfish as Sellers appears to have been. However, even the more 'average' Mercurius can be a little slippery when it suits him. He will tell a white lie rather than be found out, and he can be so clever with words that he almost convinces himself that it is the truth. Pamela Tyler says in her book 'Mercury', "The air con is the subtlest of them all. Here pretence hides insincerity. Another airy tactic is mental intimidation, the difficulty being that it is usually carried out with a high degree of finesse. This form of hoodwinking is the most refined and invidious of all; persuasive tongue-twisting and pedantic sophistry form the basis of the intellectual dodge. Doubletalk, whatever its purpose, is the tool of air'. She is referring to the astrological Mercury and the Air types in general. However, her remarks might just as well have been referring to the Mercurius constitution. It is indeed one of the main 'Air types' (see appendix), being a highly mental type. Mercurius can express himself so confidently, or so nonchalantly, that a lie sounds true. He may also deceive by staying silent. My Mercurius friend on several occasions met me for lunch in a restaurant, and long after ordering he pointed out in passing that he didn't have any money on him. I knew him well enough to know that he was not intending to pay me back.

One of the best popular examples of the Mercurius trickster is Jack (the Lad) Nicholson. One only has to look at those devilish eyes to know that he is up to no good. Nicholson sometimes appears sympathetic, both in real life and on screen, but much of the time he is being the subtle, self-serving trickster that we love to love and hate. Being a powerful, enigmatic Mercurius, Nicholson mesmerises his audience, and delights them so with his confident cunning and his unashamed self-love that they will him to succeed. He is the most charming of bad guys, and frequently he is half good, half bad. (Who better than this arch-trickster to play the Joker in the third Batman movie). Jack Palance is another good example of this type. His stare is at once sinister and mesmerising, although in recent years it has also become self-mocking. There are more extreme kinds of Mercurius trickster who are almost wholly bad guys. A good screen example (there are no end of screen examples of Mercurius, since he excels at portraying his own brilliant flexibility on the silver screen) is Dennis Hopper. Hopper plays mercurial madmen who are sinister because they are brilliant, evil and totally unpredictable. They have the detachment of a psychopath. Another equally mercurial example is John Malkovitch. He tends to play very clever, scheming villains who are as slippery as they are heartless. Malkovitch' eyes have an eerie detached quality that is often seen in Mercurius.

The Trickster character merges on the one end into the Fool (the innocent end), and on the other into the Magician. The latter has a subtle and profound knowledge of the workings of the unconscious, and can manipulate it at will. This is a rare type of Mercurius, who has devoted his energy to esoteric practices, and who generally has a love of power. I suspect that the great magician Aleister Crowley was Mercurius constitutionally. His love of ritual, his depth and subtlety of esoteric learning, and his amoral attitude all tend to conform to Mercurius.

The trickster can also embody Mercurius in a different form, as erratic and repetetive thoughts. The more nervous Mercurius is prone to repetetive thoughts which may be negetive, or merely nonsensical. This is the dark side of the mental focus of Mercurius. One man of about thirty years came to see me for this very problem. He was an intense man, who was very philosophical in his thinking, being drawn to esoteric thought. His eyes were dark and 'beady', and flitted nervously around the room. He said he had always been a nervous type, and when he was tense his mind would repeat strings of numbers over and over again. He was a little psychic, and could sometimes see auras around people's heads. He was tall, but his posture was very stooped, such that he had to extend his neck to look straight. His keen mind which played tricks on him put me in mind of Mercurius, which I gave in 10M potency. Within a couple of days the repetetive thoughts had almost stopped, and they remained more or less quiescent afterwards. Another Mercurius patient said that his mind would never slow down, and was prone to negative thinking when he was tired. He found he could counteract this by us-ing positive thinking such as the repetition of aphorisms. I have come across several Mercurius patients who used positive thinking like this to control obsessive thoughts. Natrum Muriaticum uses positive thinking to avoid sad-ness, whilst Mercurius uses it to avoid negative or obsessive thoughts. It is not surprising that Mercurius makes use of aphorisms to fight negative thinking. It is apt that a constitutuion that is so at home with the medium of words, and one that indulges in magical thinking (see later), should use mental phrases to banish the gremlins of obsessive negative thinking.

## *Detachment and Alienation*

Mercurius is one of the purest examples of an airy type, that is, one who functions primarily from the mind rather than the senses or the emotions. Only Lycopodium is as mental as Mercurius, and he is a very different type. Unlike Lycopodium, the Mercurius mind has tremendous plasticity and flex-ibility. However, it is the air element that gives both of these types their de-tachment. Mercurius is even more detached than Lycopodium, since he does not have to bother with the highly personal struggle for self-confidence and self-respect that occupies the minds of many Lycopodium men.

There is something very attractive about the detachment of Mercurius. It enables him to see all sides of a situation, and to remain calm and unaffected by personal emotions which would normally interfere with both perception and performance. It is all the more attractive because it is punctuated by flashes of excitement and inspiration, or by sudden laughter. Mercurius is such an enigma, being both highly detached and highly spontaneous. This may be hard to imagine, and so a few mercurial examples may help. The comedian Steve Martin is a good example. Although he can appear to ex-press any emotion readily, there is an impersonal, detached quality to him. Another good example is the enigmatic actor Kyle McLochlan, who played the philosophical detective in the cult TV series 'Twin Peaks'. His characters are ever so cool and in control, and yet they are not cold in the sense of without feeling. This is true of most Mercurius people. Mercurius has a cool, detached resting state which is empty of thought and feeling. He can usu-ally enter this state quite easily. From this neutral resting state he will react very spontaneously to his environment, both with emotion and with intel-lectual assessment. His emotions are usually short-lived, but they can be intense. Mercurius can swing dramatically in any direction, but he will quickly return in most cases to the calm resting state. There are, however, Mercurius individuals who find it hard to find this equilibrium, and who oscillate around all over the place. Generally even here the mental quality of con-sciousness is far greater than that of other unstable types like Ignatia and Phosphorus, who are more dominated by emotion than thought. The unstable Mercurius will be prone to quite a bit of emotion, but he will also be plagued by incessant thoughts which cannot be switched off.

Many people find that Mercurius' detachment is disconcerting. Imagine looking into the eyes of Jack Nicholson and you will see what I mean. One has the impression that one is being scrutinised by an unfeeling, all-seeing mind, and this is often the case. I have heard the word 'alien eyes' used to describe the gaze of my Mercurius friend. When I asked him what he felt when he stared impassively into another's eyes he said, 'Nothing. I just feel very still inside.'

Mercurius' detachment is expressed in his love of computers and other intelligent electronic machines. He seems to find a reflection of himself in these quick impersonal gadgets, especially if they can produce words or pictures, or travel fast, like radio-controlled aeroplanes. A good example of a Mercurius-like machine is Max Headroom, the half-computer, half-human commentator on television's 'The Max Headroom Show'. This is no dry mechanical Kali Carbonicum-like computer brain, but rather a quirky, street-wise and very flippant demi-human, whose manic and staccato speech re-sembles that of several Mercurius comics, particularly Robin Williams. He is likeable because he is so sharp in his observation of human absurdity, and so clever in his humour. Even his name is a play on words. He is fascinating because of his eerie computer-like impersonality.

The medium of film is a great Mercurius favourite. It allows him to sit back and enjoy a constantly changing visual feast, with meaning as well to add interest. Mercurius has a restless mind that thrives on stimulation, and is often too restless to enjoy reading. Science fiction is a particular favourite of Mercurius. Again he seems to catch a reflection of himself in the detached vision of endless possibilities portrayed in science fiction movies. I have found that Mercurius is especially fascinated by aliens. This is probably connected to his own sense of alienation. We tend to imagine that aliens would be mentally advanced and emotionally detached, and this is how Mercurius feels. Mercurius' affinity for deep space (inner or outer) is reflected in the casting of Mercurius actors in science fiction movies. Christopher Walken is a very enigmatic Mercurial figure who starred in the film adaptation of the book 'Communion', which deals with a writer's repeated visitation by aliens. Walken is himself somewhat akin to an alien. He has an eerie and intense presence which seems like it has come from another planet. (Even his name sounds like something out of a Fifties science fiction movie—The Walken!) Another example is the captain of the U.S.S. Enterprise in the Star Trek 'New Generation' series. Captain Jen-Luc Picard has the same cold steely stare as Walken. He is very cool and controlled in command of the Enterprise, and he seldom talks about private feelings, yet he has none of the emotional 'heaviness' of a Natrum Muriaticum, nor the ego of a Nux commander.

Although he is very much in command, he is flexible and will listen to his crew with concern and kindness.

The Mercurius detachment results from his lack of the earth element. He is like a mind unconnected to the ground or too his body. This can make him ignore his body and abuse it. It also accounts for the instability of his mind in many cases. It is the earth element that grounds us. Without it we tend to lack stability. I have seen Mercurius individuals who were unable to stand still, not because of restlessness or neurological damage, but because their muscles were not used to being physical at all. The effort of standing still was too much for them. Mercurius' detachment from the earth element also results in a disinterest in many cases towards the countryside. Many Mercurius people feel either bored or anxious in the country. They feel at home in the artificial stimulating atmosphere of the city, and don't know how to relax in a rural setting. In keeping with this, Mercurius often has a need for highly refined or adulterated food, and feels unsatisfied when he eats simple wholesome fayre. One can imagine a whole race of 'Mercurians' who flit about the universe in space ships, eating synthetic food, and creating any vista they like in their ship with advanced computerised projection techniques. They have no nuclear families, but rather couple at will, and their offspring are brought up in stimulating virtual reality parks back on the home planet, which is itself rather barren.

It can be lonely being a Mercurius. Few people can relate to the Mercurius individual, and he can relate to few people, hence he is often a loner. This does not suit him, since the emptiness he often feels inside can feel desolate, and he may long for companionship. One Mercurius patient said that he had a recurring nightmare of being the last human alive in landscape desolated by alien space ships. In the dream he would watch them land and try to hide from them. He was prone to feelings of paranoia from time to time. Not the paranoia of the psychotic (Veratrum, Stramonium, Belladonna, Hyoscyamus), but rather an overreaction to any social or official antagonism he experienced. The more alienated Mercurius feels, the more liable he is to feel unsafe in this world. It is the anxiety of the stranger, the one who is different. Perhaps this is why I have had the impression that Mercurius constitutions are more common amongst Jewish people, who have always been minorities around the world. The Jews are renowned for their sharp intellects, their adaptability and their aloofness, which at times borders on arrogance. These are all features characteristic of Mercurius.

Sometimes, the alienation of Mercurius gives rise to despair and a desire for death. This is seen in all syphilitic types, including Aurum and Syphilinum. The young woman whose identity was so fragile that it was easily scattered into a hundred fragment-selves would often feel such despair. She gradually brought her scattered fragments together using two highly

Mercurial techniques. One was writing. Through journalling she was able to make sense of her own psyche by analysing and describing it. The other technique was ritual (see later).

The above case introduced me to a fascinating phenomenon that I have come to realise is highly characteristic of Mercurius, the phenomenon of 'twinning'. There is a curious relationship between the Mercurius individual and the attributes of both Mercury and its astrological sign Gemini. Gemini is depicted as a pair of twins, and is said to have a 'split personality'. The Mecurius individual often has a sense that half of himself is missing. This is accompanied sometimes by a longing for a twin brother or sister, and a fascination with twins. The Mercurius woman who struggled to piece together her fractured self talked frequently of her tendency to treat other people as her twin. In fact she described how she would feel engulfed by the other, to the extent that she could not tell where she ended and the other began. The 'twin' was both a source of comfort, since he or she provided a sense of wholeness, filling in the missing parts, but also a sense of anxiety and powerlessness, since my patient felt utterly dependent if she gave into her tendency to project the twin upon the other. This young Mercurius woman actually felt convinced that she had been a twin in utero, and that her twin sibling had died before she was born, even though she had never been told this. She felt acute grief when she allowed herself to dwell on this topic. (It is a fact that the vast majority of twin conceptions become single births, with the other twin somehow dissappearing, usually in early pregnancy, so my patient's intuition is not all that far fetched). Several other Mercurius individuals have told me that they had a desire to merge wholly with someone who would be similar enough to them to enable such a deep union. In some cases they had been in relationships which had felt unfulfilling on some level even when they had been 'good' relationships, since the partner was not similar enough to them to fulfill their need of the twin. In one sense this need for a twin can be seen as an aspect of narcisism. Not that the Mercurius individual is necessarily in love with himself. He may or may not be, but he does seem to have a need to gaze at his own reflection in some way, whether it be in another person who is similar, or literally into a mirror. Several Mercurius patients have told me that they find looking into a mirror comforting, or even a neccessity for psychological stability. It is as if Mercurius needs some objective confirmation that he exists. This is in keeping with the theme of 'the medium', the messenger of the gods who has no discrete identity of his own.

In his detachment Mercurius tends to analyse everything. He is forever putting things and events and people in boxes. He becomes wise through this process, but remains cut off from others. Even on a mundane level the discrimination of Mercurius tends to separate him from other people. He tends to see himself as either above or below other people, and acts accordingly. As a result, he cannot meet them on his own level. It is ironic that a person who has the flexibility to experience so many different states of being that he can instantly recognise them in other people, is unable to connect with them. Instead he acts as a mirror. Like the Bard's Fool he can reflect other people back to themselves, but he cannot develop a relationship with them. It is only through the growth of love that Mercurius can reconnect with humanity, and some do succeed in this endeavor.

### Ritual and Magical Thinking

The attraction to ritual is one of the most unusual aspects of the Mercurius mind. I have seen it repeatedly and found that it is a characteristic aspect of Mercurius. Ritual can take many forms for Mercurius. It can be a compulsive ritualistic action, particularly seen during childhood. For example, Peter Sellers had to do everything five times when he was a child. He would knock on the door fives times, stir his tea five times and so on. Numbers often feature in Mercurius rituals (as they do in his obsessive thinking). On a more conscious level, Mercurius may seek to take part in rituals. The Mercurius poet who was once briefly possessed by two entities told me that as a child he was obsessed with taking part in the ritual of Mass as an alter boy. He would go into a trance-like state during the ritual, which according to his girlfriend was more demonic than spiritual. She had known him since childhood and had attended the same church. She told me that there was something 'sickening' about the way he looked during Mass. She said it felt as though he were sucking in energy from the ritual and empowering himself. Another Mercurius patient said that he had always been fascinated by ritual, and when he was offered the chance he went on a ceremonial magic weekend. He said he felt very much at home doing rituals of all kinds on the weekend, and strangely empowered. He did not follow up these activities afterwards, but he felt that they had been an important part of his psychological growth. The young woman who responded so well to Mercurius, who was struggling to re-establish a solid sense of self, relied heavily on ritual to reunite her disparate parts. She was very familiar with symbolism and mythology, and she used this knowledge to help structure her rituals. A simple example of one of her rituals was to make shell sculptures whenever she was faced with a new situation in her life. The sculpture would represent the meaning or essence of the situation for her. She said that it helped her to 'contain the energy of the situation' and thus feel less threatened by it. As her own attitude to the situation changed, she would either move the sculpture to a different location in her room, or else change it. This kind of ritual sounds crazy to many people, but it performed a vital function for this woman. Her own sense of self was very easily taken over by or surrendered to her environment, leaving her feeling either terrified or confused or both. She used the ritual object as a kind of mental scaffolding to contain the meaning of the situation (e.g. an encounter with a possible partner), and thus to keep some separation between herself and the situation. Mercurius has a very fluid consciousness. It seems that both conscious and automatic rituals are one way in which Mercurius holds on to some kind of psychic structure.

Closely connected to Mercurius' attraction to ritual is his penchant for magical thinking. Primitive tribes engage in magical thinking, which attributes special meaning to apparently ordinary or chance happening, and so do children. Astrology is a form of magical thinking, and one that seems to be popular with Mercurius individuals. The Mercurius individual may see the symbolic significance of the bird in his tree in the garden, (generally a significance pertaining to himself), or of the numberplate digits of his new friend's car. He is liable to interpret his dreams symbolically, and to attach significance to particular colours, and particular names. Often there is a great deal of subtlety and wisdom in this magical thinking. It is not merely a case of psychotic delusion, as more pragmatic minds might imagine. Rather, there is an ability to see the interconnectedness of inner and outer events. It is interesting to note that Hermes was the mediator between the inner world (Heaven, or the unconscious) and the mundane world. It is also pertinent to note that he was given a staff by Zeus which enabled him to interpret dreams. The magical thinking of Mercurius appears to be a real ability to recognise the inner significance of events. However, it can be taken too far. Some Mercurius individuals are so mesmerised by the symbolic connections between things and events that they find it hard to act using common sense. They may surrender their common sense to their symbolic sense, and this is not always a good idea. For example, one Mercurius patient of mine would not take any decisions without consulting the I Ching, the ancient Chinese book of divination. He was so intent upon interpreting omens that he could not function sensibly in the world. Generally, however, the magical thinking of Mercurius tends to greatly enrich his life, and to bring him wisdom rather than delusion. Indeed, many Mercurius individuals are blessed with lives which are rich with meaning to themselves, and with a strong sense of the magical flavour of life itself.

### Megalomania and Cruelty

It is not hard to imagine why Mercurius can be prone to megalomania. First of all, there is the Puer tendency to have everything ones own way. When the Puer doesn't get it, he creates havoc. When the dictator doesn't get his own way, he kills. It's only a question of degree. Secondly, there is the peculiar detachment of Mercurius. Some Mercurius individuals are so detached that they don't care about the feelings of others. Thirdly, there is the sense of being someone special, an infaltion of the ego which is accompanied by real mental agility and perceptiveness. This inflation can be fuelled in the case of Mercurius by his intuitive psychic sense. Combine the above and one can have a recipe for a person who thinks that he is invincible. Magicians who seek power through ritual could belong to this type of Mercurius. So could dictators. It is interesting to note that several of my Mercurius patients were fascinated by dictators. The nervous man who came for relief from obsessive 'numbers on the brain' had studied German. He became fascinated with the Nazis, and said he felt a psychic affinity for them, despite the fect that he was a spitualy orientated man who recognised their evil. Something about their evil deeds drew him in. Peter Sellers was apt to dress up in SS uniform and parade himself in public for a laugh (or for a sense of personal power?) He longed to play the role of Adolf Hitler, and relished playing the role of Napoleon in one of his films. Indeed Sellers behaved like a little Hitler throughout his life (Lewis: 'he had the intemperence and caprice that traditionally goes with being a king'). The more confident Mercurius can be very good at dishing out orders. The idiot played by Steve Martin in the film 'The Jerk' becomes very wealthy, and lords it over his attendants much as Sellers did. Other Mercurius individuals catch themselves behaving in this manner and soften up before it is too late. I have, however, come across a fascination with both power and cruelty in several of my Mercurius patients, none of whom appeared like unpleasant characters. Napoleon is said to have been a Mercurius constitution. He was known to have had the habit of pinching his soldiers' noses, a gesture which somehow found its way into the materia medica of Mercurius. A psychological and physical profile of the great general has been compiled from the writings of those who knew him, and repertorised. Mercurius was the leading remedy indicated.

A good contemporary example of a (probable) Mercurius would-be dictator is Vladimir Zhirinovsky, the Russian ultra-nationalist who was swept into parliament with the largest share of Russia's first democratic vote. Zhirinovsky is as charming and clever as he is erratic and dangerous. He will promise anything, and play upon the people's weaknesses, and their hankering after glory and self-respect. He is quite sane, and yet he impulsively emits ludicrous threats and promises, such as marching the Russian army to the Crimean and reclaiming Russia's former imperial lands. His vision of a Russian state from the Mediterranean (!) to the Indian Ocean is reminiscent of the kind of drive for power that Napoleon had. He has not yet gained leadership of the state of Russia, and he is already dreaming of a much wider dominion. Zhirinovsky's impulsive threats to 'nuke' Japan, and his volatile antics around the world, do not seem to have made him any less popular at home. Mercurius can be theatrical, and this is one of Zhirinovsky's greatest assets as a politician.

One may ask why Zhirinovsky and Napoleon could not belong to other dictatorial types, such as Nux Vomica, Veratrum or Stramonium. The reason is, that neither are as sensible and as sane as Nux, and yet neither are mad enough to be Veratrum or Stramonium. Another dictator who could well be Mercurius constitutionally is Saddam Hussein. There is something boyish and charming about Saddam, for all his brutality, and he is probably not insane enough to be one of the truly psychotic types. His habit of surrounding himself with Saddam look-alikes is curious, and reminiscent of Mercury's vanity, and also of its love of mimicry and illusion. Furthermore, his foray into Kuwait was quite foolish and impulsive, almost the action of a wicked child, rather than a sober practical general. Saddam's apparent indifference to the suffering he causes is quite in keeping with Mercurius, who can cleverly justify whatever action he has taken, and quickly forget any aspects he would rather not remember (Lewis on Sellers: 'By regularly emptying out his conscience, Sellers could rid himself of such human weaknesses as, say, guilt').

My mercurial friend (who has responded clearly to the remedy), said once that he would like to be the President of the United States, but only if he had real power to change things. Mercury could not abide the tedious toing and froing of democratic institutions, with the slow pace of change that they produce. He likes quick fixes, sudden sweeps of dramatic change, and constant innovation. Mercurius would make a terrible civil servant. The propensity that Mercurius has for cruelty is related to his ability to switch off from human feelings like love and remorse at will. In fact, Mercurius is so skillfully selective in his feelings that he is able to feel, say, love, but not remorse. He can allow in whatever he likes, and screen out whatever he likes as well. It is this extraordinary mental and emotional plasticity of Mercurius that led Roger Lewis to write of Peter Sellers, 'Heartless and sentimental, generous and stingy, violent and crying easily...Sellers would have worn out teams of mind-doctors'. Sellers could be whatever he wanted, and this made him a monster. The Mask figure that Jim Carrey plays is eerily half-human and half demon. Similarly, the robotic TV personality Max Headroom is fascinating because he can make jokes and particularly subtle puns and clever satire quicker and more entertainingly than any human. He sees all, including the absurdity and the hypocrisy of human beings, but he feels nothing. The Mercurius individual looks out from his bubble at an alien world, a world he feels separate from, and which he tries to manipulate, often very successfully. A two-year-old child learns to manipulate its physical environment, and then goes on to learn the human qualities of sharing, understanding and loving in human relationships. Some Mercurius individuals never really master this later stage of social development, but instead continue to try and manipulate human beings as if they were inanimate objects.

## Physical Appearance

The majority of Mercurius people are male, but both sexes appear relatively androgynous. Being a highly mental type, the face is angular, and is usually youthful in appearance. The eyes are often penetrating, and the eyebrows tend to be strong and straight. The hair is usually dark and straight, but can be any colour, and tends to be either thin or unruly. Most Mercurius people are slight in build, but some become fat through over-indulgence.

## Summary

It is not easy to summarise the diversity of Mercurius. He can be as light as Phosphorus, but far more detached and intellectually sharp. He can be as penetrating as Nux, but lacks the latter's one-pointedness. He can be as inspired as Sulphur, and also as selfish, but he is far more flexible, and he is as restless as Tuberculinum, and even more adaptable. Some Mercurius people appear childlike and innocent, like Michael Jackson and Dudley Moore. Others are often detached and withdrawn, and even paranoid, like Peter Sellers. A few Mercurius people are cruel and despotic, and many have some fascination with violence. Mercurius tends to be fascinated with himself, and hence is usually selfish, although he is quite capable of being loving and friendly as well. He is an unstable character, whose moods change as quickly as he changes his mind, a person who thrives on change, and cannot bear predictability and routine. Mercurius' ability to reflect and adapt to his environment (like a chamelion) is unique and is due to the relative absence of personal identity. His rapid changeability is accompanied by a love of illusion, and of magic and the supernatural. Mercurius can be so impersonal that he feels very lonely, and his impersonality results in a love of city life, of anonymity, and of semi-intelligent machines. Some Mercurius individuals mature sufficiently to be relatively stable, and these are the most likely to be mistaken by the homeopath for other types. An analysis of their habits, their gifts, and their previous characteristics, and a deeper investigation of their psyche, will reveal the diversity, the fluidity and the internal 'neutrality' of their personality.

# Natrum Carbonicum

*Keynote:* Natrum, but more 'earthy'

After Natrum Muriaticum, the Carbonicum is by far the most common Natrum constitution. It occurs principally in women, and is about as common as Sepia, and more common than the adult Pulsatilla. The task of differentiating between Natrum Muriaticum and Natrum Carbonicum is a frequent difficulty in homeopathic prescribing, since there is such a lot of common ground in both the physicals and the mentals.

The main impression one gets of the personality of the Carbonicum is that it is like the Muriaticum, only less so. In other words, the Carbonicum possesses many of the same traits as the Muriaticum, but in a milder form. Thus she is generally conscientious, but is less likely to be a perfectionist. She is rather private, but is able to be open with those she loves, and to express her affection. She prefers to give, but has no difficulty in receiving. This would imply that the Carbonicum is more healthy emotionally than the Muriaticum, and in general I find that this is the case, since there is less emotional suppression, and hence less need for avoidance mechanisms. However, there is one pathological trait that is generally stronger in the Carbonicum, and that is anxiety. Whereas the Muriaticum tends to be more prone to depression than anxiety, the reverse is true of the Carbonicum. Most are nervous people, who lack self-confidence (Kent: 'Timidity'), and are often mistaken for Lycopodiums, especially as the Carbonicum suffers from very similar digestive symptoms, and has a similar physique. However, the tendency to hide negative feelings, to be rather self-deprecating, and to put great store by the opinions of others, identifies the patient as a Natrum of some sort.

Natrum Carbonicum's anxiety is especially related to meeting people and socialising (Kent: 'Dread of men'). Like some of the Muriaticums, the Carbonicum tends to feel uneasy in unfamiliar company, sometimes to the point of panic. She also tends to worry about anything and everything, again like Lycopodium (Kent: 'Mood-anxious'). Anticipatory anxiety may be present, hence this can not be used to distinguish the latter. One fear that is very characteristic of Natrum Carbonicum is a fear of thunder-storms, or rather, anxiety during thunder storms. This also occurs in some Muriaticums, but not many, and not to the same degree. Most Carbonicums feel very uneasy during thunder-storms. Natrum Muriaticum may be frightened by the thunder and the lightning, but the Carbonicum individual is anxious as a result of the 'charge' in the air, an anxiety that is felt before the first clap of thunder is even heard. Also, the physical symptoms of the Carbonicum tend to be worse during and before a storm, which is not common in Muriaticums. (Natrum Muriaticum often has the curious trait of feeling angry on a windy day.)

The other mental pathology that is very common in Natrum Carbonicum is irritability. A Natrum person who is both very anxious and very irritable, but not prone to depression to any great degree, is more likely to be a Carbonicum. It is quite surprising to find that such a timid person is also very irritable. Her irritability is usually taken out upon her family, since this is the safest option (Kent: 'Quarrelsome'). Noise in particular irritates the Carbonicum (Kent: 'Sensitive to noise'), and she is generally very easily startled by sudden loud noises (Kent: 'Starts at trifles').

Since the Carbonicum is more open than the Muriaticum, and also less prone to depression, she tends to have a lighter, more natural air about her, which is quite close to the quiet naturalness of Calcarea Carbonica (and also Sepia, a remedy closely related to Natrum Carbonicum). Like Calcarea, the Carbonicum tends to be down to earth rather than imaginative or dramatic. Her personality is like a hybrid of Calcarea, Natrum and Lycopodium. She is sensible, quiet, and unlike some Natrum Muriaticums, she would never seek the limelight. Equally, she would not put herself down as much as many Muriaticums do. She tends to be a loving person, who enjoys giving, but is more able to give to herself than her more repressed cousin. However, a good many Natrum Carbonicum women become martyrs to some extent, because they find it difficult to stand up to stronger personalities. They do not feel guilt as much as Natrum Muriaticum, but timidity is more of a problem. 'Mildness' is a term which suits many Natrum Carbonicum women very well, despite their tendency to feel irritated. 'Sensible' is another. Natrum Carbonicum is generally more tense than Calcarea, and less analytical than Lycopodium. She has a 'dryness' to her personality that is quite similar to that seen in the Kalis, a reflection of her down-to-earth, unimaginative mind.

The generals and physicals are very helpful in distinguishing the Carbonicum from the Muriaticum. The Carbonicum tends to be more sensitive to heat, and also more sensitive to cold and to draughts. There is usually a marked aversion to, or aggravation from milk, which is seldom seen in the Muriaticum. (A great many Muriaticums avoid milk because it makes them more prone to mucus, which is not the same thing.) There is also often an aggravation from acids, such as vinegar and citrus fruits. Apart from the frequent complaint of post-nasal discharge, most of the Carbonicum's pathology tends to centre around the intestines and the joints, unlike most Muriaticums. Natrum Carbonicum is prone to bloating and non-specific abdominal pain, as is Natrum Muriaticum, but the latter may also suffer from the more severe inflammatory conditions of Crohn's Disease and Ulcerative Colitis, which I have not seen in the Carbonicum. One very characteristic symptom of the Carbonicum is the sensation of burning, especially on the soles of the feet, but also in the joints.

Physically, the Carbonicum has a more predictable appearance than the Muriaticum. Most are skinny and bony in physique, and this applies to the face as well as the body. The face is usually lined by numerous tiny creases, reflecting anxiety, and the complexion is nearly always freckled, although the hair is generally a medium brown, rather than red or blonde, and is generally straight.

# Natrum Muriaticum

*Keynote:* Suppression of emotional pain

Natrum Muriaticum is by far the commonest constitutional type, at least in modern industrialised societies. From my experience as a homeopath in England, North America and Australia, I would estimate that about one-third of all the people in each of these countries are Natrums. This compares with about one fifth for Lycopodium, and less than two percent for most of the other constitutional types. Natrum Muriaticum is the predominant type in modern times, a reflection of the suppressed emotional pain that is engendered by the average upbringing in today's society. So common is the type that most homeopaths mistake half of its mental characteristics as 'normal', and hence fail to spot the remedy in their patients. Furthermore, most Natrums are so good at disguising their inner pain and vulnerability that many a homeopath sees a patient as being open and well-balanced, when the latter is hiding from his emotional pain. To add to the problem, many homeopaths are Natrum Muriaticum themselves, often without realising it, and hence cannot see the remedy because it is too close. No remedy type is as often and as easily missed as Natrum Muriaticum, yet it is one of the first types to be learned, and is generally assumed to be easy to identify.

Tradition has it that Natrums are introverted people who hide their feelings, avoid company, and hate sympathy; who cannot cry and cannot show affection. This is true as far as it goes, but it is a gross over-simplification, and those homeopaths who can only recognise this 'archetypal' Natrum will miss the majority of the type.

## Origins

There were no Natrums in the Garden of Eden until Adam and Eve evoked the wrath of the Creator. From then on they were ashamed, and led difficult lives far from the gates of Paradise, where they considered themselves sinners, and longed to return home. This little allegory is very appropriate for describing the origins of the Natrum psyche, which now is the psyche of the majority of Humanity.

The emotional pain that is at the centre of Natrum's pathology originates early in childhood, when the unconditional love that the child needs is not received. The parents usually mean well, and are loving in their own way, but their love is not unconditional and freely given, since they are hiding from their own emotional pain. Sometimes the parents are openly cold and hos-

SPECTRACELL LABORATORIES
ADVANCED CLINICAL TESTING

Visit us at www.spectracell.com or call us at 800.227.5227

tile, and the children of such parents are likely to grow into the most closed and unhappy Natrums, the typical textbook version. More often the parents are simply average Natrums, who are afraid not only of showing emotions, but also of feeling them. Natrum's emotional suppression goes much deeper than an inability to express emotion. It involves a determined forgetting of painful emotions, many of which the average Natrum is no longer aware of. In deep psychotherapy these emotions resurface, to the amazement of the patient, who thought that he had had a happy childhood. It is only when these suppressed emotions resurface that they can be cried out and gotten rid of. Until then, the Natrum individual is forever sitting on a time-bomb of sadness, anger and fear, which tends to either explode sooner or later creating a 'breakdown', or trickle out as frequent or continual moodiness.

Even if the child is cuddled and treated lovingly, he can sense if his parent is actually feeling love, or fear, or anger. Babies are incredibly sensitive to the emotional atmosphere at home, and cannot be fooled. So, the average Natrum child senses that he is not receiving a free flow of unconditional or pure love (since his parent has partially closed off her heart to protect it, or is as needy of the child's love as it is of hers). This deficiency of love is felt keenly by the child, and is so painful that he soon learns to shut down his heart to some degree, to make it less sensitive. The more emotionally starved the child, the denser the protection around the heart, and the less the growing child will feel emotionally. Natrum children often refuse hugs and kisses, partly because they do not feel the implied affection, and partly because they are afraid of opening up the safely closed heart, which does not hurt quite so much so long as it is covered.

There are two common types of interaction between Natrum parents and their child. One is the type predicted by the traditional view of Natrum; the parents are relatively undemonstrative, and the child soon protects itself by becoming emotionally unresponsive or cold. Such children will grow into closed Natrums, and will actually be unaware of most of their feelings. The other type of interaction appears to be the very opposite. The parents show a great deal of love and affection, to the point of being over-concerned and smothering, and the child becomes clingy and very dependent upon the parents. Let us analyse these two scenarios in turn.

## Closed Parent, Closed Child

Closed Natrum parents are often very conscientious in providing for their children materially and educationally, but they cannot provide what the child most needs, which is unconditional love, unequivocally given. The emotional pain that the child feels cannot be stifled completely, and the result is a serious and moody child. He cannot say what he is feeling, since any show of unhappiness is greeted with horror by his parents, who are used to pretending that everything is alright. When he does complain, he is met with either incomprehension, and an assurance that everything is alright and he is just being silly, or with hostility. He soon learns to keep quiet about his feelings, which is what his parents unconsciously want. There is another reason why he keeps quiet, and that is guilt. Many Natrum children are full of guilt from a very early age, and never grow out of it. The origin of Natrum's lifelong guilt can be illustrated by the following reasoning, which occurs unconsciously (and often consciously) in the child; "I am not loved, therefore there is something wrong with me. I must be bad. It must be my fault." Deep psychotherapy reveals these conclusions at the very heart of many people, and most Natrums. It is very sad to see the number of disturbed children who are brought for a consultation, who are forever telling their parents that nobody loves them. Usually this is untrue, but the relative lack of love experienced in its earliest years is greatly exaggerated by the Natrum child. Once the child has come to this conclusion, every little criticism reinforces it, and since the parents do not feel unconditional love, there is often quite a lot of criticism. Criticism is felt by the Natrum child like a knife stabbing the heart (Kent: 'Oversensitive', 'Ailments from scorn'). In psychotherapy many Natrum patients actually experience pain in the chest when they contact this early grief, often of a stabbing nature.

Grief then is the first painful emotion that the average Natrum child has to face, and it is buried deep. When in future the grown Natrum loses someone dear to him, it feels unbearable, since it activates the most unbearable pain of all; the memory of feeling abandoned as a child.

The closed Natrum child usually does not know what is wrong, since he has buried the original pain deep inside. All he knows is that he is not entirely happy, and that he hates to talk about how he feels. His parents see a normal child, a little aloof at times, but no different from what they expected. The closed Natrum child feels a terrible sense of loneliness at times, but he does not talk about it. Later in life he will still feel it, even when he has a family of his own, and will wonder where it came from.

The closed Natrum child does not talk about how he feels, since he knows that he will not be understood—and he is right. He has not learned to cut off from his feelings entirely yet, and so he tends to seek solitude, rather than have to pretend that he is happy. He begins to develop a tough image, since he does not want to admit either to himself or to anyone else that he hurts inside. It hurts even more when he admits it. Eventually he appears immune to criticism and rejection, and may outwardly laugh it off, but inside it still wakes up the old pain.

The oldest child is often a closed Natrum. His closed Natrum parents often learn with subsequent children to be softer and more open, but with the first they are still closed. Furthermore, financial conditions are often hard in the early days, and the oldest child may see very little of his hard-working father, and even his mother is too busy to give him 'quality time'. If he is part of a large family the problems are compounded, since he has to grow up fast in order to look after his younger siblings, a task that his exhausted parents are glad to get help with. The average closed Natrum is not very sociable, and tends to have serious interests like reading, or constructing models. If he has to look after his brothers and sisters, he will not even be able to do this, and so he learns to accept a life of service. The only reward he receives is a little appreciation from his parents, and the respect and love of his younger siblings. These eventually become the most important things in his life, and when he is deprived of them, he feels utterly lost and hopeless.

The eldest Natrum child is even more likely to be closed if one parent is absent. The remaining parent usually has to struggle to make ends meet, and to cope emotionally. Such a struggling parent often relies a great deal upon the eldest child to help out, both practically and emotionally. The child is exposed to serious matters far too soon; matters that would normally be shared with the other parent, such as financial problems, and the tears of his remaining parent. In these situations the child feels he must be strong, and not complain or cry when he is upset. Not only does crying open up the heart, which has more pain stored away underneath, it also adds to the problems of the parent, who is as likely to despair as to comfort the crying child. A great many children will not cry because they do not want to upset their already suffering parent. The child learns to equate being strong with being unemotional, and in later life he will hide from his emotions, and hence be unable to form an intimate bond with another person.

### The Rebellious Child

The closed Natrum child may be polite, surly or insolent, depending upon the training and example he has received from his parents. A great many Natrum children rebel against their parents, particularly the closed ones. The rebellion may be brief and occasional, or virtually constant, depending upon the degree to which the child feels hurt, and the degree to which he is afraid to express himself. A child who has an aggressive or intimidating father may never dare to rebel, and will grow up a meek person, who cannot stand up for himself. This is especially common amongst Natrum women, who feel that they are not 'allowed' to get angry.

When the Natrum child does rebel, it can be a great shock to the parents, unless the latter are aggressive people, in which case they do not find it very unusual. The average Natrum parents, who are closed emotionally, but care about their child, and are not overtly aggressive, cannot understand what has gotten into the child (after all they have done for it). The middle-class parent who has provided materially, given sound moral teaching, and hidden her own unhappiness and worry from the child, is mystified and horrified to find the child angry with her. And yet angry he is, very, very angry.

The rebellious Natrum child is actually responding in a psychologically healthy way to the 'abuse' that he is suffering. All his life he has been deprived of the love he needs, and since both he and his parents are closed emotionally, neither understands the other. When parents have poor communication with their children, they tend to impose conditions upon them without checking to see if these conditions are appropriate for the child's temperament, and how the child feels about them. A perfect example is sending children to boarding school. Unless the home life is especially unhappy, nothing could be more threatening or more unnatural for a child than being sent to boarding school, and yet parents have no idea what it does to their children, who are already feeling unloved inside, but dare not say it. So, a child who is repeatedly treated in a manner that imposes undesired conditions upon him will eventually get angry, unless his parents are so threatening that he remains in a state of fear. Anger is the first step to overcoming fear for most Natrums, and the rebellious Natrum child is simply making a bid for his own rights and needs. He is saying "I've had enough, and I'm not going to take any more." The rebellion may be as little as being slow to obey his parents commands, or more dramatic, like running away from home, or swearing obscenities at his parents. In most cases the rebellion is simply punished, and the parents never realise that their child is naughty because he is angry, and he is angry because they have (unknowingly) abused him.

Naturally, punishment only increases the child's anger, and the result is either more violent rebellion, (Kent: 'Rage') or a stalemate in which the child avoids further punishment by bottling his anger, and withdrawing even further into himself. In this case, he will eventually explode and let it out, perhaps years later, when somebody abuses him, and even then he may get angry with his family rather than the abuser, since it is safer.

I have found in my own practice that angry children (and most are Natrums) respond very well to being listened to sympathetically. They are delighted to find an opportunity to express their grievances and their unhappiness, (providing the parents are not present), and usually the reasons for their anger become clear very quickly. One angry Natrum girl of about fourteen years said that her mother was always accusing her of being aggressive. She was very upset by this, because she didn't want to be aggressive, and only felt so with her mother. It turned out that her mother never listened to what she wanted, and put a great deal of importance upon the child's appearance, her academic performance, and her politeness. After telling me her grievances she broke down and sobbed. I tried to explain to the mother why her daughter was moody, but she did not want to know. The truth was simply too threatening. Most angry Natrum children will cry when they say why they are angry. The anger is sitting on top of a well of unhappiness.

## Indulgent Parent, Clingy Child

This second version of Natrum family dynamics is just as common as the first. It occurs when the Natrum parent is more open and more loving. The parent may still be closed towards other people, including their partner, but is open and loving towards the child. Very often the Natrum parent, particularly the mother, seeks to feel needed in order to feel loved, and for this reason the child is terribly important to her. The child becomes the focus of all her hopes, and all her love. The other parent may collude in this, or resent it. And this 'special' relationship between parent and child may include or exclude the other children in the family.

The child who receives this 'smother-love' does not get what it needs either. Smother-love is part love, part need, and this unhealthy mixture is not entirely satisfying. It is rather like giving the child vitamins mixed with caffeine, or milk from an infected breast. The child grows up feeling wanted, yet also feeling that something is wrong. What is wrong is that the mother is not relaxed; she is emotionally intense. The child is being fed with a sticky, sugary goo that is too sweet, and although it is soon addicted to this food, it is not healthy. Unconditional love produces strong healthy children. Needy love produces dependent, guilty children.

As the child grows up, it is rewarded whenever it responds positively towards its dependent parent. It learns to derive its greatest pleasure from pleasing. The other side to this coin is the subtle (and from the parent's point of view unconscious) punishment that the child receives when it is not behaving lovingly towards the parent. The child is aware on a subconscious level of the emotional tension in the relationship, a tension that derives from the mother's terrible need for love, and her subsequent terrible fear of losing the child (and hence her love). Whenever the child is not affectionate, the mother feels threatened, and this tension affects the child, who also feels threatened. Later on the child will also feel guilty, since his mother has done so much for him, and yet he is not always grateful, and causes her pain.

Since the child is not receiving quality love, and yet is totally dependent upon its parents, it often develops a terrible fear of losing them. The child already feels half abandoned, and fears total abandonment. This situation is especially mystifying to both the parents and outsiders. Here we have loving parents and an apparently healthy child, who is terrified that she is about to be orphaned. Her fears attract even more frantic cosseting from her parents, which does nothing to allay them. Later on in life, such clingy children will always be afraid of losing the one they love, and will lavish affection on them in the same way that their parents lavished it upon them. Homeopaths who expect Natrums to be unaffectionate will miss at least fifty percent of them.

The clingy Natrum child loves to look after others. She has been taught this by her dependent parent. She will play mother to her doll, to her pet dog, and to adults who are suffering or dependent in some way. Her ambition in life is 'to help others', and as she grows up she will fulfil this ambition, often to her own detriment. Just as her parents have an investment in keeping her dependent (which encourages sickness and weaknesses of all kinds), so she enjoys it when her pet is sick, and she can look after it. Of course, this enjoyment is only partial, since it is mixed with a fear of losing what she loves.

In the consulting room the clingy Natrum child is easily confused with Pulsatilla, especially if he is blonde. He will look to his mother for help whenever he is asked a question. Clingy Natrum girls still do this at sixteen years of age, and later on they will look to their husband to help them. Their indulgent parent tends to be very proud of them, and also over-protective. She will worry excessively when her child is out with someone else, and when the child finally leaves home, she will be both worried and grieving. Natrum does not let go easily, either of people or of negative emotions.

Naturally, the clingy Natrum child is very loyal to his parents. They are everything to him, just as he is everything to them. He will go to great lengths to defend them, and tends to be blind to their shortcomings. This is very soothing for the parents, but later on it can produce a lot of problems, when the clingy Natrum has a wife of his own, and still puts his parents first. Very often he will be torn between his allegiance to his own family, and his allegiance to his parents, who may now be interfering and possessive of him. True to his past form, he is still wracked with guilt at the thought of upsetting his parents, even though they are threatening his marriage.

A great many clingy Natrums put their parents before their partner, and when they have children, they become the indulgent parent, who puts the child before the partner. Only the other day a woman consulted me for a variety of complaints, the most pressing of which was her inability to let go of her son. She had long since separated from her husband, and her nineteen year old son lived with his father. She had a new love in her life, a devoted man who lived hundreds of miles away, whom she saw once a month. She wanted to move and live with this man, but she could not leave her son. She said that he needed her, since he was looking for work, and she was able to help him do this. She said that as soon as he found work, she would join her new partner. However, her son had been looking for work for months, and showed no sign of finding any. She eventually admitted that she needed him more than he needed her, and more than she needed her new partner.

It is likely that she secretly did not want her son to find work, and didn't try very hard to help in this regard. It is also quite likely that her son avoided finding work so as to keep his mother close. This kind of morass of interdependency is very common amongst Natrums. The remedy in high potency can help a great deal in allowing Natrum to let go, and face the pain that this entails.

### Control

The Natrum adult is a controlled person. The more closed he is, the more controlled he is, since it takes a great deal of self-control to avoid showing feelings, and also to avoid situations which may elicit feelings. Even the more open Natrum is somewhat controlled. Certain subjects are taboo, and people must be pleased, so as not to attract their disapproval. Natrums tend to stage-manage their lives. They like to leave nothing to chance, no loose ends, since something may go wrong, and that would be upsetting. There are several reasons for this. Firstly, they might upset other people. This makes them feel guilty, and they cannot bear this guilt. (It derives from feeling at fault as a child when they did not receive love.) Secondly, they may become emotional, which is to be avoided at all costs, since it opens up the wounds inside, and thirdly, they may be seen to be lacking or foolish, which they cannot bear, since it is a form of rejection, which revives both their sense of abandonment, and their sense of being unworthy.

Natrum is a constitution that is a direct result of civilisation. I expect there are relatively few Natrums in uncivilised Pacific Island communities, until the white man arrives. In such idyllic primitive paradises women love their children in a natural, unemotional way. They spend a great deal of time with them, without being suffocating, and they touch a great deal, especially when the child is young. The father goes out to hunt or to fish, but he does not put his work before his family. His work is for his family, and he keeps this perspective, unlike a great many civilised men, who give more and more of their energy to their job, thinking about it even when they are at home.

Once man becomes civilised, he becomes unnatural. He is expected to adhere to certain codes of behaviour, irrespective of how he is feeling, and there are severe punishments for failing to do so. He learns to suppress his feelings, and to give appearances more and more importance. He loses touch with his loved ones, and gives more and more time to winning prestige, respect and safety. He learns to lie, first to others, and then to himself, in order to fit into the constraints of his unnatural world. On a global scale Humanity has followed a similar course to the Natrum child. It has gradually lost its heart, and learned to make do with poor substitutes. Society produces Natrum characteristics, and Natrum people run society.

There are a thousand and one ways in which the Natrum individual imposes control upon himself and his life. The clearest example I can think of, of all-pervasive Natrum control, is the extraordinary lengths to which people went to in Victorian England to appear 'proper', and to hide unpleasantness under the carpet. Politeness was the highest virtue, and etiquette was an absolute must if one was to 'get on'. The relatively well off members of the 'ruling classes' around the world still put a great deal of store upon ceremony, manners, and a stiff upper lip. Such people are almost always Natrum Muriaticum constitutionally, although the social system is so institutionalised that a good many others comply, especially Kalis and Arsenicums.

Natrums impose control on themselves by not allowing themselves to express their emotions. This can make then very uptight and unnatural. They also impose control upon the other people in their life, usually without realising it. Certain subjects are not allowed to be discussed, and will be dismissed by Natrum in a variety of ways. There is the nonchalant brushing-off with a laugh, or a 'don't be silly', or a deft change of subject. Then there is the quietly insistent denial, which gets ever more insistent the more it is ignored; 'Now we know that's not the way it is, don't we?'. This may eventually give way to the veiled threat, which is usually a form of blackmail, uttered through clenched teeth, "Darling, I'm sure Mrs Huntsford-Smythe would rather know about your latest literary interest," referring to the pile of Playboy magazines that she has just found in his study. (This kind of threat is quite comical when parodied, as it is in the hit comedy series 'Fawlty Towers', in which Sybil, an extremely typical Natrum woman, terrorises her husband Basil into maintaining appearances at their guest-house.)

When one walks into the house of a highly controlled Natrum, especially a reasonably wealthy one, there is often a clinical feel to it. It is so clean, and so tidy, that it is hard to believe that anyone actually lives there. Children growing up in such environments soon get the message that they are to be seen but not heard, and are strictly brought into line if they disturb the fragile peace by making a noise or a mess. Such houses are like show-pieces, immaculate, but devoid of heart.

The tendency of Natrum people to impose control on their environment tends to make them rather conservative. Change is seen as threatening, since it does not initially feel in their control. This can be seen very clearly in the more conservative political and religious organisations, which cater predominantly to Natrum members and supporters. The British Conservative Party is a good example. Almost all of its M.P.s and ministers have been to public schools (which, for the benefit of non-British readers, means private schools), where they learned to be very rational, and keep their feelings to themselves. Their speeches are delivered in a very controlled, dignified manner for the most part, and appeal to the traditional (essentially Natrum) values of Law and Order, Morality and Stability. The etiquette of Parliament is itself a reflection of the controlled Natrum heritage of the majority of its present and former members. Members are called 'Honourable Gentlemen' by opponents who hate them, and it is an offence to accuse anyone of lying. This is very much the same setup that one finds in many Natrum families, where respect must be shown, whether it is earned or not, and everyone must support each other's half-truths. "Mustn't let the team down" is a very Natrum attitude. And the surest way to let the team down is to show your feelings. (The way in which conservative political parties stage-manage their conventions is another classic example of the Natrum need to control.)

The Church of England is commonly referred to as 'the Conservative Party at prayer'. Whilst this is a little exaggerated, it contains a lot of truth. The Church has had a tendency in the past to avoid hard truths, preferring instead to function as a provider of services which give the congregation a sense of security, and relieve them of their burden of guilt. This is a very attractive package for many Natrums, who use the Church as a surrogate parent, one who forgives them, and yet forever reminds them of their sin. The weekly outing to church on Sunday leaves Natrum feeling cleansed of the darkness within, and also gives a sense of belonging, which he craves.

(The Church of England is not the only Church which has been moulded from Natrum's hopes and fears. All Churches have been, whether Catholic, Evangelical or dourly Presbyterian.)

Having now inadvertently alienated a good proportion of my readers, I had better get on. In a society composed predominantly of Natrum Muriaticum people, there is no shortage of material!

There are many other ways in which Natrum people maintain control, and fear loss of control. They may avoid getting too close to people, since this would arouse feelings that they could not control. Independence is extremely important to many Natrums, since it brings with it a degree of control over their lives. Situations in which they place themselves at the mercy of others are particularly to be avoided. An example is the Natrum woman who will not fly in an aeroplane, or who feels afraid when someone else is driving her. Another situation that makes many Natrums feel out of control and hence threatened is the homeopathic interview. Nothing could be worse for them than being made to talk about themselves, in a situation where the homeopath is in control.

### Giving and Self-Denial

Many Natrums, especially female Natrums, are addicted to giving. Natrum is a very addictive type, since it is an emotionally needy type, and giving is one of its principal addictions. An addiction is a means of avoiding emotional (and physical) pain, and this is exactly why Natrum needs to give. The young Natrum learns to win approval by pleasing other people, and this habit is reinforced by the lack of self-worth that many Natrums feel. The strategy goes something like this; "I'm a bad person (I must be because I wasn't loved), but by giving I can be a better person, and can earn some approval and maybe even some love." Of course this strategy is largely unconscious in most cases, but in deep psychotherapy this pattern arises in almost every Natrum person, becoming fully conscious for the first time. When this happens, the patient realises that they don't have to give, they have to feel their own pain until it has all been cried away. After that has happened, they are free to act in accordance with the dictates of their heart, which sometimes prompts them to be giving, and sometimes doesn't. Most Natrums feel guilty when they don't give, because they have been taught that one must be unselfish, by other Natrums who also feel deep-down that they are bad people. One can hardly give from the fullness of one's heart when one's heart is not full. Instead many Natrums give out of duty, and a fear of being a bad person.

Selfishness is the ultimate sin for many Natrum people. Not only is it the thing they try hardest to avoid, it is also the accusation that Natrum parents use most 'successfully' to control their children.

During psychotherapy feelings of hostility often arise towards one's parents, and these are very distressing to most Natrums, since they have been taught that such feelings are selfish and are forbidden. It can take quite a while before the patient allows himself to feel such feelings, and even longer before he stops accusing himself of being selfish.

Many Natrum people justify their avoidance of their feelings by saying that they don't want to wallow in self-pity, that to do so would be selfish. They would rather be cheerful and help other people. If only it were as simple as that. Avoiding one's feelings by hiding behind a facade of cheerfulness, and a life of service, is avoiding the truth. Only by facing the truth can Natrum heal the pain within.

One can spot the more severe 'giveaholics' very easily, because they cannot say no. They are always trying to look after somebody, and being taken advantage of by others. This need to look after another has been given the term 'Codependency', and much has been written about the codependent personality, and how to grow out of it. The vast majority of codependents are Natrums, and if the remedy were given in high potency to the thousands of people who now attend codependency support groups, their recovery would be greatly hastened. (I have found that the remedy in a dose of 10M greatly facilitates my psychotherapeutic work with Natrums, opening them up emotionally so that they can face their past and deal with it.)

It is mainly the Natrum women who become addicted to giving. The expectations of society reinforce the tendency to a horrible degree. It is very hard trying to convince someone that their giving is not healthy, when the whole moral basis of society is based on the Christian ethic, and the attitude that women in particular should care for others. Emotionally healthy women do care for others quite spontaneously, but they also say no without feeling guilty, and indulge themselves without feeling selfish.

Ask a Natrum woman why she gives and she will tell you that she gives out of love. This is not true for the most part, but it is a lie which she believes. The previous example of the woman trying to help her son to find a job is a good example. At first she said she did it out of love, and she believed what she was saying. On closer examination, however, it became clear to both her and myself that she gave to her son because she needed him. In this case there is certainly love there as well, but it is not the cause of her compulsive giving. Love does not make one compulsive; need does.

As well as constantly trying to help others, Natrums tend to put themselves down, and to deny compliments. This is because deep down they don't think very much of themselves (Kent: 'Reproaches self', 'Shame'), because they were not shown enough love as a child. Even the relatively open Natrum person, who had apparently loving parents, tends to put himself down, and feel guilty when he is 'selfish'. This is because the parents were as needy as the child, and hence gave conditional love.

Natrum women in particular put themselves down in a thousand little ways. They tend to think that they have done awful things to other people, when they haven't. As a result, they are always apologising. "Aren't I terrible?", "Aren't I silly?", and "I'm sorry for being such a nuisance" are typical ways in which they put themselves down. Of course, there are always people who will reinforce this attitude. First of all there are the parents, who call the child selfish when she doesn't do what she's told, or even worse, call her useless or stupid. (A softer form is calling one's child 'silly', which if done too often has exactly the same effect as calling her 'stupid'.) Then there are the brothers, who arc allowed to be more selfish than the sisters, and who put the latter down. And finally there is the husband, who takes over the role of the parents in putting the woman down, either overtly and consciously, or by more subtle patronising and jesting. Even those Natrum women who are fortunate enough to have supportive friends and family who constantly try to reverse this self-denigration cannot be convinced that they are good people. No amount of compliments will undo the damage that was done in those early years, when the child didn't feel worthy of love. However, the power of love is very healing once Natrum is able to let it in. Many Natrums gradually acquire self-respect and self-love, partly by allowing themselves to feel the hurt inside, and partly by neutralising it with love.

Natrums are often very stoic people. They think that self-denial is good for their soul. It makes them strong and unselfish, or so they think. The mother who cooks for all and sundry, but won't sit down at the table and eat, is usually a Natrum. The social worker who gets involved in his work to the point that he gives his free time to it is usually a Natrum (social work attracts Natrums like moths to a flame). In fact, martyrs of all kinds are usually Natrum Muriaticum, irrespective of their conscious motivations. (A few martyrs are Phosphorus, Staphysagria or Natrum Carbonicum, but these are not common by comparison.)

When the emotional pathology of Natrum is severe, self-denial turns into self-destruction. The man who works eighteen hours a day, seven days a week is usually a Natrum. He doesn't feel he is worth very much, and as long as he keeps busy, and preferably productive, he can avoid the sense of wretchedness inside. Of course his self-abuse eventually kills him. The alcoholics and drug-addicts who flee from their pain are also killing themselves, as are the anorexics and the bulimics. All of these people are Natrum more often than not. The prostitute who does it to make ends meet lost her self-respect long before she took to the streets, and is now almost past caring whether she lives, or dies of AIDS. Death is not a very frightening thought for the most damaged Natrums. It is often comforting, and is hastened in a variety of ways.

The more healthy Natrum can be hard to spot in the consulting room. Many of the pathological features of Natrum will be missing or very subtle. In these cases, particularly in women, the question "Is it easier for you to give or to receive" may be helpful. Many relatively healthy Natrum women will reply that it is easier to give, and when asked how they feel when they receive they will say that they feel embarrassed, or if they are less healthy, that they feel guilty. Don't be fooled by embarrassment. It is a milder form of shame.

### Perfectionism and the Workaholic

Our society is full of perfectionists. Many are given Arsenicum by homeopaths who do not realise that Natrum is by far the commonest perfectionist. But Natrum is not listed in the books under fastidious, and homeopathic students are seldom taught this aspect of Natrum Muriaticum.

Natrum's perfectionism has a different motivation to that of Arsenicum. Arsenicum feels insecure when things are not in order, and it is this which drives him to be meticulous. Natrum, however, felt as a child that he was not good enough, and one way of countering this is to do his absolute best at everything. It does not matter that he cannot remember feeling inadequate, or that he was praised for his achievements as a child. He did not feel inadequate because his performance was poor. He felt inadequate because he was not loved enough, and hence felt he must be lacking in some way. (Other constitutional types also receive inadequate loving as children, but it seems that Natrum Muriaticum is more acutely sensitive to this lack from the start, and is more damaged by it.)

Many perfectionist Natrums have perfectionist Natrum parents, but not all. Some have quite 'laid back' parents, or even sloppy ones. It is not simply a copying of parental traits that produces the perfectionist. It is intimately tied up with a lack of self worth.

Natrum's perfectionism may be global, or only apply to certain things. Typically Natrum's own performance must be perfect, especially at school or at work. If it falls below his own high standards, Natrum is very self-critical, and sets about getting it right next time. Extreme tidiness is one aspect of Natrum's perfectionism, in both men and women. This is not surprising, because not only do Natrums tend to be perfectionists, they also tend to put great importance on appearances. Many a marriage has been strained or broken by the obsessive fastidiousness of a Natrum spouse.

The quest for the perfect appearance that occupies many a Natrum woman's time is of course fuelled and aggravated by the insane advertising industry, which implies that women with perfect looks will find the perfect mate, and live happily ever after. Unfortunately for many Natrum women their efforts to look perfect are constantly thwarted by acne, particularly in their younger days. This acne is itself an expression of the fact that the woman feels ugly inside, and is a constant reminder to her. Many Natrum women use a lot of make-up, in order to present the perfect image to the world. Women that feel they could not go out without 'their face on' are nearly always Natrums. They fear that the world will see how ugly they feel. Natrums of both sexes tend to dress immaculately, unless their self-esteem is very low, in which case they neglect their appearance. The latter occurs especially in very poor and very obese Natrums.

Natrums do not impose their high standards on others to the same extent as Arsenicum, but they do tend to do so with their family. The saddest expression of this is the Natrum parent who pushes his child to excel, and is never satisfied with anything less than perfection. The child grows up tense and unnatural, and terrified of failing to reach her usual high standard.

I always ask about perfectionism in the homeopathic interview. Most Natrums know if they are perfectionists. A great many, when asked in the interview if they are perfectionists, reply, "I try to be."

Natrum perfectionists are often workaholics as well, but the two characteristics do occur in isolation. The Natrum workaholic cannot bear to be idle, and passive pursuits like reading are seen as idle by many. Like so many other aspects of the Natrum personality, this trait is an attempt to avoid feeling their feelings. The restlessness that the workaholic feels when he is idle gives way to guilt, sadness and despair if felt for long enough, but this seldom happens. The workaholic Natrum hates holidays, unless they are very active, and dreads the thought of retirement. When he does retire he either keeps very busy with one project after another, or he falls into depression. The Natrum housewife may be just as addicted to keeping busy, and the more tense she becomes, the more furiously she works to keep the feelings at bay. Of course, many Natrums will justify their addiction to activity (especially productive activity) with all sorts of sensible and laudable explanations, but the truth is that they are avoiding their feelings.

Natrums are workaholics for two reasons. Firstly it is a way of avoiding feeling, and secondly a means of feeling 'worthwhile' in some way (i.e. avoiding the feeling of worthlessness). When Natrum cannot work, he is liable to get both irritable and depressed. This happens whenever he is sick, and also when he is unemployed. Both situations are unbearable to many Natrums. So many Natrum patients report that they hate being sick, and yet very often they attract sickness unconsciously, as a means of healing themselves emotionally. Only by feeling the suppressed feelings can Natrum be healed, and this is exactly what starts to happen, albeit reluctantly, when he is sick. I have treated a great many patients with M.E., otherwise known as post-viral syndrome, chronic fatigue syndrome, and Yuppie Flu. Almost all have been Natrum, and have responded to the remedy. This disease is peculiar in that it robs the patient of all energy, without producing any significant measurable physical pathology. It makes the Natrum individual stop virtually all activity, and yet their body remains 'whole', and the effects are entirely reversible. It is the perfect sickness to catch if you are a workaholic and need to stop and feel your feelings.

Some whole societies appear to be workaholics. I am thinking in particular of Germany and Japan, and also Switzerland. These societies are particularly suppressed emotionally, and the vast majority of their people are Natrums. They are very controlled societies, as are many of the countries of the Far East. I am sure that most of these Oriental people are Natrum Muriaticums, and my experience of treating people from the Far East supports this. The traditionally subservient position of women in these countries also supports my hypothesis. When women are taught to behave and to serve without complaint, they very often end up as Natrums, if they were not to start with. Where such chauvinism and repression is traditional, it produces a whole society of people who are constitutionally Natrum from birth.

### Positive Thinking

The traditional view of Natrum is one of pessimism and fixation upon past unhappiness. Whilst this is certainly one side of the Natrum psyche, it is not the whole story. The majority of Natrum people resort to positive thinking to help them avoid the bad feelings inside. Many take it to such an extreme that they will not admit to a single negative thought. In the past some of my patients have appeared so positive that I at first gave them Phosphorus, which did not act. On deeper inquiry I discovered that this positivity was an attempt to flee from past unhappiness, and from feelings of worthlessness. Upon giving Natrum Muriaticum these patients did very well.

Part of Natrum's positive front involves smiling a lot. Someone who smiles all the time is either insane or a Natrum Muriaticum. Women Natrums in particular put on a cheerful front. They smile when they are unhappy, and when they are happy they exaggerate it by smiling even more, and by talking effusively about how happy they are. The more brittle the smile, the greater the unhappiness underneath, and the easier it is for the homeopath to burst the bubble, and bring forth the tears. Very often the Natrum woman will chat happily about 'safe' subjects, smiling all the while. It is very characteristic of Natrum to smile at the end of sentences, irrespective of how sombre the content of those sentences are. But when the homeopath asks the woman if she is happily married, tears will appear in her eyes in many cases, and the smile will look less convincing. If he persists in looking beneath the surface the tears will become a flood, and the smile will be dispensed with.

Even more pathological is the Natrum who is always laughing (Kent: 'Laughs immoderately'). He gets a reputation for being a jovial person, who is always fun to have around. He knows that he is very unhappy, but he does not let on. One day he commits suicide, and nobody can believe it. Many Natrums laugh when they admit to serious matters which upset them (Kent: 'Laughs over serious matters'). In the initial consultation about half of my patients laugh when I ask them to describe their personality. They are all Natrums, who are embarrassed and threatened at the prospect of revealing themselves. During psychotherapy I ask these Natrums to stop laughing, which invariably produces a lot of tears.

The positive thinkers have often read 'New Age' books which encourage them to use affirmations. Some go to great lengths with these affirmations, writing them down, and putting them up on the walls of their home. Unfortunately, no amount of messages proclaiming 'I am worthy of love', 'I am attracting what I need into my life' and 'I am beautiful' will convince the Natrum psyche, which feels exactly the opposite. The person may in time believe these affirmations, but this belief is often fragile, and does not match the feelings inside very well. Affirmations are like antidepressants. They cover up the bad feelings, but do not always succeed in getting rid of them. Eventually they have to be felt, in order to be released, and when the Natrum person realises this, she drops both the affirmations and the antidepressants, and allows herself to cry.

The Natrum positive thinker will often become quite evangelical in her desire to dispel gloom and despondency. She (they are usually female) becomes preachy, in an attempt to convert others to her system of positive thinking. It is not enough that she is thinking positively. You must think positively as well. Such women are usually addicted to giving, and to looking after other people, and in positive thinking they think that they have found a pearl that they can share with the world. Like all zealots, their in-

tensity is a sign of their insecurity, and they can feel quite shaken when someone challenges their preaching. At such times, they often fall back upon a
kind of spiritual arrogance, saying such things as, "It's only because you hurt
that you are saying that," or "Let the good in like I have. Love yourself and
you will be amazed at what a wonderful human being you are." Naturally,
religion lends itself as a vehicle of such evangelism, and the vast majority of
preachy believers are Natrums, especially those who have been born again.
Professional do-gooders of a moralistic kind are also nearly always Natrum
individuals. Examples include the British campaigner for moral decency, Mrs
Mary Whitehouse, and the 'Right to Lifers' who campaign to put an end to
abortion and mercy killings.

Natrums love to believe in something, especially female Natrums (the men
are often more cynical). Given the amount of pain inside, hope is very precious to a good many Natrums. Witness for example, the Negro spiritual.
These terribly sad songs grew out of decades of suffering, which could not
be expressed or resisted without danger. The negro spiritual is as full of hope
as it is of sadness, hope for tomorrow, and especially, hope of returning home
to the Heavenly Father. Oppression produces Natrum people, and Natrums,
unlike Aurum, will not give up hope.

Another variant of the positive thinker, is the Natrum who becomes fascinated with the psychic world. This is really a vicarious route to exploring the
depths of her own psyche. It has the advantage of being glamorous, and of
promising a great deal for the future, and it is not as threatening as facing
her own pain directly. The old style involved seances, in which the concerned
Natrum could be assured of a more beautiful life in the hereafter, and could
hear something positive about those she had lost. It also involved psychics
and Tarot readers, who nearly always speak more of the positive than the
negative (and are nearly always Natrums themselves). The 'New Age' has
added the channeller, who speaks directly with the voice of an ascended
master, and puts the client in touch with her spirit guides. (I once had the
honour of having one of my guides speak to me, through the services of a
Natrum acquaintance who was a channeller. The guide told me that his name
was Dempsey. At this I struggled to keep a straight face, not wishing to offend my acquaintance, and waited for Makepeace to speak up.)

'New Age' Natrums have a habit of calling their children names like Spirit
and Sky. I once spent a few weeks at a 'New Age' centre in California, as part
of a working holiday. It was here that I really became acquainted with what
I call the 'Sweetness and Light Brigade'. Unlike other centres I have visited
which focused upon the real feelings inside of the participants, and hence
promoted psychological health, this centre was a haven of denial. The therapists were all Natrum Muriaticums who were hiding from themselves by trying to heal others. They used a variety of techniques, many of which involved

ceremony, and also visualisation. The latter is a favourite tool of the 'New Age' Natrum. It enables the client to imagine a beautiful outcome to his problems, (and may also increase the likelihood of this outcome), but it does little to eradicate the suppressed pain at their root.

### The Rebel

As a contrast to all this talk about being positive, let us consider the Natrum rebel, who is very angry. He doesn't want to hear that he is a beautiful person. He would rather bash somebody's head in. It would feel more therapeutic.

Some Natrums begin their rebellion during childhood. Others are grown up before they overcome their fear sufficiently to feel their anger. A good example of the young Natrum rebel is the difficult boy who is always starting fights, defying his teachers, and swearing at his parents. Such children have usually been quite obviously starved of love, and are often the victims of parental abuse. They pride themselves on their ability to withstand the strap without flinching, and their favourite word (apart from a couple of unprintable ones) is 'hate'. Such children are very uncomfortable when the talk comes round to family, love and intimacy. They like to pretend that they don't hurt, and to do this they jeer at such talk. Some rebels who are not so deeply wounded will talk about their pain if they think you will understand, and may even cry in doing so.

Unfortunately, the future is not very rosy for the hardened Natrum delinquent. He is likely to attract greater and greater punishment, eventually ending up in remand centres, and then gaol. Such children do soften on receiving the remedy in high potency, but they need a lot of caring support if this change is to be more than a brief thawing.

The Natrum rebel suffers from a kind of paranoia. He is always looking for insults and ulterior motives, and finds it very hard to trust. This is hardly surprising in view of the difficult life he has led. Rather than give you the benefit of the doubt, he will start a fight if he thinks you may have insulted him. This kind of 'attitude problem' is very common in New York, especially in the rougher parts like the Bronx. (New York cab drivers are notorious for their rudeness, and I am sure that the majority are Natrums.) The Natrum rebel is hurting inside, and can still be reached by a consistent caring approach, providing he is not offered sympathy, which he cannot bear.

Adult Natrum rebels often focus all of their anger upon a particular section of society. So for that matter do young Natrum rebels who become Punks and skin-heads (the former rebelling against the middle-classes, the latter against foreigners and Jews). This is really a projection of anger that is felt towards the parents, who hurt the child more than they can imagine. Feminists are usually Natrum rebels (though some are Sepia and Ignatia). Having received a hard deal from their fathers, (and often from other men who sexually abused them) they proceed to systematically attack him through every man they come across (Kent: 'Hatred of persons who have offended'). They are unable to see the goodness in a nice man when they come across it, so soured are they by the past. Many become lesbians in an attempt to seek safe sexual and emotional contact. When such feminists enter into deep psychotherapy they eventually locate the source of their rage, which is usually their father, or some other man who abused them. Once the original abuse has been relived (it has often been forgotten many years previously), and the rage has been expressed towards the man who engendered it (in therapy rather than in real life), the anger can be dispersed once and for all, and is no longer projected upon men in general.

Some rebels make use of their anger professionally. A great many sportsmen fit into this category, especially boxers, who have often had tough childhoods. Policemen and soldiers are also often Natrum rebels, which is unfortunate, since they are liable to take their anger out on innocent victims. The brutality with which soldiers and policemen sometimes beat their charges is evidence of the hatred that exists inside the Natrum rebel (Kent: 'Violence', 'Malicious'), a hatred that grows out of a childhood deprived of love.

The Natrum rebel exists in some form in a great many Natrum people, who nurse their grievances for years, and are angry much of the time (Kent: 'Discontented with everything'). Sometimes the angry Natrum knows that he is projecting his anger on innocent scapegoats, (such as his family) but cannot help himself. At other times he is totally blind to the projection. The more hurt the angry Natrum is, the more dangerous is his anger. It is all the more dangerous because it is bottled up most of the time. The longer it is bottled, the more violently Natrum's anger explodes. Many a case of wife bashing and impulsive murder could have been prevented by a dose or two of Natrum Muriaticum 10M.

One subtle version of the Natrum rebel is the cynic. A great many Natrum people become cynical, and in particular, about half of Natrum men are cynical to a significant degree. Cynicism is actually a form of aggression. It sees only the negative in a situation. It is a form of protection that Natrum people in particular use to help keep their heart sealed. When one's heart is open, one feels either love or hurt. The cynic retreats from his heart to his head, where he proceeds to demolish all that is beautiful, since if he were to allow in its beauty, his heart would be opened, and his hurt would be felt. Other highly rational types may also become cynics, particularly Nux Vomica and Kali Carbonicum, but also Sulphur, Ignatia and Tuberculinum. However, Natrum is not only far more numerous than these other types, but also more liable to be cynical, because he is more open to being hurt.

## *Morality and Sexuality*

Most Natrums have rather high morals, compared to opportunists like Lycopodium and Nux. They feel that they have let themselves down when their behaviour falls below their own high standards. Consequently, one can usually trust a Natrum's promise. Even tough Natrum rebels keep their word more than one would expect, which is presumably the origin of the criminal's 'code of honour', which states that it's O.K. to lie to the police, but not to one's fellow criminals. The tendency of Natrums to stick together and support the team, which originates as a protective mechanism, is thus one reason behind Natrum's morality. Another is that Natrum has suffered, and thus can empathise with the suffering of others. Most Natrums are very sensitive emotionally, and feel for other people a great deal (Kent: 'Sympathetic'). A third factor which promotes morality is the sense of guilt that lies within the subconscious of most Natrum individuals, a guilt that is entirely undeserved. The moral codes of society give Natrum a framework by which he can do the right thing and avoid reactivating his guilt.

Morality is a strange animal; part noble and part motivated by fear. The more fearful Natrum is, the more rigid is his morality likely to be. Thus the guilt-ridden, acquiescent Natrum woman couldn't possibly be impolite to anybody, whereas the more healthy Natrum has a far more flexible code of ethics, and is less worried about what other people think. Natrum's code of ethics is reassuring to her, in a world so full of uncertainty. She feels steadied and vindicated when others share her principles, and especially when they win a moral victory. This attitude is taken to extremes by some Natrums, such as the militant anti-abortionists and animal liberationists, who feel that they must impose their morality upon other people.

Given the stabilising influence of Natrum's moral code, it can be very threatening for a Natrum to have to question her ethics. For example, if she has derived her moral principles from a particular religious organisation, and then discovers that her religious elders are corrupt, the effect can be shattering. A similar but more fundamental shock sometimes occurs during psychotherapy, when Natrum realises that many of her high principles have been based on a reaction to her own fear and guilt. Such realisations, although distressing, bring with them relief, since they allow Natrum to 'loosen up' a little, and reject those values that come from weakness. Her remaining values are then based on love and practicalities, and are generally both more flexible and more individual than before.

Rigid moralists are usually Natrums (although they may also be Arsenicum), who seek absolution from their own guilt without realising it. The more rigid they are, the more out of touch they become with other people, and also with their own feelings. They usually adopt religious codes to justify their principles, but there is nothing spiritual about their morality, based as it is not on love, but on an absence of love. Good examples of this are the Pharisees in the New Testament, who object to Jesus working on the Sabbath, and mixing with prostitutes and other sinners.

Sexual morality tends to arouse the strongest feelings of all, particularly amongst Natrum people. Since there are so many diverse types within the Natrum constitution there are many attitudes to sexuality, but one or two are more common than the others. Natrum men tend to be far more suppressed emotionally than the women, and hence less sensitive. As a result, their sexual morality tends to be looser and more variable. Some see nothing wrong with being promiscuous (although they may not accept this behaviour from their girlfriend), and will in fact seek sex rather than love because their heart no longer knows how to feel. Others avoid loving relationships because they know that they couldn't bear the pain involved, as many Natrum women do. Some have close, loving relationships, and are able to be loving during sex (by which I mean 'feel love', not just be gentle), whilst others choose monogamy because it is safer, and some are morally against promiscuity and sex before marriage. In general, the most highly sexed Natrum men are the most repressed emotionally. They use sex as a means of releasing emotional tension, and as a substitute pleasure for love.

When we come to Natrum women we find their sexual morality tends to be stricter and more consistent. This is not surprising, in view of social expectations, and also the fact that Natrum women are far more vulnerable emotionally than the men.

Most Natrum women want sex to be loving, and will not enjoy casual sex. It makes them feel cheap more than any other type, since they already have a sense of guilt and lack of self-worth inside, which is only aggravated (or made conscious) by loveless coupling. It is in part this tendency to feel shame very easily (Kent: 'Emotion—shame') that results in most Natrum women having high sexual morals. Of course, there are less pathological reasons as well in the relatively healthy Natrum woman, who respects herself too much to debase herself with animalistic sex, and who simply does not feel physically attracted to a man until she loves him.

Many Natrum women are quite prudish about sexuality, especially those of 'the older generation', who are often appalled by the lack of modesty they see in younger women. I am inclined to think that their attitude is in part pathological, a reflection of the shame they associate with nudity and sexuality, but also in part a healthy reaction to the sexual obsession that has infected the whole of society, and makes young women dress up like vamps to hook lusty men. Love has come under a terrible assault in our society by sexual obsession. When the word is used in the media it means sex most of the time, and many young people are confusing the two. The more emotionally healthy individuals of all constitutional types are able to recognise the damage that this global sexual obsession is doing, and tend to feel repulsion at the grosser forms of sexual flaunting, both in the media and in casual conversation. Since Natrum women are emotionally sensitive, a great many deplore being seen as sexual objects. Unfortunately just as many 'buy into the system', seeking to arouse men in order to 'win' their approval, and hopefully their love. Eventually they find that sex does not lead to love in most cases, and they feel cheated and abandoned.

It is such a normal thing for women today to try to win men's love by making themselves look seductive, that it is done by women of all constitutional types, but Natrums have a particularly strong need to feel loved, and hence are more likely than most types to seduce. Some Natrum women take this to extremes, trying to hook men with sex, and settling for just sex if they can't find a man who loves them. The majority of vamps are Natrums (but then the majority of people are Natrums too). They have always been deprived of love in their childhood (more so than the average Natrum) and use sex as an easy substitute. Naturally, it is not very satisfying, and leads to an increasing sense of worthlessness inside. The Natrum woman who has been deprived of love in childhood is often easily manipulated by men, who give her approval in return for sexual stimulation. She pretends not to mind, since she is afraid of losing this approval. In the most unhealthy cases she really doesn't mind, since she has cut off from her deeper feelings. If she gets moody she doesn't associate this with the abusive situation she is in, because she doesn't even realise that it is abusive. Such is the power of sexual conditioning on those with little self-respect.

Most Natrum women enjoy sex so long as it is loving. However, quite a few are unable to experience orgasm, even with a loving partner. This is because they cannot totally 'let go' and be vulnerable emotionally, since they are afraid of getting hurt. Some Natrum women feel sad after intercourse because they do open up, and uncover the old hurt inside (Kent: 'Sadness after coitus'). Others have difficulty relaxing during sex because of previous traumatic sexual experiences. (There is one response to sexual abuse that is highly characteristic of Natrum women in particular. Many gain a lot of weight, in an unconscious (and often conscious) attempt to make themselves unattractive to the opposite sex, and hence less likely to be abused again. In my experience, the majority of very fat women are Natrums, and a high proportion are using their weight to avoid sex. (Fat Calcareas and Graphites are not usually fat for this reason.)

### Actors and Actresses
All Natrums are actors to some extent. They tend to put on a bright face when they are unhappy, and for some the mask becomes constant. The emphasis of many Natrums upon the positive is itself an act, especially when it is brittle

and inappropriate. Some Natrums, principally women and homosexual men, dramatise their emotions. This is the last thing that many homeopaths expect of sober Natrum, but it is the hallmark of a particular subset of the type. Wealthy Natrum women in particular often go in for this acting out of emotions. The society lady who comments at a dinner party, "Daarling, this wine is simply ghaastly!" is almost certainly resonating to the wavelength of salt. When she does have a real cause for sadness, she will dramatise this as well; "Daarling, I feel so awful, you have no idea how miserable I am!" Such people use this emotional dramatism to avoid real feelings. They are invariably very unhappy inside, but they manage to avoid feeling it most of the time. Natrum will help their physical symptoms, and may bring up some real feelings, but most have invested too heavily in avoidance to give it up.

The dramatic Natrum loves to talk about emotions, rather than feel them. Even your average Natrum woman has something of the dramatist in her. She will feign shock when hearing of an acquaintance's infidelity, during gossip with her friends, and will enthuse about how wonderful her favourite man is, or how fabulous her next holiday is going to be. Young Natrums of both sexes tend to overuse superlatives, and generally exaggerate those feelings which they feel are socially acceptable, whilst hiding the rest. Thus the teenage Natrum boy will announce to his mates, "Jeez, I hate these stupid cigarettes," but fail to tell them that he is sad because his father broke a promise to take him fishing.

When the Natrum woman wants to be liked by someone, she will often dramatise the things which she likes. For example, she may say to a prospective mate on their first date," I do love pasta, it's so yummy!", followed two minutes later by, "I just love jazz, it's so free!", and so on. She does not realise it, but she is trying to appear more attractive by exaggerating the joy she experiences in life. For some reason, she often thinks that dramatising her negative feelings is also attractive. Thus she will say, "Don't you think it's dreadful the way the telephone charges have gone up?", and "I can't bear the way that waiter walks!" Her strategy is most likely that she will be liked if she is intimate with this person, and rather than be truly intimate, she gives an imitation of intimacy by exaggerating trivial feelings.

Some Natrum women take this 'pseudo-intimacy' to extremes. They latch onto someone whom they feel may be sympathetic, and proceed to tell him the intimate details of their life, in an emotionally dramatic fashion; "My husband doesn't like sex, you know. The years I've wasted! He got me to have my tubes tied because he was too bloody selfish to have a vasectomy, and do you know, he never came near me after that. Course, I blame his drinking. A slave to it he is," and so on. The phone conversations of Sybil in the TV comedy 'Fawlty Towers' are typical of this 'gushing' Natrum, who tries to win a friend by being intimate, and often succeeds in winning the friendship of another gushing Natrum, with whom a silent pact is made, to the effect, "You listen to me, and I'll listen to you." (Another hilarious parody of the gushing Natrum is Dame Edna Everage, the fictional Australian housewife, who is dramatically effusive, embarrassingly intimate, and very proud of her generosity in sharing her life with the public.)

The important thing to realise about the emotionally effusive Natrum is that she is doing it to avoid really feeling her feelings. When such women have deep psychotherapy (which is not very often) the therapist is faced with a constant stream of words, and no crying or other signs of real emotion. However, by forbidding the patient to speak for most of the session, and asking her to focus on her body and her feelings, the therapist can soon bypass the mental chatter and get to the real feelings underneath. Sometimes simply saying "Don't talk" is enough to bring forth floods of tears immediately.

Some homeopathic students may be confused by the thought of an emotionally effusive and dramatic Natrum. It is not so confusing, however, when one remembers that this is just another way in which Natrum avoids feeling her feelings. The old Materia Medicas do not give a subtle account of the mentals of any remedy. However, Kent does say that Natrum 'is a remedy for hysterical girls'. If Natrums can be hysterical, they can also be 'pre-hysterical', or emotionally dramatic.

Not surprisingly, many Natrum people make use of their ability to dramatise emotions by becoming amateur or professional actors and actresses. The majority of the profession are Natrums, (though many are also equally dramatic Phosphorus, Ignatia and Sulphur individuals) as are the majority of models, a profession very closely allied to acting. Elizabeth Taylor is a good example of a Natrum actress, both on and off the screen.

Just as many homeopaths expect Natrum to be discrete, many also expect Natrum to avoid the limelight. Naturally, actors do just the opposite, but so do many 'ordinary' Natrums, particularly some of the women. Many Natrum parents actively encourage their child to perform, through dance, singing and poetry recital. This is healthy as long as the child wants to, and is not pushed to excel, but often the parents are seeking to live vicariously through the child, and this produces tension in her. It can also result in a tendency later on in life to seek to be the centre of attention. Even some Natrums who were not encouraged to perform in an obvious way by their parents seek the centre-stage later on, not literally, but in the form of trying to attract positive attention and admiration. Without any prompting from her parents, the little Natrum girl may launch herself into public performances of singing or dancing in an attempt to impress, and therefore gain approval and love. All children do this to some extent, but some never grow out of the habit, and many of them are Natrums. Those who do not become performing artists find other ways to attract admiration. One of these is boasting, or letting slip little pieces of personal information that are meant to impress. Many of the more dramatic Natrum women do this, particularly with men they are attracted to (so do many Ignatia women). They have a need to feel special, because they feel neglected deep down. A good example is the wealthy aristocratic lady in the film 'The Sound of Music' who almost becomes Baron Von Trap's wife. She does not feel secure in his affections, and so is constantly praising herself, and also fishing for compliments. The harder she tries to impress, the less impressive she appears, and the more frantic her attempts become. Feeling threatened by her fiance's new governess Maria, she persuades him to throw a banquet in her honour, at which she parades herself before the local elite in her finery, and generally plays the gracious hostess and Maid of Honour. Alas all this is to no avail, as he falls instead for the more natural charm of the Phosphoric Maria.

### The Natrum Expert

Whereas many insecure Natrum women resort to being emotionally dramatic in order to feel special, many Natrum men (and some Natrum women) develop an inordinate pride in their intellectual knowledge.

The Natrum man has just as great a need to feel special as the Natrum woman, and like many Lycopodium men, he will often become a specialist in a particular area of knowledge, and take great pride in presenting his expertise to the world. The more intelligent Natrum does this with some subtlety. Nevertheless, he still injects a certain flourish into his pronouncements, as if to say, 'Look how clever I am'. Not all Natrum experts are like this, but those that are can be quite tiresome. Typically they are very keen to express their own opinions, and not very interested in listening to the opinions of others. This is the exact opposite of the common Natrum who is a good listener and speaks relatively little. The proud Natrum expert will grab any opportunity to show off his knowledge, and will wait expectantly at the end of his discourse for signs of praise. This is in contrast to the enthusiastic Sulphur expert who is equally keen to share his knowledge, but is not looking for praise. He already feels good enough inside, and is sharing his knowledge purely out of the love of doing so. The Sulphur expert does not wait expectantly for praise, and is happy so long as his audience understands him, and especially if they share his joy in their discovery.

The proud Natrum expert can be very difficult to distinguish from the proud Lycopodium expert. Both are seeking to bolster their self-esteem by impressing others with their knowledge, and both are very keen to elicit approval from their audience. In general I have found that the true Natrum intellectual is seldom proud in an overt way. It is the non-intellectual Natrum who gains a little knowledge in a particular area who is liable to put on airs and become puffed up with self-importance. It is difficult to describe the differences between the Natrum pseudo-expert and his Lycopodium counterpart. One generally has to rely on other aspects of the personality, such as fears, ability to relate to others, and the degree of emotionality, to separate the two. Often the physicals and generals are of more help. One difference that I have found is that the Lycopodium pseudo-intellectual is often a know-all, he has something to say about everything in most cases, whereas his Natrum counterpart tends to stick to his pet topic. Another is that the Natrum pseudo-expert comes across as emotionally more intense than Lycopodium, which makes him feel somehow 'heavier'. As long as the homeopath knows that these two types tend to produce men who are inordinately proud of their knowledge and loquacious with it, then with experience he can learn the subtle differences between the two.

### The Snob

One version of the Natrum who seeks to impress is the snob. The snob may come from a wealthy, cultured background, and in this case he usually does not try very hard to impress, since his 'breeding' and his money are impressive enough. He is a snob because he looks down on other people, who are less sophisticated than himself, and enjoys parading his finery, and boasting subtly about his noble qualities. Natrums are not the only ones to do this. Arsenicum is often a snob, and so sometimes is Nux. The aristocratic Natrum snob is appalled by the vulgarity of more common folk. He presents himself as an upholder of decency and nobility, and to this end he may favour a charitable trust. Being a Natrum, he is very closed emotionally in most cases, preserving the stiff upper lip of a bygone era. (Not all Natrum aristocrats are snobs, but it is a tendency that is hard to avoid.) He maintains a cordial distance from his family, hiding behind etiquette, his hobbies, and his authority. He is very proud of the public school he went to as a boy, (despite the fact that he was bitterly unhappy there half of the time), and enrols his own son there as soon as he is born. To the snob, appearances are all-important, and his children are not allowed to forget this. The genuinely aristocratic Natrum snob tends to be fairly stable emotionally (ie. shut down), especially in the case of the man. The female snob may have bouts of depression, histrionics or panic, but is very careful to keep these moods out of public view. She is likely to be quite demanding at times, in the manner of a spoilt child, and she sees to it that she always gets what she wants. (Well, nearly always.) Such people live an extraordinarily unreal existence, that is superficial and utterly devoid of real self-understanding. Unfortunately, they used to rule a good part of the globe, and their influence is still strong.

The other kind of Natrum snob has illusions of grandeur. She is most often female, but not always (Basil Fawlty is a notable male example, albeit fictional). Since she is not from aristocratic stock, she must do her best to acquire the trappings of wealth and elegance. If she does not manage to marry wealth, she will at least marry a man who will give her her own way, often another Natrum who if not a snob, is at least aiming for wealth and social respectability. These 'Nouveaux Riche' snobs (and also the 'pre-riche' ones) are far more insufferable than the aristocratic ones, since they feel the need to go out of their way to emphasise their superiority. To this end they put on a very affected accent (often paying for elocution lessons), and if they are not very well educated use long words incorrectly. Nouveaux snobs are terribly self-obsessed, spending much of their time and money on attending to their appearance, and reading magazines like 'House and Garden' to keep up with the latest in haute couture. It is particularly sad to see the way in which such people bring up their children. If they can afford it, they send them to boarding school. If not, they either treat them as social showpieces, or whipping posts, or both. Such children grow up bitterly unhappy, and either submit to their parents' conditioning, growing up into snobs themselves, or rebel, which is healthier and more hopeful.

The origin of the mentality of the Nouveau snob is interesting. In some people it is a case of 'Like father, like son', but in others the Natrum child grew up in a poor family with no sophistication, and was deeply ashamed of her origins. In this case she attempts to disown her family as soon as possible, or to return in splendour to lord it over them. Such children have presumably been denied quality love in their childhood, otherwise they would not feel so ashamed. They have an inferiority complex which derives secondarily from their humble origins, but initially from that old Natrum feeling of abandonment. It is quite likely that their parents were indulgent, and spoilt the child, but indulgence is not the same as unconditional love, and does not prevent the feeling of abandonment and emptiness inside. The Nouveau snob is rigidly defended emotionally, and will not even consider that she might be unhealthy in some way, unless she is forced to by crisis and severe losses. The latter, if they come, are blessings in disguise, since they force her to face reality.

## Depression

Natrum Muriaticum is more prone to depression than any other type except Aurum, and Aurum people are uncommon. By far the majority of depressed homeopathic patients need the remedy, in very high potency if they can take it physically. The response of a depressed Natrum to the remedy in 10M potency is one of the most dramatic and satisfying responses of all to homeopathic treatment, providing the patient is not taking antidepressants as well, which will antidote the remedy. After a day or two of aggravation the heavy weight of sadness and despair begins to lift, and within a couple of weeks the patient is usually improved beyond recognition. (It is about time such treatment was verified by double-blind controlled trials, as it is so reliable, and so effective.)

Natrums become depressed as a result of suppressing sadness. If all the sadness that they had ever felt was given release through crying as it originated, there would be no depression, and also no sense of worthlessness, and all the myriad defence mechanisms which Natrums use to avoid such feelings. That is why Natrums feel better when they cry. Crying releases a layer of sadness, which brings relief, until the next layer of sadness begins to surface. (Each of these layers can be released until emotional health is achieved, but this requires deep psychotherapy, which is practised by very few therapists worldwide. More about such therapy later.)

The bulk of Natrum's sadness is usually acquired during childhood, when the psyche is most vulnerable. Much of it is then suppressed, pushed out of consciousness, and stored in the body as a chemical and energetic memory. When the Natrum individual encounters prolonged periods of adversity later on, or sudden intense suffering, more sadness is suppressed, until eventually the subconscious store is full, and the excess pours into consciousness, resulting in the continual sadness of depression. It is important to realise that the sadness the depressed person feels is only the tip of the psychic iceberg. That is why depression is so difficult to eradicate, not because it results from some chemical imbalance. Deep psychotherapy eradicates the sadness through crying, and with it goes the chemical imbalance caused by storing all that sadness in the body. It is a process which takes years of regular therapy, but it works. The origins of depression are so well hidden in the patient's past that they have not yet been discovered by mainstream medical science, which uses 'the medical model' of mental illness, based on the assumption that mental illness is essentially a physical, biochemical problem.

The correct use of homeopathy in the treatment of depression is a big step forward from the medical model, since the remedy is energetic, and hence works on the emotional as well as the biochemical level. Nevertheless, the remedies alone will only end a relatively superficial depression, or palliate a deep one. They will enable the uppermost layer of sadness to be discharged, thus bringing relief. However, sooner or later another layer of sadness will be 'activated', and the process must be repeated.

There are many common precipitants for Natrum's depression. The most potent ones are related to loss of love, since this reactivates the early grief. Thus bereavement, separation and estrangement from a loved one can all tip the scales and initiate a depressive episode. The commonest situation of all is that of the Natrum wife who has a relatively loveless marriage. Often the husband is neglectful or abusive, and the woman tolerates this abuse because she is afraid of losing him. She may take it silently, slipping gradually into despair, or she may become aggressive, taking out her anger on both her husband and her children. The latter is decidedly more healthy. Those women who cannot get angry will remain in the abusive situation for most of their life, and will forever be slipping in and out of depression. Sometimes the remedy in high potency is enough to mobilise the woman's confidence, and she expresses her anger for the first time in her life. I once treated an acquaintance for emotional problems. She was a middle-aged woman who had always had trouble standing up to men, and tended to live under a perpetual shadow of fear. Her father had been very strict, and had beaten her for relatively trivial misdemeanours, thus inducing a permanent state of helplessness in his daughter. I gave the woman Natrum Muriaticum 10M, and a couple of days later received a message that she was very angry with me. I contacted her and she told me that after she had taken the medicine she suddenly felt outraged that I had hoodwinked her by charging her money for a couple of sugar tablets. I pointed out that she was behaving rather out of character, and she agreed, commenting that she had also told a work colleague who had intimidated her for months what she thought of him. I then pointed out that the remedy was increasing her self-confidence, and bringing feelings of suppressed anger to the surface. She then understood what was happening, and said that she was amazed that she didn't feel guilty about being rude to her colleague.

Sometimes the remedy is enough to help a woman to stand up to her neglectful husband and either push him into listening to her, or give her the courage to leave. More often psychotherapy is needed in addition, and the remedy alone will simply help her to cope with the unhappy situation.

Some Natrum women are so 'codependent' that they become depressed when their alcoholic or invalid husband makes a recovery. He is then no longer dependent upon her, and hence she feels she is no longer of any use, and fears that he will leave. (The whole codependency movement arose as a result of the wives of men in Alcoholics Anonymous who grouped together for support when they became depressed as a result of their husbands' recoveries.)

For many Natrum women depression suddenly appears out of the blue, with no apparent precipitating factor. Usually there is one, but it is subtle, and missed by the patient. For example, she may become depressed after marrying a man who is loving and attentive. Closer questioning reveals that she has difficulty relaxing during intercourse, and after she takes the remedy she remembers that she was sexually abused as a child, a memory that had been totally suppressed for decades. In this case the precipitating factor for the depression was sexual activity. Without the remedy she may never have identified the cause of her depression, which may have continued for the rest of her life. (Many will not identify the cause despite the remedy).

The most intractable cases of depression occur in those Natrum individuals, mostly women, who have suffered a multitude of traumas, starting at birth. (It is extraordinary how often such people report that they had very difficult births). These tragic people have been victims all of their lives, going from one abusive situation to another. They are generally utterly lacking in both confidence and self-esteem, and they react to all abuse and all threats with fear and sadness, rather than anger. They tend to latch on rather desperately to therapists who offer some hope to them, and apart from their stubborn tendency to put themselves down and accept abuse silently, they are 'model patients', following every instruction to the letter, turning up in good time for their appointments, and thanking the therapist enthusiastically each time. They tend to smile or laugh inappropriately, and to cry profusely when they talk of their past sufferings. Such patients can be helped along by the remedy, but only the deepest of psychotherapies can exorcise their pain, and even then only after years of therapy.

The most characteristic thing about a Natrum depression is that it is silent for the most part. The feelings of sadness and anxiety are not expressed verbally to anyone, and very often tears are fought back. They are resisted for several reasons, but the main one is that the patient senses the mountain of sadness beneath the surface, and is unwilling to face it by crying. Other reasons for suppressing tears include the guilt that Natrum feels when she upsets other people, and the belief that crying is a weakness. Some depressed Natrums cannot cry at all, especially some of the men. Their previous emotional wounds were so painful that they covered them up with an impenetrable shield, maintaining a stiff control of feelings at all times. This shield is a barrier to true recovery, and it often cracks as a result of taking the remedy.

Natrum is a remedy for retention of all kinds; fluid retention, retention of salty tears, retention of sadness and anger, and retention of attachment to loved ones. Letting go is the hardest thing for Natrum, on so many different levels.

During periods of depression, all the old demons lurking in the patient's subconscious mind tend to resurface. Depression results from a flooding of psychological defence mechanisms, and the flood agitates the murky waters of the depths, waking sleeping monsters which then rise into full awareness. These monsters include guilt, fear, and the sense of worthlessness that lies at the root of Natrum's insecurities.

Some Natrum depressions are more active than others. The defence mechanisms which keep suppressed feelings at bay may be only slightly leaky. In this case a prolonged but 'low grade' depression occurs, characterised by apathy (Kent: 'Dullness, sluggishness'), and mild feelings of irritability, sadness, anxiety or guilt. This apathetic depression can be difficult to differentiate from a Sepia depression. Generally the depressed Sepia cries more, but this is not a reliable differentiating factor, and more helpful hints will often be found in the patient's physical symptoms, and especially in the pre-morbid personality. With few exceptions, Sepia people enter into Sepia depressions, and Natrum people enter into Natrum depressions.

The apathetic depressed Natrum tends to sleep a great deal. For once she can't be bothered keeping up with her perfectionist standards, allowing housework to accumulate, and she no longer even cares what people think, or whether she is upsetting anyone. She is liable to eat a lot, constantly nibbling on high calorie snacks in order to fill the sense of emptiness within. Comfort eating is especially characteristic of Natrum and Sepia, and it results in a great many obese Natrums.

Unlike the more deeply depressed Natrum, the apathetic Natrum may feel better for company, since it can stimulate her into forgetting her feelings for a while, and she may also respond positively to affection.

More serious rifts in Natrum's defences result in deep depressions, as suppressed sadness pours in. The deeply depressed Natrum becomes very withdrawn (Kent: 'Averse company'), deliberately isolating herself, because she feels that nobody could understand how she is feeling, and she can no longer pretend everything is alright. She will only cry if she is alone, or with somebody she feels very close to, since she feels at her most vulnerable when she is crying. Consolation makes her feel worse, and can precipitate tears, because it touches her heart, which is still protected to some extent, and hence opens it up.

The deeply depressed Natrum is assailed by painful memories which had been suppressed for years. She will agonise over them, reliving a trauma again and again, quite unable to stop the replays in her mind (Kent: 'Thoughts—tormenting'). At such times she may be overwhelmed with remorse for things she regrets doing, or things she should have done, and may feel responsible for a great many problems of other people which were not her fault at all (Kent: 'Anxiety with guilt').

Although many depressed Natrums cannot cry, others cannot stop crying (Kent: 'Causeless weeping'), and the slightest thing can set them off, particularly contact with people. This can happen to both superficially and deeply depressed Natrums. The resulting bouts of crying are generally short lived, and do not relieve like the more hearty ones.

Depression in Natrum men is much like that of Natrum women, with the addition sometimes of tremendous rage, which the patient struggles to keep under control. One depressed Natrum man vented all of his aggressive feelings on his wife. She would wake up in the night terrified to find him punching her pillow next to her head. Occasionally he punched her instead of her pillow. He'd had a loveless childhood, and he knew that his wife was not the problem, but he could not help himself. He felt terrible remorse after bouts of violence, but this did nothing to prevent subsequent loss of control. He needed to find a safe way to release his anger, but was not willing to try. However, his nocturnal spasms of rage gradually became less and less frequent after taking Natrum Muriaticum 10M. (This man was one of those Natrum pseudo-experts who become obsessed with a given topic and talk about it at any opportunity. He had wanted to be a pilot, but his father would not support him financially to learn to fly, so he became an aeroplane mechanic instead. Every day he would watch the planes go up, tortured by regret that he was not flying them. He would learn everything there was to know about the planes, putting in many hours of overtime just to be around them. In the consulting room he would constantly bring the conversation around to planes, and quote endless technical details which had no interest whatsoever to me. It is Natrum men such as he who had poor relationships with their parents who are most prone to both depression and to obsessions. The obsession becomes a substitute for the affection and pleasure he missed out on as a child, and actually helps to keep him out of depression.)

The Natrum woman is particularly likely to experience depression during times of hormonal instability. This includes premenstrually, post-natally, during pregnancy and post-menopausally (Kent: 'Sadness before menses', 'Sadness in pregnancy'). The majority of women who experience emotional problems at these times need Natrum Muriaticum. There is nothing wrong with their hormones. It is just that a rapid change in hormones destabilises Natrum's emotional defences, allowing suppressed emotions to surface. If there were no suppressed emotions, there would be no premenstrual or post-natal depression.

Suicidal thoughts are common when Natrum is deeply depressed. Those who do seek release from suffering through death usually do it quietly, using sleeping tablets or car exhaust fumes. However, some Natrums with a strong anger component to their depression slash their wrists.

Manic depression is a hereditary illness characterised by alternations of depression and euphoria. In my experience, the vast majority of manic depressives respond to high potencies of Natrum Muriaticum or Natrum Sulphuricum, and have Natrum personalities in between the two extremes of mood (Kent: 'Mania'). The manic stage tends to have similar characteristics irrespective of the constitutional type of the patient, including a great acceleration of thought processes and activity, increased sexuality, delusions of grandeur, and a tendency to go on wild spending sprees. Since these features are characteristic of the disease rather than the patient, they are not useful distinguishing symptoms. The personality outside of manic episodes is a better guide to the indicated remedy. (Aurum and Veratrum Album are occasionally indicated). When treating manic depression the indicated remedy is effective irrespective of which phase of the illness it is given in. It can curtail a manic episode as effectively as a depressive one, providing the patient is not on anti-depressants.

## Disappointed Love

Natrum is very similar to Ignatia, in that most Natrums have a sense of abandonment deep inside, and are extremely sensitive to loss of love. For these reasons, both types tend to suffer greatly when they lose someone close to them, whether through death or separation. Such situations resonate with the childhood memory of emotional pain, bringing the old feelings back to the surface that had been suppressed at the age of (say) two or three. Severe grief is a replay of an old suppressed emotion. It is never new. Most Natrums who undergo deep psychotherapy experience a profound sense of grief when they re-experience what they felt as a small child.

There are two common 'abnormal' grief reactions in Natrum individuals. The first is a complete lack of reaction. The person feels nothing, except perhaps a sense of numbness. This is a common feeling when one first hears of a bereavement, but with Natrum it may never be followed by the usual sadness and tears, because the injured heart is determined not to feel. Another layer of sadness is pushed into the subconscious, insulating the heart even more heavily from feeling. As a result, Natrum may feel a permanent loss following such silent grief, without being able to pinpoint it. There is just that much less joy in his life, and that much less meaning. The remedy in high potency can sometimes reverse this suppression, and bring forth the tears that were never shed.

The other common reaction is a prolonged and particularly deep version of the 'normal' grief process. The bereaved individual is at first in shock, which quickly gives way to profound sadness and heavy sobbing. During this initial unstable stage Ignatia will usually stabilise the patient, bringing him back to his senses. After the Ignatia stage, the patient may remain in a state of grieving for months or even years. During this time the departed one keeps reappearing in the mind, and reactivating the pain like another knife in the heart. Any reminder of the lost one will precipitate tears in the eyes, and a heavy load of grief inside. These Natrums, on losing a partner, will declare that they could never love another, and indeed they usually remain single until the pain has subsided, which can take many years. If they re-marry before they have stopped grieving, they are often unable to give their heart to their new spouse, and remain obsessed with the departed one. A dose of the remedy in high potency is usually very effective in completing these protracted grief reactions.

Exactly the same reactions occur in Natrums after being left by a loved one, and even after leaving a loved one themselves. Whether the loss is through death or separation, the process is the same, and the remedy can be used effectively to help the patient to let go.

It is very common for Natrum to agonise over unfinished business with the lost one. He may be racked with guilt because he never said he loved them, or worse, feels responsible for their death. This is just another replay of the guilt the Natrum child feels, when he concludes that it must be his fault that his parents don't love him.

It is quite common for Natrum to suppress his grief deliberately, because he feels that he has to be strong, either for the sake of his family, or to prevent himself falling into a depression. Unfortunately, he does not realise that such tactics backfire in the end, since they result in further suffering down the line. Many Natrum patients have told me that as children they were not allowed to grieve when they lost a favourite relative (or parent). Often, they were not allowed to go to the funeral, and were distracted by being given some task or other to perform. This is a result of their guardian's own fear of emotion, and it is very damaging to the child, who never finishes the normal grieving process, because it was artificially frozen and pushed under the surface of consciousness. Later on in life it will reappear, and the sadness will have to be faced.

### The Clown

Everybody knows that the clown has a broken heart. What they don't know is that a dose of Natrum Muriaticum could help to mend it. I have come across several amateur and professional clowns, and all have been Natrums. The clown's act has a dual purpose. It helps Natrum to forget that his heart is aching, and in the process it attracts approval from others, which Natrum uses as a substitute for love.

There are a great many comedians who do the same. The earlier in life the person became a comedian, the more likely it is that he is hiding from great emotional pain. Children who compulsively play the fool at school are usually Natrums, and are usually very unhappy inside. The Australian comedian and broadcaster Clive James gives a very clear description in his autobiography of how he turned into a comedian at school, in order that people would laugh with him and not at him. Natrum cannot bear to be laughed at. It hurts him far more than he lets on, as does any form of rejection. I once treated the son of a friend of mine, who was incapable of having a serious conversation, even for a few seconds. He was very intelligent, and used his quick wits to make puns and smart remarks in reply to anything anybody said to him. His mother told me that he was very insecure, and worried unrealistically about his parents dying. He was about ten years old, but often seemed older, because his wit was so sophisticated. I told him that his compulsive punning was unhealthy, and he seemed to understand. Within a couple of weeks of taking Natrum Muriaticum 10M he was a different person. He was much quieter, and was now able to have sensible conversations without playing the fool.

Natrum comedians have all sorts of humorous styles. Many have a wry, dry wit, that is symptomatic of their cynical outlook on life (eg Basil Fawlty). Sarcasm is not the prerogative of Natrum, but it is one of his commonest defence mechanisms. It may be the lowest form of wit, but it is often Natrum's only means of expressing anger. Manic humour is also a Natrum forte, of the style perfected by comedians such as John Cleese, and Harry Secombe. It allows Natrum to indulge his dramatic tendency, and hence avoid his real feelings. Slapstick and mime are also Natrum favourites; in fact Natrums tend to be the leading exponents of all forms of humour, irrespective of its subtlety or simplicity. When confronted with a Natrum patient who appears to have a very negative self-image, I often ask "and what are your good points?." Frequently the only one they can think of is "I have a good sense of humour." Many Natrums have to laugh, or make others laugh, or they would cry.

## The Addict

Addiction to anything can be seen at its simplest as a flight from emotional pain, towards a substitute for love. The substance or activity to which the addict is addicted produces a temporary sense of well-being, dispelling the unease that is constantly there without it. Not all addicts are Natrums, but the majority are, since Natrum is so common, and is so commonly emotionally hurt. Thus the majority of alcoholics are Natrum Muriaticums, and most of them are men. Male Natrums are generally more emotionally repressed than women, which results in a greater psychological tension inside. Since the men do not allow themselves to cry at all for the most part, they tend to resort to addictive behaviour to ease the tension. Alcohol, nicotine, caffeine, marijuana and cocaine are some of the more commonly used substances by Natrum addicts. The women often become addicted to food, especially chocolate, which contains several stimulants. There is even a serious organisation in the United States called Chocoholics Anonymous, which helps obese Natrums in the main to cope with their habit.

Natrum's comfort eating progresses in some cases to bulimia, (food binging followed by either vomiting or laxative abuse to control weight). In my experience the majority of bulimics are Natrums, and they generally respond very well to the remedy. The bulimic is desperately trying to fill the void inside, but since the sense of emptiness in the body is a reflection of emotional starvation, no amount of food is felt to be satisfying.

Related to bulimia is the even more serious condition of Anorexia

Nervosa. Nearly every anorexic patient I have treated has needed Natrum Muriaticum as the principal or sole remedy. The anorexic is always severely disturbed emotionally. Typically she is a teenage girl with a very controlling parent or parents. (This dynamic is very common in Natrum households, where parents are often more concerned with appearances than with what their child is feeling.) The anorexic child decides that what she eats is the only thing in her life that is under her control. She unconsciously decides to exert control over her life in the only way available, by restricting her food intake. Her 'habit' is reinforced by her low self-esteem, which (no doubt encouraged by the fashion industry) tends to make her feel ugly, and to equate ugly with fat. Since she feels ugly, she must be fat, and this unconscious conclusion distorts her conscious self-image, so that even when she is as thin as a corpse, she sees herself as fat, and hence ugly. Anorexia usually responds well to Natrum Muriaticum 10M, combined with counselling. (Sometimes Ignatia is the constitutional remedy needed.)

Activities can serve as more socially acceptable forms of addiction than substance abuse. The workaholic is just as much an addict as the alcoholic, although the deleterious effects of this addiction to activity are less.

Addictive behaviour is by no means restricted to Natrum individuals, but other constitutional types who are prone to addictive behaviour (notably Phosphorus, Staphysagria, Tuberculinum and Syphilinum) are uncommon in comparison. Natrum Muriaticum 10M would help the majority of addicts to 'kick their habit'.

### *Emotional Intensity*

Since Natrum people tend to bottle up their emotions, they have a constant emotional tension within. The majority of Natrum women, and about half of the men, are sufficiently open to feel intense emotions quite a lot of the time. These people have a constant 'ooze' of emotion from the subconscious to the conscious mind, the tide varying with outside triggers, as well as hormonal status in the women. The result of this 'emotional tide' is that much of Natrum's experience of everyday living is coloured by emotion. It may not be expressed, but it is felt. This is why Natrum people tend to have watery eyes much of the time.

There are a thousand and one different stimuli which may trigger an upsurge of emotion in a Natrum person, stimuli which resemble in some way old experiences that elicited emotions so intense that much of it was stored away without being felt properly. In modern psychological slang, these stimuli 'press Natrum's buttons'. The most common button-pressers in this regard are; criticism or rejection of any kind, aggression of any kind, scenes and stories of tragedy or of joy after great suffering, unexpectedly being shown love and affection, and emotional possessiveness (particularly in the men).

Many Natrum people are constantly reacting emotionally to subtle triggers in the environment, like weather vanes shifting in a changeable wind. For example, the Natrum woman may awake in the morning from a dream feeling vaguely exhausted. This wears off, but over breakfast she hears on the radio that a sixteen year old girl has been abducted in her town. Immediately, she experiences a mixture of fear and sadness. Walking to her car after breakfast she passes a stranger who looks into her eyes, making her feel uneasy. On the drive to work she feels slightly panicky when a police car follows her for a mile or so, though she is breaking no laws. At work she is greeted by the other receptionist, and feels inside a mixture of affection and a sense of safety in the company of this friendly, familiar person. However, she soon feels the pressure to perform, and the tension rises as she starts to worry that she isn't keeping up. A customer looks impatient, and she feels responsible, and smiles apologetically at him, although he is being seen to by her colleague. A mother walks in with a baby daughter, and her heart reaches out to the child, and basks in a rich cocktail of love and sentiment. And so on. Natrum women in particular tend to live in a constantly changing tide of emotion. Much of it they are only vaguely aware of, particularly the background of anxiety that they only register when it becomes intense.

Natrum men tend to cut off their feelings more effectively, but even so, many are still slaves to the button-pushing stimuli of everyday life. It is this constant toing and froing of emotions that makes Natrum feel out of control, and makes him impose discipline upon almost every area of his life, particularly his potentially emotive interactions with other people. Natrums tend to be very controlled and cautious with people they do not know well, since they never know what threatening stimulus they may be confronted with. The equally emotionally labile Phosphorus, on the other hand, is spontaneous and adventurous with new company, since he is not so easily hurt, and when he is hurt he tends to get over it very quickly, unlike Natrum, who is liable to stew in an uncomfortable brew of old emotions.

The constant background emotion that colours Natrum's experience imparts a certain emotional intensity to her communication with others, particularly with those people she is close to. With strangers she gives little away, but with those she trusts she allows the emotion to slip into her voice, adding a touch of aggression, sadness, anxiety or euphoria to otherwise commonplace statements. At times the emotional tide is in full flow, and everything she says sounds emotionally intense. This is attractive and reassuring to other Natrum women, who can identify with her, but it tends to make men switch off emotionally to prevent themselves from being 'swamped'. (Other emotional types like Sepia, Ignatia, Pulsatilla and Phosphorus tend to have the same effect on men.)

Because Natrums tend to 'bottle' unpleasant emotions, the latter have a habit of building up silently, and then erupting with force. The Natrum wife will take neglect or abuse from her husband for several days or weeks, and then suddenly snap, hurling abuse at him with the ferocity of all that stored up resentment. When she does snap, she will also fling at him all the other resentments she has been storing up since her last explosion, barraging him with an avalanche of bitterness that takes him totally by surprise, and leaves him mystified as to where it all came from. Unfortunately, this style of fitful communication between partners is rather counterproductive, since it allows problems to grow to serious proportions before being aired, and the mutual hostility engendered by such outbursts of resentment makes a sensible approach to the problem much more difficult. It is this lack of easy communication that results in many Natrum parents being estranged from their children, leaving the latter feeling alienated, lonely and misunderstood, and sowing the seeds of youthful rebellion.

The Natrum men who are not shut-down emotionally live in the same emotional soup as the women, but they tend not to express it so much, since it is not socially acceptable, and their mates wouldn't know how to cope with it. The more repressed men alternate between periods of objectivity, when they feel very little, and occasional powerful emotions which break through the defences like tidal waves. At these times they may be violent, depressed or very anxious, though mostly these powerful emotions are bottled up and sent back whence they came, to the dark depths of the subconscious, without ever being outwardly expressed. Most Natrum men cultivate a cool, detached appearance, and many will go to great lengths to deny their emotions, except for anger, which men are 'allowed' to express. The more physical Natrum man indulges in the same bravado as Lycopodium to hide his true feelings, and often uses alcohol to loosen up socially, since it allows his mind to dissociate from his emotions, and to trip lightly from one piece of posturing to another. Many committed sportsmen fall into this category, as do many manual workers.

The more intellectual Natrum man is often equally evasive emotionally. He uses his intellect to avoid feeling (as do a great many Natrum women, and also Ignatia women), and enjoys being highly rational. A good example of this sort is Humphrey Bogart in the classic film 'Casablanca'. He keeps his emotions very close to his chest, presenting a cool, logical persona, and using irony to gently ridicule a woman's more emotional outbursts. The logical Natrum man can be difficult to distinguish from other highly rational types like Lycopodium and Kali. Apart from confirming some of the more characteristically Natrum attributes like perfectionism, high morals and a preference for his own company, he may also hint at being more emotional than the other rational types. For example, he may admit to the occasional periods of depression, or to feeling very emotional at farewells. Natrum men really are more emotional than Lycopodiums and Kalis, but they may not admit it, and the homeopath may have to rely on the strength of their denial, and their tendency to look uncomfortable talking about emotions, to confirm that they are more emotional than they let on.

### *Sentimentality*

Natrum is a sentimental type. Sentimentality is essentially a kind of superficial love which one can feel without making oneself too vulnerable. It is a gentle, safe emotion which generates warmth, much like a glass of sherry. It is this combination of warmth and safety that makes sentimentality so attractive to many Natrums, especially the women, and also the children. Pink is probably the Natrum woman's favourite colour, and it is certainly the young Natrum child's favourite, especially when in the form of a stylised heart. Natrum women often love enormous pink and red padded greeting cards, which their Natrum men send them, though not without some embarrassment. The Hollywood 'weepy' is sure to evoke rivers of tears from most Natrum women, and a good many of the men; tears which are gentle (Kent: 'Mildness') , and do not threaten Natrum's emotional stability.

Many Natrums confuse love with sentimentality. They become dependent upon hearing the words 'I love you' several times a day from their partner, and they cherish jewellery and other gifts given to them by loved ones, irrespective of whether they would normally like it. The fact that their boyfriend lays on a candle-lit dinner for them is enough to make many Natrum women overlook the fact that he is emotionally immature, and incapable of an open, adult relationship. As long as he 'shows that he cares', she is happy, not realising that this show is no deeper than any other based on sentimentality. Since Natrums constitute the majority of civilised people on the planet, it is small wonder that love is represented by pink hearts, padded cards and bunny rabbits.

Natrum's sentimentality is especially aroused by children and animals, since they are defenceless and very loving, and hence are safe emotionally. Many a Natrum girl has grown up closer to her horse or her dog than anyone else, and is devastated when it dies.

Religion is another source of sentimental comfort for a good many Natrums, especially children. The attachment to gentle Jesus, to the story of the Nativity, and to Christmas carols is reassuring and soothing, even though it may have little to do with true spirituality. Many young Natrum girls want to be nuns when they grow up, because they have absorbed such a sentimental version of a nun's life. Parents encourage their child's sentimentality, not realising that they are encouraging an escapist tendency, and a trivialisation of love. Of course, the more emotionally healthy Natrum does know the difference between true love and sentimentality, but she is in the minority.

## Fears and Phobias

Natrum is a more fearful type than is often realised. The principal fear of the Natrum individual is the fear of emotional pain, but this fear is often barely conscious, though it may control a great deal of the person's life, by forcing him to avoid threatening situations. Natrum individuals use a variety of strategies to avoid reactivating their sleeping sense of hurt. Some avoid intimate relationships altogether. If they don't open up their heart, they can't get hurt. Others are less closed, but they will wait a long time before they trust somebody enough to really be vulnerable with them.

I have already mentioned the common Natrum fear of losing a loved one. This fear is particularly common in Natrum children. One Natrum woman told me that as a child she used to sleep on the hall carpet in front of her parent's bedroom, much to their dismay. She did this in order to prevent her parents from leaving in the night and abandoning her. Although this behaviour is an extreme example, the fear of losing one or both patents is very common in Natrum children.

Adult Natrums have similar fears to this. Some still dread the death of their parent, to whom they are unhealthily attached, both by guilt, and by emotional dependence. Many Natrum people unconsciously feel that if their parent should die, they will have lost all chance of gaining their love. Consciously they think that they are loved by their parent, who has been somewhat distant throughout their life, but they do not really feel this love. One very attractive and sophisticated mother of two told me during psychotherapy that she felt her mother had 'an intellectual love' for her, but not a heartfelt love, and that she felt the same towards her mother. I explained that there is no such thing as 'intellectual love', that this is merely an idea and a belief which (predominantly Natrum) people use to comfort themselves when love is absent, much as others are comforted by the promise of everlasting joy in the hereafter when their present life is miserable. Being a Natrum woman, who was very well guarded from emotional honesty, she at first refused to accept this interpretation. Eventually, however, she did contact the deep well of grief inside of her, and she realised that she had never been loved by her mother. Following realisations like this, and the cleansing tears that accompany them, many Natrums are able to let go of their fear of losing loved ones.

Even more common is the Natrum parent who dreads that something fatal will happen to her child. The child is the principal source of emotional support for her, and given the fact that she felt abandoned by her parents during childhood, she cannot now bear the thought of being abandoned by her child. Similarly, many happily married Natrums secretly dread that something will happen to their spouse, and others panic just as things are going well in their new relationship, because they fear they will lose what has become so dear.

Fear of social disapproval is extremely common amongst Natrum people, as is fear of parental disapproval, which nearly always precedes the former. As a result, many Natrums go out of their way to satisfy the expectations of others, and in doing so they never really do what they want. (The pattern becomes so habitual that they often forget what they want in life, and give up all 'selfish' expectations.) An example is the Natrum patient of mine who recently injured her back trying to help straighten out a friend's back. Although her back was very painful, she couldn't bear to let her tennis team down by withdrawing from a competition. She played well despite great pain with typical Natrum stoicism, and in the process aggravated her back so much that she could not play again for weeks. Some Natrums gradually learn from such experiences that they must put themselves before social expectations, but many others never do.

Closely related to the fear of social disapproval is the commonest Natrum fear of all, the fear of making a fool of oneself in public. Natrum women in particular sometimes go to great lengths to avoid feeling foolish or embarrassed. They will not say what is on their mind, especially in public, for fear of looking ridiculous, and they will blush easily during the homeopathic interview when they say something which they think sounds silly. This fear originates in childhood. The Natrum child is extremely sensitive to being laughed at by anybody, but especially by his parents (Kent: 'Ailments from scorn'). It feels like rejection, and reinforces the feeling most Natrum children have to some degree, that there is something wrong with them. Most Natrum children hate being made fun of, and they will often avoid it by trying to deliberately amuse. Many a Natrum adult makes a joke of how foolish she sounds or appears, in order to mitigate the scorn she imagines in other people's minds. After forgetting the name of her consultant, she will laugh and say to the homeopath, "What a silly woman I am!" Such attempts to cover up usually appear more silly than the 'foolishness' they are mocking.

One classic example of Natrum's fear of looking foolish in public is the common Natrum aversion to using public lavatories. One reason for this is Natrum's fear of dirt, but the main reason is that she fears the embarrassment that she will feel when others in adjoining cubicles hear what she is doing. Many a Natrum person has developed constipation because she will not use the toilet even at home if there is anyone around who could hear her.

Unlike the social fears and fears of emotional loss, Natrum has other fears which are not so close to the underlying emotional hurt, but which nevertheless are derived from it. An example is claustrophobia. This fear often prompts homeopaths to think of Argentum Nitricum and Stramonium, and to ignore Natrum, since it does not feature largely in traditional texts under this symptom (Natrum is not listed in Kent's repertory under 'Fear in a narrow place', but is listed under 'Fear in a crowd'.) This is an example of how incomplete the old repertories and materia medicas are, especially with regard to mental features. Natrum Muriaticum is the principal remedy for claustrophobic patients, since this phobia is common in Natrums, and Argentum and Stramonium patients are very uncommon in comparison. Natrum's claustrophobia may be very specific, being experienced only in certain situations, such as small lifts, or rooms without windows, or it may be more global, threatening the individual's peace of mind in a great many different places. Some Natrums only feel claustrophobic when water is poured over their head, or if the bedsheet is pulled over them. Others panic only in crowds, or in motorcars. Natrum's claustrophobia is particularly likely to arise during periods of emotional stress, such as marital difficulty, or following a bereavement, and this hints at its underlying origins. I suspect that Natrum is prone to feelings of suffocation, because he is emotionally full to the brim with suppressed feelings. It is as though these feelings rise like a fluid level, and when they reach the throat Natrum feels as though he cannot breathe, especially when the outside surroundings mirror his inner confinement.

Closely related to Natrum's claustrophobic tendency is the tendency towards panic attacks of all kinds (Kent: 'Hysteria'). A great many Natrum patients consult the homeopath for panic attacks which seemingly arise out of the blue, and often severely curtail the patient's activities. Very often they are given Argentum, (which does not help) because the homeopath does not realise that Natrum is prone to panic attacks. There is seldom anything very specific about the attack. It consists of a sudden feeling of terror, accompanied by difficulty in breathing and a racing, pounding heart. Identical attacks are described by Argentum, Sepia, Alumina, Causticum, Phosphorus, Ignatia and Syphilinum people. It is not the characteristics of the panic attack which help in identifying the indicated remedy, but the totality of the patient's history, and especially the overall personality. These panic attacks are merely an expression of the tension within that results from a continual suppression of painful feelings. Once these feelings are felt and expressed, the panic attacks disappear. Sometimes the remedy in high potency is enough to dispel the tension. At other times, deep psychotherapy is needed in addition.

A great many Natrum women have a fear of attack by men, which they describe as a fear of robbers, or a fear of being assaulted and raped. Sometimes this is due to episodes of childhood abuse which have been forcibly forgotten, or to more recent attacks which are not forgotten. Often no such attacks have occurred, and the fear originates from the sense of vulnerability and danger experienced by the young child who does not feel loved. (To a young child, to feel unloved is to feel in danger of being killed). Such women cannot relax when alone at night, and even when they are not alone, they may check and recheck the locks on the doors and windows before retiring. The fear is often accompanied by dreams of attack, of being pursued, or of being robbed (Kent: 'Dreams of robbers, and cannot sleep until the house is searched'). Children who are afraid of intruders at night will also respond to Natrum Muriaticum more often than not.

Other common Natrum fears include fear of snakes (seen far more often in Natrum than in Lachesis, since the latter is a far less common type), and fear of insects, particularly spiders. These fears are presumably related to Natrum's fear of attack, since both spiders and snakes can be venomous, and make lightning strikes at their victims. Natrums often have a great fear of sharks for the same reason.

One Natrum fear that at first appears unexpected is the fear of death itself. Many depressed Natrums would welcome death, but others live in constant fear of this ultimate unknown. It is the unknown aspect of death that Natrum fears, just as he fears the unknown depths of his own mind. One Natrum friend of mine didn't mind talking about death in general, but the subject of her own death was very threatening, since it conjured up in her mind the image of an infinite void, an image which made her feel quite panicky.

Infirmity is another classic Natrum fear. Many would rather die than become an invalid, since as an invalid they would be totally dependent upon other people, something they have avoided as much as they possibly could, since dependency brings with it vulnerability, and the possibility of being hurt, not to mention the guilt of being a burden to others. Chronic illness is also feared because it brings with it immobility, and hence the inability to avoid suppressed emotions by keeping active.

Like claustrophobia, agarophobia (the fear of open spaces) is sometimes seen in Natrum individuals. An example is the teenage Natrum boy whose mother brought him to see me, because he felt afraid to go out of the house. Whenever he strayed from home he felt uneasy, or even downright scared, and this fear was starting to turn him into a hermit. In his case the fear appeared to relate to his earlier childhood, when his mother was forever taking him away from home to be with his father, who was a professional sportsman and travelled to competitions around the country. His parents did not get on, and he was much closer to his mother than his father. He thus felt threatened away from home, since he could not have his mother to himself, and he was reminded with each outing of the precarious nature of his family life. All he wanted to do was to stay at home with his mother, and this produced an aversion to going out at all, an aversion which disappeared with a few doses of Natrum Muriaticum 10M. Natrum children such as he, who feel insecure because of the precarious relationship between their parents, very often wet their bed regularly until they are in their teens. (Bedwetting seems to occur more in Natrum children than in any other type, and they respond well to the remedy in 10M potency in most cases.) Nightmares are also very common in these insecure Natrum children, who often try to sleep in their parents' bed to allay their fear.

### The Healthy Natrum

The truly healthy individual, who is free of past emotional trauma, and is both loving and confident, is a rarity irrespective of constitutional type. There are, however, many Natrum individuals who are relatively healthy emotionally, having either received quality love from their parents as children, or having let go of the past through deep psychotherapy. These 'healthy' Natrums are easily missed by the homeopath, since most of Natrum's characteristic mental attributes are connected to emotional pathology. The homeopath must look carefully for the remaining subtle signs of insecurity and defensiveness to spot these Natrums, and may have to rely principally on the physicals and the generals to reach the correct prescription.

The healthy Natrum is not emotionally closed. She is in touch with her emotions, and is not afraid of expressing them. However, she is still likely to be a relatively private, discreet person, not only because there are still a few hurts she is nursing inside, but also because she is sensitive enough to respect other peoples' feelings, and she has enough self-love to protect herself and her loved ones from the insensitivity of others. The healthy Natrum is affectionate, and the more healthy she is, the less clingy is her love. Truly healthy Natrums are able to let go of their children, and do not grieve indefinitely after a bereavement.

As individuals become more healthy emotionally, they lose the excesses and deficiencies of character that are such an integral part of the constitutional picture, but they do not all become the same. For example, the emotionally healthy Lycopodium man will be sensitive to the feelings of other people, but not as sensitive or empathic as the emotionally healthy Natrum man, although the latter will not be quite so objective as the former. Healthy Natrums are emotionally 'deep', without being oversensitive or tied to the past. They have warm hearts, but they are able to say 'no' when they wish, without feeling guilty. The healthy Natrum retains the efficiency and organising abilities of her less healthy Natrum relatives, but no longer loses perspective by putting control before emotional satisfaction. (Less healthy Natrums are often compulsive organisers. They run committees, become school-teachers, and generally try to organise other people's lives, without looking too closely at their own.) Gone is the excessive stoicism of the controlled Natrum, replaced by an ability for self-indulgence without regret. Relationships are entered into more courageously by the healthy Natrum, and because they have more to give, and do not hide from their partner, such relationships are more satisfying, though when they end, the healthy Natrum is sad but not devastated. The morality of the healthy Natrum is still likely to be that bit higher that that of Lycopodium or Nux, but it is flexible, and it is not imposed upon other people. Similarly, healthy Natrums do not care too much about what other people think. As long as they are living up to their own reasonable standards, they are at peace with themselves, and do need to court social approval. They may always have more respect for traditional values of decency and fidelity than some other constitutional types, but they no longer follow artificial values laid down by their parents, their church or society as a whole. This is a great freedom for Natrum, who when healthy has the best of both worlds; deep emotional satisfaction, and the freedom to be oneself.

When one is faced with a relatively healthy, open person who may be a Natrum, asking about what they were like previously often reveals more typical Natrum characteristics, since many Natrum individuals become more healthy with time. Also, asking what they would most like to change about themselves if they could can be very useful. Many people who are relatively healthy emotionally know where their emotional 'blind-spots' are, and will surprise the homeopath by replying to this question with a typical Natrum weakness.

### Conclusion

Natrum is the dominant constitutional type in the world today (I have found that in underprivileged areas up to eighty percent of people are Natrums, presumably because hardship generates emotionally suppressed people). It is so common that the homeopath is faced with a great breadth of expression of Natrum characteristics, and this variety of Natrum personalities may appear confusing and daunting at first sight. Nevertheless, familiarisation with all the different expressions of the Natrum constitution is the only way a homeopath can avoid missing the correct prescription for a great many of his patients. In order to make the study of the Natrum psyche a little less daunting, I have decided to list the principal Natrum characteristics we have already examined.

### Natrum Characteristics

Inability to let go of emotions, to let go of loved ones
Fear of expressing emotion, of losing loved ones, of rejection, of appearing

219

foolish, of losing control, of spiders and/or snakes, of death
Aversion to affection, sympathy, to talking about one's feelings
Tendency to grief and depression
Difficulty in crying
Controlled speech and actions
Need to please people
Guilt
Anorexia nervosa, Bulimia
Tendency to put parents on a pedestal
Avoidance of feelings by:
    retreating into the intellect
    smiling and laughing
    joking and clowning
    abusing food, alcohol and drugs
    keeping busy
    looking after other people
    being a perfectionist
    dramatising emotions
    positive thinking
Fascination with matters psychic
Difficulty in receiving
Rebellion
Cynicism
Appearances very important
Easily moved to tears
Premenstrual, post-natal and post-menopausal depression/irritability
Claustrophobia
Sentimentality
Low self-esteem with sense of worthlessness
Self-neglect and tendency to apologise
Panic attacks
Moral and religious evangelism
Intellectual pride

### Positive Qualities
High morals
Nurturing
Love of children and animals
Sympathetic
Sensitivity
Integrity
Conscience (e.g. social, ecological)

Organised and efficient
Charitable
Cooperative
Sense of humour
Diplomatic

### Some Natrum Types

The clingy child
The workaholic
The aloof child
The alcoholic
The cold parent
The counsellor
The smothering parent
The clown
The perfectionist
The hermit
The victim/martyr
The evangelist
The rebel
The codependent
The positive thinker
The bully
The 'gushing' Natrum
The vamp
The snob and society actress
The strong, silent type

### Physical Appearance

There are as many different Natrum appearances as there are Natrum sub-types. However, here are a few of the commoner features:

fleshy face, with smallish eyes (due to 'full' surrounding tissues)
bloated appearance to face (e.g. the older Elvis Presley)
perfect face and perfect complexion (e.g. many models)
short, fleshy nose
full lips
very thin lips if shut down emotionally
the very obese Natrum
the very skinny Natrum
acne and facial and bodily hair in women
broad, rounded face
'bullish' appearance of heavy, physical Natrum (e.g. many rugby players)

broad, high forehead of intellectual Natrum, often with balding (intellectual Lycopodiums usually have a narrower face).

the fixed smile

large hips in women

heavily built men

All complexions are seen, but dark complexions are most common.

The constitution is seen slightly more often in women than in men (due to the large number of men who are Lycopodium).

## *A Note About Psychotherapy*

Several times during this analysis of Natrum Muriaticum I have referred to 'deep psychotherapy'. Many Natrum people would benefit from the kind of psychotherapy which can help them to contact, re-experience and then let go of suppressed emotions. Unfortunately, very few psychotherapists work sufficiently deeply to allow this to fully take place. Most psychotherapy is talking therapy, and whilst this helps to some extent, it tends to keep the patient in his head, rather than his emotions. Natrums are usually very good at avoiding emotions by staying in their heads. I have found that primal therapy is the deepest form of psychotherapy available, and it is especially effective in Natrum individuals (who can be made to feel relatively easily). Other relatively deep psychotherapy techniques include breathwork, Hakomi, Reichian therapy, Gestalt and Psychodrama.

# Natrum Sulphuricum

*Keynote:* The fiery Natrum

Natrum Sulphuricum is not nearly as common as its Muriaticum sister, being about as common as Natrum Carbonicum. Whereas the latter is an 'earthy' Natrum, who is pragmatic and unimaginative, Natrum Sulphuricum possesses all the fiery attributes of Sulphur, but in a quieter way, since they are wedded to the introverted emotionality of the Natrums, and also because Natrum Sulphuricum is primarily a female type.

## The Inspired Natrum

The addition of Sulphur to the Sodium atom adds fire to Natrum, and this fire is often expressed as inspired passion. I have seen Natrum Sulphuricum individuals who were passionate in an intellectual way about homeopathy, rather as Sulphur might be, and also quieter examples of the type who possessed the assurance of unshakeable spiritual faith. Both intellectual inspiration and spiritual faith are aspects of the fire element, the element of passion, and both are to be found more frequently in the Sulphuricum individual than in the Muriaticum. There are passionate and inspired Muriaticums, and these can be difficult to distinguish from Sulphuricums, but having said that, I do feel there is a difference in the 'flavour' of the Muriaticum passion compared to the Sulphuricum passion. Fire is an impersonal element (which is why Sulphur men may feel that they love everyone, and yet they may neglect their family), whereas water is the most personal of elements, since it is concerned with personal emotion. A Natrum Muriaticum woman who is passionate tends to be less objective and more emotional in her attachment to whatever she is passionate about, when compared to the Sulphuricum. The Muriaticum woman, for example, may enthuse about the practice of Reiki healing in a very inspired manner, but there will usually be a personal need expressed in her enthusiasm which the skilled observer can detect. She needs you to agree with her. Her emotional security is intimately bound up with her passion. In contrast, Sulphur will enthuse without any sense of the personal, and if you do not agree with him, he will not be hurt in the slightest. Natrum Sulphuricum lies somewhere in between, since she is both a sensitive, watery Natrum and a fiery Sulphuricum. The Muriaticum who has a strong sense of faith in the Almighty to guide her has generally had to struggle harder to establish her faith than the Sulphuricum, since faith is a fiery quality, and thus comes more naturally to the latter. Furthermore, the emotional watery element actually encourages doubt and fear, and thus must be overcome to a certain extent before true faith can dawn. There is often a certain compensation for doubt that the Muriatucum uses, in the form of positive thinking , which gives her passion an emotional intensity greater than that of the Sulphuricum. Several Natrum Sulphuricum patients I have treated had a quiet unshakeabke faith in God and their spiritual destiny, which was all the more convincing for its quietness.

### The Caretaker

One might expect a fiery Natrum to be less patient than a watery one, and also more selfish. I have come across relatively self-obsessed intellectually inspired Natrum Sulphuricum women, but I have also come across the opposite; quiet long suffering Sulphuricum women who were dedicated carers. Here the fire element is still present, but instead of expressing itself as ego, it is expressed as fortitude and a spiritual affinity for service. I remember one such lady who I treated for bronchiectasis (a condition which nearly always requires Natrum Sulphuricum constitutionally). She was tall and slim, with broad shoulders and hips, and a squareish face which gave the impression of a serious intelligence. Her manner was modest but confident (water and fire), her intellect sharp and yet not used in any formal way in her life. She had spent the best part of her life looking after her ailing mother, and yet I caught no trace of either regret or weakness in her presence. It was as if she were born for this service, equipped with sufficient patience, love and fortitude to see it through without resentment. She also bore her own chronic illness stoically, without complaint. When I asked her if she suffered from depression, she said, 'Not really depression, but a kind of melancholy which is almost poetic, which sweeps over me from time to time'. Natrum Sulphuricum is said in the old materia medicas to be prone to experiencing 'sadness from music'. I imagine this is a reference to this soft and gentle kind of melancholy referred to by my patient, one that is reminiscent of the whimsical sadness to which Sulphur is prone.

Whilst I worked at the Royal London Homeopathic Hospital we would occasionally admit a lady for treatment of flare-ups of her ulcerative colitis and bronchiectasis. Both of these serious conditions tended to flare together. She was a very thin lady, on account of her bowel condition, and she had to endure a great deal of suffering year in and year out. What impressed me was that she was always cheerful in the hospital. She seemed to enjoy her stay there despite the seriousness of her condition, and she would have a friendly word to say to anyone who spoke to her. Her good cheer was quieter than that of a Phosphorus, or a Natrum Muriaticum who was seeking to put on a bright face, but it was consistent and convincing. She would always improve physically after a week or two of Natrum Sulphuricum 30c. It appears that cheerful stoicism is a part of the Natrum Sulphuricum clinical picture. It is sometimes seen also in Natrum Muriaticum individuals, but more often the latter are either dourly stoic, or they put on a false cheerfulness to disguise their suffgering.

## Manic Depression

I have come across several patients whose manic depressive illness responded to Natrum Sulphuricum. It is not surprising that the Sulphuricum is prone to this mysterious illness, since it is a split ilness, characterised by depression on the one hand (Natrum, water) and mania on the other (Sulphur, fire). The depressive phase may be just as intense as any Muriaticum depression, and hard to distinguish from the latter. In the manic phase I have noticed that the Natrum Sulphuricum individual has pressure of thoughts, but that these thoughts tend to dwell on the past. Thus there is a speeding up of thoughts, which crowd in upon each other (the energy of fire), and the focus on the past that is characteristic of water. Obsessive thoughts are liable to occur in the manic phase, especially involving regret, and unrealistic romantic desire. One woman came to see me for treatment of manic depression. During the manic phase she was obsessed with romantic longing for a doctor she had worked with twenty years before. She had had to cut short her nursing career at that time because she had become unstable emotionally, and obsessed with this man, entertaining delusions that he loved her. I treated her with Natrum Sulphuricum 10M monthly, which produced an immediate aggravation of manic syptoms, followed by a gradual decline in both the depressive and manic phases. The Sulphur element seems to add an obsessive quality to Natrum's depression, which should not surprise us, since Sulphur is such an obsessive type.

I have not found suicidal impulses to be any more common in the Sulphuricum than in the Muriaticum, but they certainly do occur. George Vithoulkas says that the Natrum Sulphuricum individual resists suicide on account of his strong sense of duty to his family, and I have seen this in some of my Sulphuricum patients. Many others experienced gentle melancholy without any suicidal thoughts.

Despite the differences mentioned between the Sulphuricum and the Muriaticum, the choice is sometimes a difficult one for the homeopath, since there is such a lot of common ground both physically and emotionally. Like the Muriaticum, the Sulphuricum is quite a sensitive, emotional person, with a strong sense of values. She tends to be more emotionally open than former, but less intense, since there is less supressed emotion behind her self-expression. Many common features can be seen, such as claustrophobia, stoicism, and also self-reproach in the more depressive Sulphuricums. I often find that in difficult cases the physicals and generals help a great deal in the differentiation. In this regard, Natrum Sulphuricum tends to be more sensitive to the heat, and far more universally aggravated by wet or humid weather. There is also often a history of repeated bouts of diarrhoea.

### *Physical Appearance*
Natrum Sulphuricum tends to have a more angular face and physique than her Muriaticum counterparts. The face tends to be quite broad, and the eyes appear more open than those of the Muriaticum. The physique may be either broad or delicate, but is seldom as rounded as that of many Muriaticums, and is often light and thin.

# Nux Vomica

*Keynote:* The conqueror

Nux is a fascinating and relatively uncommon type, whose character is far more rich and interesting than one might gather from reading the old materia medicas, which concentrate principally upon anger and irritability. This is unfortunate, not only because it results in homeopaths missing a great many Nux patients, but also because it underestimates the Nux individual, who generally has just as many positive as negative traits.

The most universal and fundamental aspect of Nux' character is a love of power, and an ability to acquire power and exercise it with confidence. Virtually all Nux people are powerful individuals, except those who have been crushed by severe adversity (it takes a lot to crush a Nux), and those who have exhausted themselves. Nux is more at home with power than any other type; in fact, he cannot be happy without it. It is his nature to rule, and he does so with assurance, and also quite often with magnanimity.

I have chosen six characters or 'archetypes' to represent the various qualities that characterise Nux psychologically. Most Nux people are a composite of all of these 'archetypes', but one will usually predominate.

## The Warrior

The true warrior is a Nux Vomica, and all Nux people have something of the warrior in their blood. Success is not enough for Nux. It is winning that gives meaning to his life, and at the moment of conquest he experiences his sweetest pleasure. After a victory, Nux does not rest on his laurels. He is quick to consolidate his power, and to seek new battles to fight, and new territory to conquer.

There are few true warriors today. The term warrior implies far more than a mere fighter or soldier, and it is these extra qualities that set Nux apart from the rest. The warrior is not only skilled in the arts of warfare; he is also fearless, extremely agile in mind and body, and in some sense noble. The Natrum and the Kali soldier may fight dutifully for their country, but they will be glad when the war is over, and they can get back to the security of their family. The Nux warrior, on the other hand, relishes the fight, and feels restless during peacetime. Shakespeare paints a perfect portrait of the Nux warrior in the character of Hotspur, the fiery noble in 'Henry IV Part 1' who betrays the King at the end of the play. During peacetime Hotspur thinks of nothing but the next battle, even during his sleep—(Lady Percy: "In thy faint slumbers, I by thee have watched, and heard thee murmur tales of iron wars.")

The Nux warrior is in control of his own destiny, and will not follow orders from any, except another Nux warrior whose skill and experience exceed his own. If he is part of a regiment, he will grit his teeth when he has to obey a command he disagrees with, and will rise to the top as quickly as possible, from whence he is answerable to nobody (Kent: 'Aversion to answer'—this applies not only to Nux' aversion to being interrupted, but also to his refusal to be questioned about the merits of his actions). Nux is extremely pragmatic, and tends to be very thorough in the things he does (Kent: 'Carefulness'), unlike Sulphur, who is often a mere theoretician. The Nux commander is the toughest and most capable member of his regiment. He leads from the front (or at least he used to), and would not wish it any other way.

Nux is so self-confident, and sure of his own powers, that he tends to ignore rules and regulations (unlike Arsenicum and Natrum, two other very thorough types). In any situation, Nux tends to feel in charge, and hence he regards outside rules as an affront to his natural authority. As a result of this, the Nux warrior is a maverick. He follows his own rules, and because he is so skilful and so courageous, he tends to succeed. The Nux maverick is encapsulated beautifully by the actor Clint Eastwood, and the characters he plays on the screen. Whether he be a high plains drifter, who dominates a township with his silent power, or a New York cop, Eastwood's characters do it their own way, and they always succeed. Whilst this is in part due to the script-writer, it is also a faithful portrait of the Nux warrior, who very seldom loses. Another good example of the Nux warrior is Muhammed Ali, the former heavyweight boxing champion. Unlike many of his opponents, who were heavy and lumbering, Ali 'floated like a butterfly, and stung like a bee'. His speed and agility was graceful, and mesmerised his bewildered opponents. In true Nux fashion, Ali never missed an opportunity to advertise his broad, clean good looks, and in the ring he glorified his own power, saying 'I am the greatest!', and daring his opponent to call him by his former name of Cassius Clay. Unlike dour Natrum heavyweights, the Nux warrior is like a cheetah, as graceful as he is swift and deadly.

Unlike Natrum, the Nux warrior does not fight out of bitterness, but rather because it is his role in life - it is what he does best and enjoys most. Once he has an opponent in his sights, he is totally one-pointed about defeating them, but once they are defeated, he will bear them no malice (unless the fight happened to be a grudge-fight to start with). Nux has the greatest respect for a strong opponent; the kind of respect that opposing ace pilots had for each other during the world wars, or that generals would show toward their captured enemy officers. If you cross Nux, he will either ignore you because you are small fry (Kent: 'Contemptuous'), or swiftly defeat you, with his razor sharp wit if not more tangibly. Once he has defeated you, he will forget about you, or even become your friend if he finds you interesting. It is the victory that Nux must have. He is not usually a sadist, once he has defeated his opponent.

The Nux warrior has little time for gentle pursuits such as art and romance. As the warlike Hotspur puts it; "This is no world to play with mammets (variously translated as puppets and breasts) and to tilt with lips. We must have bloody noses and cracked crowns, and pass them current too." He will not let others dissuade him from his course, and is liable to get angry if his serious business is interrupted by 'triflers'. Hotspur refuses to hand over an important prisoner of war to an emissary from the King. Later he explains to the King; "I remember when the fight was done, and I was dry with rage and extreme toil, came there a certain lord, neat, trimly dress'd, fresh as a bridegroom,...He was perfumed like a milliner, and twixt his finger and his thumb he held a pouncet box, which ever and anon he gave his nose, and took't away again. With many holiday and lady terms he questioned me; I, then all smarting with my wounds being cold, to be so pester'd with a popinjay, answer'd neglectingly, I know not what." (Kent: 'Anger with indignation').

The Nux warrior has a simplicity that is refreshing, and is shared to a great degree by most Nux individuals. To him life consists of conquest and its enjoyment. There is no need for such complications as philosophy and morality. He leaves such distractions to politicians and sophists, who he detests, because they are cowards and they lie. The Nux warrior is very forthright in his speech. He speaks his truth without regard for the feelings of other people (Kent: 'Indiscretion'), which is very attractive to some, and very threatening to others, particularly those who like to pretend they are something other than what they are. When the great Welsh commander Owen Glendower boasts to Hotspur in typical Sulphur fashion that that he can teach him to summon the Devil, Hotspur replies; "And I can teach thee, coz, to shame the Devil, by telling truth." There is nothing Nux enjoys more than bursting the bubble of another's arrogance. A particularly arrogant doctor once had dinner with a Nux friend of mine. The doctor made fun of my friend's red Porsche, suggesting it was a phallic symbol. My Nux friend calmly replied "I know why you don't have a Porsche. You're too fat to get into one."

I am sure that virtually all great military generals are Nux Vomica. Few other types have got what it takes. Men like Ghengis Khan and Alexander the Great exemplify the greatness of the Nux warrior. Not only were they brilliant military strategists, they were also utterly determined, and so hungry for power that they continued expanding their empires until they could no longer hold them. If the Nux warrior has a weakness, it is this, that he will eventually over-extend himself in his pursuit of power.

The average Nux individual ('average' does not sit easily upon Nux' shoulders) is also something of a strategist. Whether he is pursuing a pretty woman, or a company takeover, he will plan his moves with utmost precision, and when the right time comes he will strike without hesitation. Natrum and Arsenicum may have the precision of Nux, and Arsenicum can be just as crafty, but neither has the iron will that ensures Nux his success. When Nux does succeed, he shouts with the exhilaration of victory, his fists raised in defiance and self-glorification.

The Nux warrior is not only the bullet that penetrates, but also the powder that supplies the power. Nux has enormous reserves of energy, which enable him to fight on without flagging until the battle is won. This energy is in part a result of his physical strength and fitness, in part a perpetual creation of his endless determination. Most Nux individuals lead lives so hectic that they exhaust those around them. They may think nothing of working for twelve hours, and then demolishing a squash opponent or two, before going out to eat. Then on to a nightclub for drinks, before retiring exhausted but exhilarated. In order to sustain this lifestyle a good many Nux individuals invest time regularly in keeping fit. Many Nux individuals enjoy brisk physical activities such as squash and skiing, and pursue them with the same determination and enthusiasm that they pursue their careers with. I remember one Nux doctor who would swim a few miles each day at great speed, in preparation for his skiing holiday. This was not the dour stoicism of Aurum and Natrum, but simple practicality. The fitter he was, the longer and more aggressively he could ski on the slopes. In typical Nux style, he preferred to be dropped off by helicopter on the top of inaccessible mountains, and to battle his way down through virgin snow. The more sedate challenges of the piste were for softer mortals than he. Also in typical Nux style, he excelled at numerous different sports, and indeed at anything he put his attention to. His wife said it was like being married to superman.

There is a warrior trying to get out of even the mildest of Nux individuals. Those Nux people who have not yet established a power-base for themselves have a habit of fantasising about fighting glorious battles. One Nux patient told me that he had always had a fantasy about beating up a pack of thugs single handedly. He was not a very physical Nux, being more cerebral in his interests. It was this fantasy that hinted at the warrior in him, itching to get out from behind the intellectual exterior. Nux admires strength, and the young Nux in particular will model himself on other powerful Nux figures, such as his successful Nux father, and glamorous fighters like Clint Eastwood characters and historical generals.

## The Knight

Not all Nux warriors are ruthless. Many follow a code of honour, and love to defend the weak. The legendary Robin Hood is a fine example, as are the Knights of King Arthur's Round Table. Like most other powerful figures, true Knights tend to be either Sulphur or Nux individuals. The Nux knight is not quite as idealistic as his Sulphur counterpart, but he will defend his honour, and the honour of his King and his Lady to the death. (Hotspur: "From this nettle, Danger, I pluck this flower, Honour.")

The Knight represents all that is most noble about Nux. There are no Knights in armour anymore, but there are still a good many Nux Knights fighting to defend the weak. The noble Nux cannot bear a bully, and since he is powerful as well as noble, he enjoys standing up to oppressors. My Nux schoolfriend was forever standing between the class bully (who was a Natrum rebel) and a couple of the class 'weeds'. He never did fight the bully, but his steely glare was always enough to make the latter back off.

Every Nux man is a Knight to his partner and his children. Although he may be obsessed at times with his work, he is a pillar of strength to his family, and he will defend them to the ends of the earth. He may agree with equality for women, but he knows that men and women are different, and that the man's role involves protecting his family, and providing for them. There is still something of the caveman hunter in Nux. He may drag his women into his cave by the hair (metaphorically speaking), but he will defend her and his brood against all dangers. The greater the threat against his family, the more courage Nux finds inside, a courage that consists of rage in addition to Nux' usual determination.

I am reminded of a distant Nux relative, who told me once of a battle he had fought in a hotel. He was staying with his wife at a hotel, when they were disturbed in the night by the drunken revelry of a group of men in the next room. His wife had a headache, so he went next door and complained about the noise. He was wearing only a towel around his waist. Not surprisingly, he received only abuse from his drunken neighbours, one of whom he punched in the face. He was then set upon by several of these men, and fled down the corridor, pausing momentarily to yell to his wife to keep her door locked. The drunks chased him naked up stairways until he had reached the top floor and could run no further. Here he put his back to the wall and proceeded to defend himself. For about five minutes he fought with one assailant after another, repelling each attack with a karate style blow from his hands or feet. Eventually he found a fire alarm button and pressed it, and was rescued by the police, but not before he had bloodied the faces of his assailants, and left a couple lifeless on the floor. Being a Nux, he was very proud of this victory, and he clearly revelled in describing it to me, although he retained a certain nonchalance in his voice, as if to say "It was nothing really." Nux is more likely to get into such situations than any other type, since he will not tolerate abuse to himself or his family, and will often defend an innocent victim of street violence. He prefers to take the law into his own hands, than to rely on the cumbersome and unpredictable justice of the legal system.

The Knight is generally a lot more courteous than other Nux warriors. Though never fawning, he treats people with respect, and he is especially courteous towards women (There are few Nux women, but the ones I have come across do not fit the Knight 'archetype'). It is hard to say when courtesy towards the opposite sex ceases to be honourable in intention, and becomes a means of attraction and conquest. Most Nux men love women in general, (although they may be quite chauvinistic in their love), and although the Knight is somewhat purer in his attitude towards women than the others, he still wants to win an attractive woman's favour, even if he is married and has no intention of jumping into bed with her. A great many Nux men have handsome, chiselled looks (e.g. Clint Eastwood), and when these are combined with charm and a penetrating look, the combination can be irresistible to a great many women. Most Nux people are charismatic. They exude personal magnetism, which derives both from their strength and their natural grace. The Knight is particularly charismatic since he possesses all the strength of a diamond, but has polished the rough edges that often make Nux appear abrasive. Like the Eastern martial arts Master, he has a great sense of balance within. The knight is the most graceful and gracious of Nux individuals. He may have none of the temper that Nux is so famous for, and this may confuse the homeopath into giving him a more 'sanguine' remedy like Sulphur or Lycopodium.

The Knight can even be confused with the Causticum reformer. Both are very open types, who appear forthright and courageous, and both like to stand up for those weaker than themselves. The Knight, for all his gallantry, is still very pragmatic, unlike many Causticums, who dream fantastic dreams of overturning prejudice. Whilst Causticum will apply himself to large-scale projects to alleviate suffering and right wrongs, the Knight will intervene in cases of individual strife which come to his attention, indignant at the sight of bullying and cruelty, but afterwards he will get on with his own life, whereas Causticum tends to remain caught up with his 'mission'. Hero figures like Batman and Superman are based on the Nux Knight. They are practical people, who intervene in individual cases, not reformers who try to change the political and social system.

The Knight is the more spiritual pole of the Nux personality. Many homeopaths do not consider that Nux can be a spiritual person, but I have known quite a few spiritually orientated Nux individuals. Nux always aims for the top, and to some Nux people the top is perfect equanimity of mind and body, a spiritual state of great stillness and integrity. The spiritual Nux individual pursues his loftier goal with the same one-pointedness that others pursue wealth and temporal power. He will spend long hours in meditation, directing his attention within just as skilfully as a general directs his attention to the battle, and in his early years of practice, he will be just as annoyed as the general when he is interrupted. When he does achieve his goal of equanimity, or gets close, he will loosen up and start to enjoy the physical world more again, this time from a stiller, wider perspective. The tradition of the disciple eventually becoming the master is well suited to the spiritual Nux individual, who is willing to kneel at the feet of one greater than himself, but only so that he may achieve that greatness. Nux is never prepared to remain a follower forever.

### The Emperor

Leadership is what Nux was born for. Just as some Kings are noble, whilst others are tyrants, so it is with the Nux leader. Both types have their hands very firmly on the controls, and know exactly what they are doing.

I once knew a father and son (both Nux) who had achieved positions of authority. The father exemplified the ruthless tyrant, whilst the son was a firm but fair ruler of his company. The two got on remarkably well, with the son respecting his father's strength and the fact that he worked his way up from the gutter to become a millionaire, but choosing to dispense with his father's more heartless tactics. This couple illustrates very clearly the closeness of the two types of Nux ruler. It was because the father had had a very tough childhood that he became a ruthless businessman, whereas the son had his opportunity handed to him by his father. He had not needed to struggle, or to use deceit and blackmail to gain his position, and hence he was a likeable and reasonable boss. He was still his father's son, and would fire an employee without hesitation if he did not do his job, but unlike his father, he did not stab people in the back.

The Nux ruler who has clawed his way up from the bottom is the most formidable despot (Kent's omission of Nux from the rubric 'dictatorial' is most strange. It belongs here in black type.) He must have his own way in all things, and he translates the term 'compromise' to 'weakness'. This kind of Nux is really more of an emperor than a king. He is continually bent on expanding his empire, and will resort to both trickery and force to do so. The Nux father I was referring to made his business empire single-handedly, beginning as a mere clerk in a travel agency. During his meteoric rise to power he trampled on a good many people who stood in his way. His daughter told me that her father made sure he always 'had something' on anyone he wanted to influence. In other words, he blackmailed them. He did this just as ruthlessly at home as in business. If his daughter refused to indulge one of his wishes, he would threaten to have her horse sold, and worse still, he compared her unfavourably with the daughter of his mistress. In business he knew everything about everybody. Even less ruthless Nux people tend to be very well connected, and use their connections to gain influence, and avoid censure, but the Nux tyrant also uses his information to hold both opponents and underlings to ransom. Such people never do anything that appears generous without having an ulterior motive, and that motive usually involves increasing their own power, pleasure, or immunity from prosecution.

I remember the first time I met the ruthless Nux father of the more reasonable Nux son. I had heard all about his ruthlessness, but I had also been warned that he was so charming that I would like him. I considered myself a better judge of character than this, but sure enough, before dinner was half eaten I was falling under the man's charm. His wit was sharp, his knowledge was extensive and diverse, and his manner gracious. I never did doubt the reputation he had for ruthlessness, but I enjoyed the evening.

So many tyrants have a smooth, charming exterior. They remain in power partly because others are afraid of them, and partly because they are able to fool the masses into thinking that they have their interests at heart. (The great psychoanalyst Carl Jung was quite charmed by his first encounter with the Italian dictator Mussolini. He wrote of the latter's buoyancy and sheer physical magnetism, which he contrasted with the shadowy impression he received from Adolf Hitler, whose meeting with Mussolini he observed from a distance. I suspect this contrast is reflection of the differences between sane Nux dictators like Mussolini, and insane Stramonium or Veratrum dictators like Hitler.)

Like other Nux types, the Emperor is a pragmatic man. If he is a business man, he knows exactly when to buy and when to sell. He knows which luxury car to buy, and which doctors will perform an abortion with no questions asked. He is supremely in control of his life, and he will only delegate small portions of his responsibility, and then only to his most trusted accomplices (who are very often relatives. Nux tends to have a clan mentality, looking after and trusting his own). There are many examples of the Nux Emperor that come to mind. Mafia bosses are clear examples, with their respectable fronts, and their reliance on terror to run the show. Governing dictators are usually Nux, as are the heads of multi-national companies. Media tycoons are often Nux. Their lust for power impels them to take over more and more media enterprises, which they can use not only to influence the voting public, but also the politicians, with whom they are mutually dependent. Only a Nux tycoon could get away with paying ten cents income tax in the dollar.

### The King
I have called the more benign Nux ruler the King, in contrast to the rapa-

cious Emperor. The king enjoys his power, and is very efficient at ruling over his dominion, but he is not without a heart, and he generally makes a fair and even kind boss. The Nux son I mentioned earlier was such a man. He was respected by the (generally much older) workers under him, not only because he was fair, but also because he could do the job of any one of them. Whilst his father was grooming him for the job of director of a large factory, he made himself learn every job on the shop floor. That way, when he came to take over at the tender age of twenty three he could take control like a far more experienced man, and he knew when any one of his employees tried to pull the wool over his eyes. His foreman, a man twice his age who had worked for his father, told me that although he was fairer, he was just as firm as his father. The Nux King may not need to amass the enormous wealth or influence that the Emperor needs to feel satisfied, but he remains very much in control of his kingdom.

The King is far more healthy emotionally than the Emperor. He may still be a little too obsessed with his work, but he makes sure he finds time to stay close to his family. At work he is often rather stern and officious, but he has enough insight to catch himself being so, and will soften a little. At home he is usually benign and playful. Like the lion relaxing with his cubs after a day's hunting, Nux will often relish his home life, and the opportunity it provides for warmth and relaxation. He is still the King at home, but he is happy to leave the domestic decisions to his Queen. She doesn't tell him how to do his work, and in most cases, he allows her to run the home. (He made sure he married a woman who would provide a stable, supportive home life.)

Many politicians belong to the King sub-type of Nux, particularly the more dynamic and successful ones. They rise quickly to prominence, and whilst they are careful to retain the trust of their superiors, they often have their sights set on the top job. There is nothing so entertaining to the public as a gladitorial contest between rival Nux politicians, especially two from the same party. At such times Nux will use all his powers of leverage, appealing to the loyalty of some, and the fears of others. When he gains power he will not forget his friends, nor for that matter will he forgive his enemies. The King may be more benign than the Emperor, but there is really a continuum between the two, and it is a rare Nux leader who forgives his previous enemies before he has first put them in their place.

Margaret Thatcher, the former British Prime Minister, is an excellent example of the Nux King (or Queen), albeit one who leans at times towards the Emperor. Only a Nux woman could lead a party dominated by men, and not only lead them, but inspire in them a mixture of fear, respect, and motivation. In typical Nux fashion Mrs Thatcher ruled autocratically. In fact she was the most autocratic Prime Minister Britain had seen this century. Supporters were rewarded, but criticism was not tolerated (Kent: 'Anger from contradiction'), and by her third term in office she had dismissed virtually all of her original cabinet ministers, retaining only the most acquiescent of them. Despite her uncompromising style (or perhaps because of it), Mrs Thatcher remained extremely popular with her electorate for a decade. Many people did not like her, but they respected her, and recognised that few other leaders would have had the courage to take on the monolithic British labour unions and break their domination of the labour structure. Like most Nux rulers, Mrs Thatcher did not know the meaning of the word 'consensus'. She knew that she was right and saw no reason why she should listen to other opinions. In a sense the Nux ruler is more suited to a one-party system, where he can get on with the job without worrying about his popularity. Sadly, such systems tend to produce the most ruthless of all Nux leaders.

Mrs Thatcher exhibited a good many attributes of the Nux King figure. She had a great deal of respect for individual liberty, and the principal of promotion according to individual merit. Nux is a very independent type, and just as he cannot abide interference from others in his own affairs, he expects others to do likewise. Few Nux individuals have time for the welfare system. They may recognise a need for it, but they resent the dependence and passivity it generates, and the abuse it is subject to. (I am reminded here of Norman 'on your bike' Tebbit, one of the few of Mrs Thatcher's ministers who was strong enough and 'dry' enough to win her respect. His famous comment that unemployed people should get on their bikes and travel further in their search for work had a distinctly Nux ring to it.)

Another of Thatcher's typically Nux attributes was her tendency to speak bluntly, dispensing with the usual diplomatic niceties. She called a spade a spade, and this endeared her to a good many people, but it also gave her a tough, uncaring image which she spent millions trying to soften, by employing the best advertising consultants and public relations officers, who took the hard edges off both her voice and her hairstyle.

Nux leaders are quick to recognise talent. They tend to cultivate proteges, for several reasons. Firstly, it is a pleasure for them to work with someone with as much courage and skill as themselves. It is lonely at the top, and a protege is good company (especially another Nux). Secondly, they could only entrust the result of their labours to somebody they had schooled to look after it with the same zeal as themselves, and thirdly, such a protege acts as an extension of themselves, and all of their power into the future. Nux cannot bear the thought of having no heir, nobody to look after the dynasty.

Those Nux people who do not find public prominence usually do manage to carve out for themselves a position of some authority. I once knew a natural therapy practitioner who had retrained after being an officer in the Navy. He ran his clinic along the lines of a ship's captain, issuing orders to his crew of receptionists, picking them up for every little inefficiency or mistake. When he gave me a tour of his clinic, he went to great lengths to advertise his new and impressive equipment. He then gave me a little speech on the dreadful lack of recognition that his specialty suffered from, and the wonderful results that he achieved. Like many Nux people he was a great self-publicist. This tendency is especially common in those Nux individuals who are still in the early days of setting up their power-base. Once they have achieved this, their self-congratulation becomes more subtle. He eventually sought treatment for nervous tension, which gave him indigestion, and he responded very quickly to Nux Vomica.

The strict boss may belong to one of a variety of constitutional types. Arsenicum is the one most likely to be confused with Nux. Both types are very keen on efficiency, and tend to be tight with money, and both have a need to present an impressive appearance to the public, although Arsenic is more particular about the details of this public image, and unlike Nux is just as fastidious in private. The principal difference between the two is the degree of confidence with which he runs the establishment. Arsenicum often gives the appearance of confidence, but he worries far more than Nux, and this makes his confident exterior a little 'brittle'. It can be made to look shaky by adverse circumstances rather more quickly than that of Nux, who usually has great faith in himself. Both types can become very irritable with employees who fall below their standards, but Nux finds it easier to fire people than Arsenicum. (The Natrum boss may also be exacting. Many Natrums are both perfectionists and workaholics, and some apply their high standards to their employees. Other Natrum bosses are angry types who take out their aggression on their employees, just as some angry Nux and Arsenicum bosses do.)

Unlike Arsenicum, Nux is quite capable of double standards. Since he feels like a king, he tends to expect others to do as he says, not what he does. He is the least liable of the three types to be held back by principles and scruples.

Nux is most naturally suited to leadership, and he appears more calmly assured in the role than other leaders, the exception being Sulphur, who is the other natural leader. Although Nux is scratchy when things do not go well, he tends to be far more buoyant and cheerful than Arsenicum and Natrum when things are running smoothly. Nux thrives on success, and the Nux boss will often be found humming to himself and being mischievous with his staff during the good times. He is a sociable type, and particularly enjoys intelligent, confident company, and also those he considers sexy. He can be the most pleasant of bosses when happy, and the most intimidating when displeased.

The Nux ruler is often magnanimous as long as his position is not threatened. When it is threatened he can be both petty and vindictive. Furthermore, Nux has a tendency to become paranoid with respect to competition

(Kent: 'Imagines being persecuted'). Although he is very successful and established, he may get edgy when a younger and less experienced competitor arrives on the scene, even though his position may be entirely secure. His irrational anxiety may soon turn to anger, when it is expressed as an obsessive attempt to undermine the newcomer. Nux may go to great lengths to blacken the name of his 'competitor' (Kent: 'Jealousy', 'Disposition to slander'), whilst all the time pretending that he is not perturbed. These paranoid antics are in stark contrast to the calm assurance with which Nux normally goes about his business, and reveal the vulnerable underbelly of the King.

I once witnessed such a reaction in a hospital where I was working. One of my colleagues was a 'golden boy', a young Nux doctor who not only knew far more about medicine than his superiors, but was also charming and in possession of chiselled good looks. He was discreet in the way he applied his superior knowledge. On the ward round he would express a clinical opinion quietly but firmly, and the consultant would invariably adopt this opinion as his own, confirming it with a grave nod of the head. This was all well and good, since my Nux colleague's knowledge really was first rate. However, I saw a different side to my normally affable colleague when he acquired a new junior doctor on his team. The latter was probably a Nux himself, since he tended to question his superior a lot, and was indignant when he was not answered, or worse, received a condescending reply. He questioned a lot because he was keen to learn, but my Nux colleague interpreted his behaviour as insolence, and proceeded over the next few weeks to systematically persecute him, criticising his every remark, and publicly humiliating him. When it came to the time for the new doctor to renew his contract, his Nux superior put in a few bad words for him, and his contract was severed. I was amazed at the transformation in my Nux friend, until I realised that he was a Nux, and felt both threatened and furious with the questioning of his bright young junior. Nux enjoys competition in sports and other games, but at work where the stakes are higher, he can be very heavy handed in protecting his position of supremacy. (I am reminded of the habit of Mafia bosses to eliminate any underlings who show the slightest tendency towards thinking for themselves.)

Unlike the Lycopodium strutter, whose pride is a rather obvious reaction to an inferiority complex, Nux tends to have a more convincing air of superiority. (Arsenicum lies somewhere in between, sometimes resembling the strutter, and sometimes appearing genuinely aristocratic.) The experienced observer can spot Nux from the way he holds himself. Like a true King, his proud bearing is relaxed rather than stiff, (cf. Lycopodium and Arsenicum). His gait is either a confident stride, with head held rather high, and eyes fixed in front, oblivious to the various distractions in the street, or a relaxed lope.

The lope is very characteristic of Nux (and also of Sulphur, whose pride is equally natural). It is a very casual, very confident gait, which is often seen in tall Nux individuals. The best example is the on-screen lope of the Clint Eastwood gunslinger, who wanders round a new town as if he owns it. Note how both shoulders and hips swing effortlessly as he walks, and how the confident Nux gunslinger looks as if he has all the time in the world. He is the best and he knows it, and as such he feels he has the right to say and do exactly as he pleases. A great many Nux individuals behave like this, and it earns them both admiration and a reputation for arrogance and anti-social behaviour.

In keeping with his kingly persona, Nux tends to have the attitude that only the best is good enough for him, and if for some reason he can't afford the best, he usually knows somebody who can help out, or else he will buy now and pay later. After all, his abundant skills and his effortless self-promotion ensure him a profitable future, or so he reckons, and he is usually right. (A good example is the Nux entrepreneur who actually owes more millions than he earns. Thanks to his self-confidence, his credit is seen as so good that he can go on borrowing to finance his extravagant lifestyle, and nobody seems to mind that he owes several fortunes.) Nux sees nothing wrong in buying the most expensive luxuries, since he feels himself to be a King, and hence it is his natural due. (Again I am reminded of Paul Keating, who caused an uproar by ordering a teak table from Thailand for the parliament house which cost several thousand dollars, and which happened to be supplied by a friend of his. He also raised eyebrows by using public money to buy prints of Australian birds for his office, totalling about seventy thousand dollars.)

### The Expert

Many Nux individuals become experts, often in more than one field. Nux has a natural love of excellence, and when this is combined with a sharp, penetrating intellect, as it very often is, the result is a person who becomes extremely knowledgeable about those subjects he is interested in. A great many Nux people become experts in their line of work. I once treated a man in his early forties for tinnitus. The first thing that struck me on meeting him was the clarity and directness of his steely blue eyes, and his resemblance to the actor Clint Eastwood. During the interview he told me that at school he had been determined to be the best at whatever he did, and he had fulfilled his wish by becoming a prominent astrophysicist, and had worked with NASA amongst others. He invited me to his home one day, which turned out to be a lovely ranch-style house on top of a hill overlooking the ocean. By this time it came as no surprise to me to learn that he had designed and built the house himself. He knew a great deal about a great many other things, but unlike some Lycopodium and Natrum experts, he never sounded either condescending or proud of his knowledge. It was just something he enjoyed. His tinnitus did respond very well to Nux Vomica 10M. It did not disappear, but after the remedy it stopped distracting him from his work and his play.

The Nux expert really does know a great deal, but he is not always right. Nevertheless, he often acts as though he is. He has supreme confidence in his knowledge, and this confidence extends to those areas where his understanding and experience is limited. (I was once given a lecture on homeopathy by a Nux doctor who knew only a thumb-nail sketch of each remedy. When I tried to point out that there was more than one remedy for bronchitis he ignored my remarks, since they did not fit in with his scheme.) This is an example of that common Nux mistake of over-extending oneself.

I have come across two Nux homeopaths, and both were more knowledgeable than most. Also, both thought that they are always right, and became rather heated when another homeopath questioned their prescriptions.

There are those Nux experts who study endlessly to acquire their comprehensive knowledge, and also others who are more relaxed about their study. The former are just as bright as the latter for the most part, but they are more obsessed with their particular subject. One of the Nux homeopaths I know fits the first type. He reads materia medica in bed, much to his wife's dismay, and would rather talk homeopathy than anything else. The other is just as capable, but less obsessive. He achieved his skills gradually without a great deal of study, and is just as interested in other favourite subjects as he is in homeopathy, and also just as interested in having fun and playing sports. Many Nux people are so bright (Kent: 'Ideas abundant, clearness of mind') that they do not have to try very hard. They then have the choice of putting all of their energies into becoming a world authority, or settling for being a mere expert, and spending the rest of their time having fun with other things.

Like that other intellectual omnivore Sulphur, the Nux expert is generally very happy to share his knowledge. Indeed he loves to. Both types are show-offs, and the expert has no qualms about showing off how knowledgeable he is. Unlike the Kali expert, the Nux expert usually has a good rapport with his audience, since he is confident socially, and is a man of the world, not a mere bookworm. After he has explained the mechanics of the jet engine, he is liable to pat you on the back paternally, and invite you to dinner, where he will reveal his extensive knowledge of Shang-Hai brothels, or some other fascinating diversion. Like Sulphur, Nux is often a good raconteur. With his wide experience, his confidence, and his love of being the centre of attention, he is as comfortable telling a story as he is giving a lecture. When he gives a lecture he sometimes sounds a little pompous, and takes himself too seriously, but as a storyteller he is laid-back and laconic.

Although Nux may occasionally fill in the gaps with a calculated guess (which is usually correct), his knowledge can generally be relied upon. Nux takes facts very seriously. He is as intellectually accurate as Kali Carbonicum, but even more pragmatic. Whereas Kali will know the exact design of his car's engine, Nux will go one step further, pulling the engine apart and re-assembling it just for fun. When his car breaks down he will usually be able to diagnose the fault, and more often than not will have both the know-how and the tools to fix it himself. However, he is not likely to bore you with unwanted information. (He leaves that to Lycopodium, Sulphur and Kali Carbonicum.)

The Nux expert differs from others in being interested in knowledge principally for its practical application. Virtually everything about Nux is orientated towards concrete results, and his specialist knowledge is no exception. Sulphur and Lycopodium experts love knowledge for its own sake, and as a result, they will enjoy investigating minute details and peripheral information which has no practical relevance. Kali, Arsenicum and Natrum experts tend to be very thorough, and gather every little detail together, partly out of a fear of missing something important. Nux tends to go for the bare essentials, and to ignore supporting information which is not necessary for the outcome he is interested in. For example, the Nux homeopath may develop a system for identifying remedy types using a checklist of a very few essential criteria for each type. If he feels that a case fits one of these sets of criteria, he will ignore the hundreds of other features of the case, since he does not need them to identify the remedy. In contrast, the Kali or Natrum homeopath is likely to record all available information, and use it in deciding upon a remedy.

Despite his relatively brief consultations, the Nux homeopath is likely to get just as good results as the others, if not better. Nux is the expert at honing down information to its bare essentials. This does not mean that he is superficial in his approach. On the contrary, he can usually go straight to the heart of the matter. The Nux homeopath will go straight to the deepest pathology of the case, and pay little attention to peripheral problems. In doing so, he will generally make the correct prescription, in a very short time.

Just as the Nux warrior will favour a lightning attack straight for the heart of the enemy stronghold, so the Nux intellectual hones in with unusual precision upon the crux of the matter. He is able to scan information quickly, and then dive for the required material, spotting it instantly amongst a jungle of distracting details. In this sense his focus is like that of a hawk circling above a field, broad in scope, but extremely sharp when it comes to identifying the material he is searching for. This is very different from the plodding, reductionist approach of Kali and most Lycopodium intellectuals. Nux does not have the intellectual inspiration and originality of Sulphur, nor the latter's love of abstract ideas, but he is quicker to grasp the crux of the matter than any other type.

Just as Sulphur is prone to paroxysms of inspiration of an abstract intellectual nature, so Nux may be equally consumed by ambitious plans to apply the knowledge he has gained. He will lie awake at night in a lather of excitement as he constructs the mental foundations for his future projects (Kent: 'Ideas abundant in the evening'). These plans may be as modest as choosing the type of music centre which he plans to purchase in the morning, or as elaborate as his plan to design a space-station capable of operating independently from the Earth. Nux experts tend to achieve a great deal, since their knowledge is accompanied by a passion for getting concrete results, and the practical know-how to do so.

There are some disadvantages to the speed and rather exclusive nature of Nux' intellectual focus. At times, the Nux expert will fail to appreciate the ramifications of his very narrow field of interest. For example, a Nux chiropractor may be extremely proficient at identifying and realigning spinal subluxations, and in his enthusiasm to do this, he may ignore the fact that his patient has a high fever, and needs to be medically investigated before being manipulated. A more commonly encountered example of the Nux narrow focus is the surgeon who pays no regard to the patient's psychological status, and is only interested in his overall health to the extent that it renders him fit or unfit for operation. Such Nux surgeons are generally very good surgically, but their insensitivity can be harmful to the patient, and exasperating to other medical colleagues. (A good many surgeons are Nux constitutionally. It is very satisfying for Nux to exercise power by achieving fast results through the precise use of a scalpel.) Nux' arrogance makes him doubly inclined to rely upon his own perspective, when a broader one may be needed. He tends to feel that he can get by without relying on any one else's expertise, and this is one of his greatest weaknesses.

### The Playboy

Any constitutional type can become a hedonistic playboy, but the four who most commonly do so are Nux, Lachesis, Tuberculinum and Lycopodium. For all his precision and determination, Nux is a self-indulgent sensualist. His appetite for excitement, food, alcohol and sex are almost as insatiable as his lust for power (Kent: 'Excitable', 'Dipsomania', 'Libertinism'). Arrogance is one of Nux' biggest weaknesses. Sensual indulgence is another. People are often surprised to find that the dynamic businessman, who demolishes rivals on the stock exchange and maintains the utmost discipline amongst his staff, will order the biggest ice-cream sundae they have ever seen, and devour it unselfconsciously before their eyes. Nux is very innocent about his appetites. Like a child he tends to satisfy them without giving it much thought. He takes a break to puff on a cigar, or drink a glass of whisky, and then he is back to satisfying his first love; practical achievement, and the influence it brings.

Many Nux individuals have a high revving nervous system, and a corresponding high metabolism, which they keep supplied with enormous amounts of food and drink. Some are snackers, who grab junk food on the run, whilst they are absorbed in either work or play. Others are gourmands, who prefer a feast at least once a day, and often more. The latter are liable to become obese eventually, despite their high metabolism, and Nux' tendency to be slim and wiry constitutionally. Kings are traditionally great feasters, as are Emperors. The Roman Empire in particular seems to have been based around Nux ideals, and no doubt was led by Nux warriors and Emperors. It eventually succumbed to decadence, just like many Nux individuals.

Many Nux people are addicted to stimulation. They live on the 'buzz' of victory, the buzz of danger, the buzz of rich food and intoxicating liquor, and the thrill of adventurous sex. They drive fast cars, earn great deals of money, and spend it on a luxurious and stimulating lifestyle. One of my Nux patients was a retired Casino owner. He had suffered from insomnia ever since he had left the Casino business. For thirty years he had stayed up till the middle of the night, part working, part playing in his Casino. When he gave it up, his nervous system was so used to running in top gear that he couldn't slow it down, and he quickly became exhausted (Kent: 'Prostration of mind'), but remained unable to sleep. When I asked him why he had never married, he replied that in his line of business there were always willing females available, and he did not relish the commitment of marriage. (Many Nux people overindulge in sex, and then become impotent—Kent: 'Sexually exhausted'.) Like many Nux patients, he was loath to admit to any weaknesses of character, and this characteristic itself led me to prescribe Lycopodium initially, along with his playboy lifestyle. When this did not act I gave Nux 10M, and within a week his sleep was restored almost to normal.

Nux plays just as hard as he works. He is likely to get restless at the prospect of an evening by the fireside, unless it includes some mental or sensory stimulation, such as wine, music and food. Nux does not like to be quiet and still for long, because at such times he becomes aware of the uncomfortable restlessness within. This is also true of Tuberculinum. Both types are hedonists, and their nervous systems remain 'stoked' at all times with stimulating experience. Nux does not like silence (unless he is one of the rare Nux individuals who has done a lot of meditation). He tends to turn a radio on wherever he goes, and he will even carry one with him to the bathroom. Similarly, he may snack constantly whilst he is working, and feel jittery if he runs out of supplies. Nux' aversion to silence is similar to his aversion to salads, drinks of water, and immobility. He requires stimulation, and anything as pure as lettuce can't quite be tasted by his over-excited palate. Ironically, after decades of overindulgence, many Nux individuals 'burn out', and can tolerate only the blandest of diets, and the quietest of surroundings (Kent:

'Sensitive to noise'). Reading tends to be too sedate for the average Nux, who is far more likely to lose himself in a film than a book. When he has been over-revving for a long time his nervous tension is simply too great to allow him to concentrate on reading material (Kent: 'Averse to reading'), and he will choose some effortless distraction such as watching a film, preferably with a stiff scotch to help him unwind.

Nux can be very playful when he is relaxing. He often has a fascination for games, and will play them as enthusiastically as his children. His favourite toys are often electronic gadgets, and powered vehicles, whether self-driven or remotely controlled. Nux loves speed, and is likely to be almost as captivated by electrically driven toy racing cars as he is by driving his own fast car. The latter is often his most prized toy. It gives him freedom, adaptability, and the thrill of tangible power. Most Nux people enjoy driving, and will often drive to unwind.

Computers are also Nux favourites, both as information collators, and as toys. Like Nux himself they are quick and versatile, and Nux takes to them like an extension of himself. He is particularly stimulated by the computer graphics now available. Perhaps as a result of his warrior ancestry, Nux is very visually orientated, not in the sense that he likes to look at old masters in the art gallery, but rather that he enjoys rapidly changing visual feasts, such as the computer screen during a video game, or a display of fireworks.

Not surprisingly, Nux is often very fond of war games. Whether he is shooting a rifle at the gallery, or attempting a world takeover on the playing board, he is in his element, and takes the game almost as seriously as his warrior brothers fought their battles. Nux loves to wage war, and when he wins a contest, he will let out a triumphal yell. I once played tennis regularly with a Nux friend who did this after every winning shot he hit.

Like most hedonists, Nux requires company to have fun (Kent: 'Desires company'), and like those other two playboys Lycopodium and Tuberculinum, he tends to prefer the company of the opposite sex. One reason for this is that Nux sees most other men as rivals (or as inferior). Like the bull walrus, he surrounds himself with admiring females, and he tends to be distinctly cool with members of his own sex. Even when he is married he will prefer the company of other women to men, although he may be quite capable of fidelity, so long as his wife is stimulating. If she is not, he may like to keep her as a stabilising influence in his life, and seek stimulation elsewhere. Like your typical Clint Eastwood character, the average Nux man is something of a chauvinist. He is also very charming and intelligent, and usually manages to acquire a partner who is more than just a pretty face.

Nux gets restless and lonely if he is without company for long, like his closely related brothers Phosphorus and Tuberculinum. When he is concentrating upon his work he may hate interruption, and if he is of an intellectual (or especially, spiritual) frame of mind, he can become quite reclusive at times, but when he wants to enjoy himself, he looks for convivial company. The majority of Nux people have no difficulty finding playmates. The more ruthless, hardened Nux may buy them, but most Nux people are good fun to be around when they are playing, and have no need to resort to such inducements. Like Sulphur, Nux has a spirit that is larger than life, and his enthusiasm is quite infectious. He is generally the ring-leader when it comes to merrymaking, particularly if he is the more physical Nux type. Some intellectual Nux people are more subdued in company, but even they have flashes of playful inspiration, which prompt them to sing, play practical jokes, or do adventurous things on the spur of the moment, (Kent: 'Impulsive') like diving into the ocean fully clothed, or stealing a police-car's number plate (Kent: 'Mischievous'). More often, the more intellectual Nux plays with words. He is generally an expert when it comes to dry humour, particularly ironic one-liners, and sometimes he gets carried away with this, making fun of everything and everyone he comes across. This is not usually malicious, but it can give offence unintentionally.

In all matters Nux is impatient when it comes to satisfying his desires. This is just as true at work as it is at play. If he is hungry, he may send his secretary out for pastries in the middle of the morning rush, or jump out himself at the traffic lights to buy a bar of chocolate. He spends money as fast as he earns it, and relishes the luxuries he buys. A grown Nux man is every bit as excited as a child when he buys himself a new car, or a new mountain bike. Of course, many Nux people tire quickly of their new toys, and so they are constantly on the look-out for novel forms of stimulation. The Nux astrophysicist to whom I referred earlier told me that in his younger days he had taken part in very high dose experiments with the hallucinogen LSD, taking huge amounts over long periods, in carefully controlled conditions. It is so typical of the Nux intellectual to take serious interest in an experiment that is at once intellectually expansive (literally!), and also highly stimulating to the senses. This is one difference between Nux and Lycopodium. Whereas Lycopodium is likely to take LSD simply to escape into psychedelia, Nux will take it seriously, as fascinated with the new insights it delivers as he is euphoric with its pleasure. Even in the midst of wild orgies of sensual indulgence, Nux tends to retain his alertness, and to see more than the other revellers. In this he is like the warrior who relaxes with a flask of ale and a wench after the battle, but is ever ready should the enemy launch a surprise counter-attack.

Because Nux lives on stimulation, he is more prone than most to nervous exhaustion. After years of late nights, dietary overindulgence, excessive alcohol and nicotine consumption, and nightly sexual gymnastics, he may eventually burn out. When this happens he becomes simultaneously tense and exhausted, like an alcoholic in withdrawal. He cannot relax, because his nerves are so jangled, but neither can he act effectively, because his mind is muddled (Kent: 'Prostration of mind'), and his body is weak. A shorter version of this is the hangover, which has been treated with Nux Vomica by homeopaths for generations. Like one hung over, the exhausted Nux individual is generally rather irritable, and prefers to be left alone (Kent: 'Aversion to company'). He is oversensitive to stimuli of all kinds (Kent: 'Senses hyperacute'), particularly to noise, light (hence the dark glasses that so many Nux people wear) and rich food.

Insomnia is nearly always a problem for the overwrought Nux. He will lie awake for hours with his mind racing, generally occupied with trivia, or the affairs of the coming day. Often the Nux insomniac will have a restless sleep, in which he tosses and turns and remains somewhere between sleeping and waking, in a no-man's land full of shifting thoughts that are anxious but incoherent. In the morning he feels wretched, and drags himself around the house. In such a state he will often turn to coffee, tobacco or alcohol to brace himself, and these may temporarily make him feel brighter, but in the long run they put his system further out of balance. Nux' nervous system is more robust than that of Lachesis, but even Nux cannot take the kind of punishment he often dishes out to himself, and eventually he must either dry out, or fall apart completely.

### Relationships

As one would expect from an emperor and a playboy, Nux tends to be a little imperious in relationships. The more crude and ruthless physically orientated Nux individual uses everybody, including his wife and children. He has very little heart, and may keep up the pretence of family life in order to retain social respectability, whilst spending most of his nights with his mistress. Even more human Nux individuals tend to be rather selfish in relationships. The average Nux husband will love and respect his wife, but tend to think of his own needs first, and hers as an after-thought. As a result, most Nux men are familiar with the truth session, in which their aggrieved partner points out to them how selfishly they are behaving. Nux is often rather shocked by these home-truths. He tends to see himself as a wonderful provider and lover, and he usually doesn't even notice when he is being insensitive. Many Nux men are rather innocent in their insensitivity, and will make a genuine effort to be more considerate when it is pointed out. However, these efforts are often short-lived, since Nux can only concentrate on one thing at a time, and his search for power and stimulation tends to win out in the end.

The more sensitive Nux individual (they do exist) plays the role of the knight in his relationships, at least some of the time. He chooses a sensible caring partner, who provides a steadying influence in his life, making sure he eats properly, and gets enough rest. Most women who are married to Nux men become secretaries to their husband to some extent, since this is often the only way that they can share in his first love, and see something of him. In return, the Nux (part-time) knight will treat his partner like a queen, when he is in a good mood. He will enjoy dressing her in the finest clothes, taking her to the best restaurants, and treating her with courtesy and admiration.

Nux sees his family as an extension of himself, and usually takes great pride in them (even if he abuses them as well). He is often very indulgent of his family, and tends to treat his daughter as a princess, and his son as the heir to his throne. The son who is sickly or effeminate is likely to be a great disappointment to his Nux father, who will tend to ignore the boy, and focus all of his attention on a stronger sibling, or even on an unrelated youth who becomes the surrogate heir. Nux can tolerate 'weakness' in a women; he expects it, but in a man, or in his own son, he cannot abide it.

Because he is a self-indulgent man, Nux tends to look to his partner for comfort and support. If he has had a hard day, he may collapse in her arms, and become quite childlike. He may even exaggerate his physical discomfort when he is ill, so that he receives more mothering. The Nux warrior has a soft underside in many cases. He may wrestle fearlessly with his opponents on the battle-field, but when the fight is over, he is liable to show off his wounds to his woman, and enjoy her fussing. If he has no battles to fight, he is liable to become even more self-indulgent, and to bring her his scratches to be dressed.

Nux respects strength, and if his partner is a strong woman, he will willingly share his throne with her. He will not only leave the domestic decisions to her in the main, but will also encourage her to make her mark upon the world. Many a Nux wife lives in her husband's shadow publicly, but some are able to match his energy and his ability, and manage to avoid losing themselves. Others fall prey to Nux' dominating personality, and end up as his chattel.

Because Nux has strong appetites, and is possessive of his spoils of war, he is more prone than most to jealousy. Even though he may be unfaithful to his wife, he is liable to explode with rage if she favours another, and to punish both his wife and her other man. Emperors do not take kindly to competition when it comes to sexual love.

### The Nux Woman

Nux women are rare, but they do exist. They are very similar to Nux men in temperament. Most become careerists, and excel in their chosen field (eg. Margaret Thatcher). The Nux woman is decidedly more masculine than most, and has little time for frivolities like crocheting and reading women's magazines. She is likely to find a strong man to marry, but if she cannot find a strong one, then she may settle for a wealthy or influential one. Like the

Nux man, she is usually very concerned with establishing her power-base. Those Nux women who do not have a career often become bitter and frustrated, and turn their attention to manipulating whatever power they can from their associates and family. Nux people of both sexes are born to lead, and do not do well when they are denied the chance, whether through circumstances or through poor judgement.

The homeopath who is faced with a tough career woman in the consulting room must chose between Nux, Ignatia and Natrum Muriaticum in the main. Natrum is by far the commonest of the three, and Nux is rare in comparison to Ignatia. Nux is not a sentimentalist, unlike the other two. She has not become hardened as a response to emotional pain, and hence her actions tend to be less 'reactive' than those of the other two types. The tough Natrum or Ignatia career woman tends to be very defensive when criticised, for example. The Nux woman may become angry when criticised, but her anger is not mixed with fear, and like her male counterpart, she will either ignore her opponent, or crush him. In deciding between these three types, the homeopath may do well to enquire into the childhood personality. Here the emotionality and vulnerability of Natrum and Ignatia usually becomes apparent, in contrast to the calm determination of the Nux girl.

### *Physical Appearance*

In keeping with the penetrating nature of the Nux psyche, most Nux people have a 'pointed' appearance. The face is generally a little longer than it is wide, and the features are sharp, particularly the nose, which tends to end in a point. The facial features are angular rather than rounded, reflecting the sharp intellect, and the jaw is firm and definite, reflecting determination. The eyes have a penetrating stare that tends to be disarming.

The Nux physique tends to be slim and wiry or muscular. Many Nux people are taller than average. The hair is straight, and is generally dark or reddish, though any shade can occur. The appearance of the actor Clint Eastwood is a good example of the type, as is that of the Australian Prime Minister Paul Keating.

# Phosphoric Acid

*Keynote:* Emotional numbness

Phosphoric Acid is generally thought of as an acute or sub-acute remedy for the effects of grief and exhaustion. I have come across several patients who appear to have resonated to this remedy for most of their life, and since they had a number of common features mentally as well as physically, and they responded to the remedy, I have come to regard Phosphoric Acid as a rare but distinct constitutional type, as well as an acute remedy.

The most characteristic feature of the mentals of Phosphoric Acid is a peculiar emotional neutrality. This is a more profound, more abnormal state of emotional numbness than we see in the apathy of Sepia, the temporary exhaustion of Phosphorus, and the unemotional rationality of Kali. The sense of neutrality is so complete and continuous that the patient reports 'It is as if I were not alive'. No emotions at all are experienced (except fear at times), and the patient feels like a ghost, drifting through an unreal life in which he performs almost automatically (Kent: 'As if in a dream'), with no motivation, and no sense of satisfaction. Although the intellect eventually becomes affected, Phosphoric Acid's pathology is initially on the emotional level. He may function effectively in the world for a long time, and yet feel nothing inside; no happiness, no love, no sadness - just an emptiness where his feelings should be, which he knows is unhealthy and abnormal.

## Grief and Disappointed Love

In every case of Phosphoric Acid I have come across, the pathological state was preceded by a profound grief of some kind (Kent: 'Ailments from grief'). A couple of patients had felt reasonably normal until they separated from their partners, since which time their emotions gradually shut down. (The same thing can happen to Natrum Muriaticum, but the emotional shutdown is never so absolute as it is in the case of Phosphoric Acid.) They could thus remember the time when they had felt joy and sorrow, and were consequently aware that there was something very wrong with them. This awareness gen-erated a sense of uneasiness, an anxiety that they were vaguely conscious of at least part of the time, which added a sinister feeling to their state of 'limbo'.

Grief can come in many forms. Phosphoric Acid is listed in Kent's Reper-tory under the rubric 'Homesickness'. A young person who is constitution-ally Phosphoric Acid, but who has never experienced profound emotional trauma, may have mild but tangible emotions. On leaving home, especially

249

if she moves far away from her parents, she at first pines for her loved ones, and then gradually drifts into the state of emotional numbness that is so characteristic of the pathology of Phosphoric Acid. This is really the same process as that which occurs after separation from a partner, bereavement, and loss of love in any form.

I suspect that it is only when an individual is constitutionally Phosphoric Acid, or perhaps Phosphorus, that grief can result in this lasting state of emotional numbness. (The vast majority of long-term grief reactions require Natrum Muriaticum.) It thus appears that there is a 'pre-traumatic' state of Phosphoric Acid, which in my experience with patients closely resembles that of Phosphorus but is more subdued, and more delicate. After treatment with the remedy, my Phosphoric Acid patients did not change into different constitutional types, but their emotions gradually reappeared. They then appeared like Phosphorus - sensitive, gentle and impressionable, but generally quieter and more introverted. (I did not give Phosphorus to these patients, since there were no longer any clearly pathological symptoms to treat, hence it is possible that some of them did change to Phosphorus constitutionally.)

One patient, a young woman of about twenty five years of age, came to see me complaining of apathy, emotional numbness, and difficulty in concentration. She reported that she seemed to have 'no personality at all'. When I asked her how long she had felt like this, she replied 'All of my life'. She then told me that her mother had died when she was three months old, and she had been told that she became very passive after this, whereas before she had been a normal, active baby. It thus appears that the pathological state of Phosphoric Acid can appear soon after birth, and can last indefinitely without treatment. As with my other Phosphoric Acid patients, this woman gradually came to life emotionally after taking the remedy in 10M potency, and her mental confusion disappeared.

### Mental Confusion

Kent notes in his Materia Medica that the mental pathology of Phosphoric Acid usually precedes the physical ('In every case we find the mental symptoms are the first to develop'). What he does not do is differentiate between emotional and intellectual impairment. In my experience the emotional pathology of Phosphoric Acid is the first to appear, followed later by intellectual impairment, and lastly by physical problems (none of my Phosphoric Acid patients had significant physical problems). After a period of emotional numbness the patient may start to forget things (Kent: 'Forgetful'). Gradually, as the memory deteriorates, the thought processes start to freeze up, just as the emotions had done previously. The patient will comment that his mind goes blank in the middle of a train of thought. In the consulting room he may stop speaking in mid-sentence for the same reason. The thoughts have just disappeared. As the mind gets 'filled up' with more and more blank spaces, the patient finds it harder and harder to think straight. When asked a question, he will take a long time to answer (Kent: 'Answers slowly', 'Answers-reflects long'). This is because it takes him a long time first to comprehend the question, and then to respond to it. This is not a lack of intelligence as such, but rather a random freezing of the thought processes. Eventually the effort to think may become so great that the patient simply answers 'I don't know' to most of the questions he is asked. Naturally, this kind of mental pathology has profound consequences for the patient. He is able to function less and less in the world. At first he will withdraw socially (which has happened to some extent already, as a result of the emotional numbness), declining invitations, and sitting passively in company (Kent: 'Inclination to sit'). At the same time practical performance deteriorates, as the mind becomes more muddled. Reading becomes impossible (Kent: 'Concentration difficult', 'Unable to think long'), and soon he is unable to keep down a job. Eventually he will either be supported by a relative or friend as an invalid, or he will end up in an institution, most probably diagnosed with either pre-senile dementia, or 'passive schizophrenia'. (None of the patients I have seen had reached this stage, and some had functioned for decades with no emotions, but passable mental skills.)

The intellectual deterioration seen in some Phosphoric Acid patients resembles that of Alumina and Argentum. In Argentum, however, mental deterioration is more marked than emotional pathology, whereas the reverse is true of Phosphoric Acid. However, like Alumina and Argentum, Phosphoric Acid patients can become increasingly anxious as their thinking deteriorates, and anxiety seems to be the one emotion that most Phosphoric Acid patients do experience. This is usually a realistic anxiety about coping, and about how far their mental deterioration will progress (Kent: 'Anxiety about the future').

Although most Phosphoric Acid patients who experience mental pathology complain of a slowing down of their mental processes, or a vanishing of thought, some become hurried, at least some of the time. This seems to be a universal reaction to mental deterioration, since it also occurs during the mental breakdown of Alumina, Argentum and Medorrhinum individuals. Panic sets in as a result of inability to think coherently, and this panic drives the person into rushing, in an attempt to compensate. This hurriedness only results in even less effective functioning, unlike the hurriedness of Nux, Natrum and Lachesis, which is often focused, and results in more rather than less being accomplished.

## *Miscellanea*

One result of the emotional impoverishment of Phosphoric Acid individuals is that they may rely on others to 'feel for them'. I once treated a young man for apathy, irresolution and psoriasis. His mental and emotional problems had developed after separating from his girlfriend, even though it had been his decision to leave. He was a very open, impressionable youth, and had a Phosphoric appearance, but he complained of confusion emotionally in the sense that his emotions were so vague that he didn't know what he felt. He also had a few characteristic physical symptoms suggestive of Phosphoric Acid, including chronic, profuse and painless diarrhoea, which was associated with anxiety. He told me that even before he separated from his girlfriend, his emotions had always been very vague and hard to identify, and that he tended to feel whatever his girlfriend felt, but much less intensely (Phosphorus would feel it just as intensely). He commented that he seemed to use his girlfriend's emotions to help him to feel anything at all. His history put me in mind of the stories of discarnate spirits, who lacking a body with which to feel, fed off the feelings of living people. He resembled Phosphorus in many ways, including the fact that he was a gifted artist, and painted in a very imaginative, visionary style. Nevertheless, both his psoriasis and his emotional confusion responded to Phosphoric Acid, and I never did find out whether or not he was Phosphorus 'underneath'.

Kent lists Phosphoric Acid in his Repertory under the rubric 'Gestures - reaching or grasping for something'. I have seen something similar in the history of one of my Phosphoric Acid patients—the young artist mentioned above. He told me that as a child he would always touch the stair rail at a particular point on descending the stairs. As he grew older he tried to stop doing this, but found the compulsion to do so almost irresistible. Phosphoric Acid is a Syphilitic remedy with a relatively severe picture of mental pathology. In keeping with other remedies of this type (Argentum, Alumina, Veratrum, Stramonium), the mental picture appears to include compulsive behaviour, which the individual resorts to automatically in an attempt to preserve some mental stability. One other example of compulsive behaviour which I have seen in a Phosphoric Acid patient is bulimia, or compulsive food bingeing. One can easily imagine a patient with such emotional emptiness trying to fill the void inside with food.

## *Physical Appearance*

Most of the Phosphoric Acid patients I have seen had a relatively 'Phosphoric' appearance, being skinny, with angular, open facial features. However, there were a number of differences which confirm to me that this is a separate type from Phosphorus. Firstly, many were dark in complexion, whereas most Phosphorus people are fair. Secondly, the eyes had a very characteristic and unusual appearance in many cases. Whereas Phosphorus has large, attractive, healthy looking eyes, most of my Phosphoric Acid patients had bulging eyes like goldfish. This is characteristic of thyroid overactivity, but it appeared in these patients in the absence of thyroid pathology.

There are many physical symptoms which help to confirm Phosphoric Acid. Two I have come across most frequently are painless profuse diarrhoea (especially associated with anxiety), and numbness of the extremities.

# Phosphorus

*Keynote:* Lack of boundaries

Phosphorus has had a very good press up till now. Homeopaths generally regard Phosphorus as the nicest of people, and the type that everyone wishes they belonged to. Many Phosphorus individuals really are radiant, loving and spiritual, but the truth is never that simple, at least not when it comes to psychological types. Just as there is a progression from the least conscious to the most conscious Sulphur individual, the former exhibiting all the negative characteristics of the type, the latter all the positive, so there is the same kind of progression amongst Phosphorus individuals. Not all Phosphorus people are giving or spiritually inclined. The less developed Phosphorus may give when it suits him, or when he is in a good mood, but he is just as likely to be self-centred and inconsiderate.

The essence running through Phosphorus is a lack of personal boundaries, and it is this lack of boundaries that accounts for both the positive and the negative characteristics of the Phosphorus psyche. The vast majority of people develop in childhood an ego-identity which separates them from the rest of the world. Before this happens, the infant feels at one with his surroundings, and especially with his mother. This ego-identity is made up of hundreds of boundaries or conditions, which determine who the child thinks he is, and how he relates to the world around him. It is made up mostly of opinions and beliefs, and hence it is essentially intellectual in character, since it is the intellect which distinguishes and analyses, rejects and approves. Gradually, most children come to live more and more in their intellect, and as this happens, they become more and more separated from the world around them, since it is no longer experienced directly, but through the filter of the ego or intellect. The ego also includes emotions, which initially were impersonal in the infant, since there was no person for them to attach to. Hence the infant bathed in waves of contentment or fear, without knowing why he was contented or afraid, or even that he was. These were just feeling tones that pervaded his whole experience. Once the intellect has been established, there is a person who can identify with the feelings, and say, 'This is my anger, and my fear'. The person can also escape from feelings to some extent by dissociating from them.

The process of identification with the intellect is partial and incomplete in the Phosphorus individual. Phosphorus tends to experience the world like a young child. Sensory stimuli are more vibrant and immediate to Phosphorus, because they are not filtered by the intellect to the same degree as in others (Kent: 'Sensitive to external impressions'). As a result, they have more effect on him. This is equally true of pleasant and unpleasant stimuli. A beautiful sunset will send Phosphorus into a rapture that few other mortals ever experience, a rapture that totally bypasses the intellect. By the same token, Phosphorus will be acutely distressed by the ugliness and squalor of a slum district. This is not the outraged concern of Causticum, and not only the sympathetic suffering of Natrum, but an absorption by psychic osmosis of the 'vibes' of the place, which all of us experience to some extent, but are insulated from by layers of insensitivity, and by being firmly rooted in our ego. Phosphorus is like a sponge, absorbing all the impressions that are in the immediate environment, and then experiencing waves of emotion, both pleasant and unpleasant, which they produce.

To Phosphorus, the worlds of intuition and feeling are very alive and real, and this includes the feelings that exist in other people. Phosphorus can pick up on another's feelings, and sometimes does this without realising it. For example, a Phosphorus woman may suddenly become anxious without knowing why, because she sits next to someone who is very afraid. She may also become anxious because her loved one is in danger hundreds of miles away (Kent: 'Clairvoyance').

The romantic poet John Keats describes Phosphorus' impressionability very clearly in a letter to a friend when he writes 'as to the poetic character …it has no self; it is everything and nothing; it has no character; it enjoys light and shade. A poet…has no identity—he is continually in for and filling some other body—the Sun, the Moon, the Sea. When I am in a room with people if ever I am free from speculating on creations of my own brain, then not myself goes home to myself, but the identity of everyone in the room begins to press upon me, that I am in very little time annihilated'. (This could also apply to Mercurius.)

As a result of the extraordinary 'openness' of the Phosphorus psyche, reality is a far broader and richer experience for Phosphorus than it is for most other mortals, but it is also more confusing and bewildering. Although Phosphorus is capable of remarkable intuition or second sense, he is just as likely to misinterpret emotion and wishful thinking as intuition, and to be led astray by it. His intuitions are not reliable, because they get lost in a sea of sensual impressions, emotions and imaginings. The Phosphorus individual floats in the ocean of these constantly shifting currents, (Kent: 'Chaos') marvelling at its beauty, shrinking from its terrors, and struggling to keep afloat, and avoid being swallowed up completely.

### Innocence

No type is more innocent than Phosphorus (though Pulsatilla, Baryta and

255

China come close). Phosphorus is open to the point of being transparent, and this gives him a childlike quality that is endearing to many, and infuriating to some. A perfect example of the innocence of Phosphorus can be seen in the character of Maria, played by Julie Andrews in the film 'The Sound of Music'. All the nuns love her, but they are exasperated by her flighty sense of fun, and her inability to take adult conventions like modesty and propriety seriously (Kent: 'Heedless'). Innocence is as much a strength in Phosphorus as a weakness. Like children, many Phosphorus people remain uncorrupted by a corrupt world. They are idealistic in the extreme, but they can see the cruelty of the world far more clearly than most, and it feels very alien to them. Maria cannot bear the severity with which the Nux captain marshals his brood of children, and whilst he is away she teaches them to sing, and re-introduces them to the wonder of life. Upon his return (in true Nux style) he orders her to pack her bags when he sees the lack of discipline she has fostered in his children, but his heart then melts when he hears them sing for the first time. Phosphorus can melt the heart of the coldest tyrant. Her love is so innocent and unconditional that only a robot or a devil could resist it.

The innocence of Phosphorus can get her into trouble, since it makes her gullible. Most Phosphorus individuals are very trusting, especially when they like somebody, and although like children their sensitivity usually warns them away from negative people, they may be persuaded by an appearance of kindness to ignore their intuition, and give a manipulative person the benefit of the doubt. Phosphorus is terribly optimistic, and would far rather think well of somebody than ill. She is likely to be charmed by the travelling Lycopodium salesman into buying something she would never have dreamt of spending so much money on, and to be frightened by the insurance agent into buying far too much cover.

Phosphorus is very vulnerable to scaremongering. Because she is gullible, and has a relatively poor understanding of material reality, she is not able to assess risks realistically, and is liable to over-react to threatening impressions (Kent: 'Frightened at trifles'). When Orson Welles broadcast his mock news flash on American radio claiming that aliens had landed in space-craft, hundreds of people fled to the hills in a panic. Many of them must have been Phosphorus constitutionally.

Related to Phosphorus' gullibility is her tendency to jump to conclusions. Her mind tends to be imprecise and impressionable, and her imagination is vivid. As a result, Phosphorus often finds it difficult to differentiate the real from the illusory. In particular, she will often interpret the facts before her in the light of her fears and desires. I was once on holiday with a Phosphoric friend, who spotted a middle-aged man paying a lot of attention to a pretty young girl in a swim suit. My friend's interest was aroused further by the observation that the man was on holiday with his equally middle-aged wife, who seemed not to have noticed her husband's interest in the girl. I suggested to my friend that she was jumping to conclusions, but she insisted that this man would soon 'blow his cover', and that we were about to witness the spectacle of a scorned and outraged wife venting her fury on her heartless husband, a prospect that my Phosphoric friend anticipated with a mixture of excitement, dread and enthusiasm. It turned out that the pretty girl was the daughter of the middle-aged couple, a discovery which punctured my friend's mounting imaginative bubble, but also relieved her, since she couldn't bear the thought of the pain that she had expected to arise in the heart of the scorned wife (Kent: 'Sympathetic').

The Phosphorus patient is often a delight to have in the consulting room, but her assessment of her health must be taken with a pinch of salt. She is just as likely to exaggerate her symptoms as she is to ignore the more serious ones (especially if she is afraid that she has some life-threatening disease, or indeed if she has one). Because she is gullible, and also frightened by illness (Kent: 'Fear of impending disease'), the Phosphorus patient will often try a number of different traditional or fashionable cures in addition to seeing a doctor and a homeopath. She may then attribute either her improvement, or her failure to improve to these other remedies, and treat her homeopathic medicine as just another of her medicinal 'crutches'. This is just another example of the woolly thinking that is common amongst Phosphorus people. It results from a failure to differentiate, and whilst it is often quite charming, it can lead to considerable practical difficulties.

### *Irresponsibility and Avoidance of Reality*
Responsibility is not one of Phosphorus' stronger points, since it requires the voluntary boundary of self-discipline. This goes against the grain of Phosphorus' natural spontaneity, and requires the kind of mental focus that Phosphorus finds either boring or a strain. Phosphorus has a flighty, evanescent quality, which enables him to glide lightly over Life's great pageant, taking things on appearances, and in the process skirting superficially over matters that require more commitment and more depth of attention, such as the details of contracts, or the repayment of debts. Phosphorus is notorious for borrowing money to finance some passing enthusiasm, (whether it be the purchase of alcohol or a Ferrari, or a donation to children in need), without paying any regard to his ability to repay the loan. He neither looks back to previous experience, which could warn him of the dangers of his present actions, nor forwards to the likely repercussions of his impulsive behaviour. He simply trusts that things will work out, and then becomes bewildered and panicky when they do not. He is generous to those in need (both because he cares, and because he doesn't understand the value of money), and he

expects others to bail him out when he is in trouble, even though the trouble is entirely due to his own short-sightedness. Such is the charm of Phosphorus, and his ability to look forlorn and pathetic when he is upset, that he often does succeed in finding someone to bail him out. At such times, he may garnish genuine distress with a good deal of play-acting to win sympathy and support. Exaggeration and emotional dramatism is a common trait amongst Phosphorus individuals. They use it in story telling to make their tale more dramatic and interesting, but it is when they are in difficulty that they are especially liable to 'gild the lily', both verbally in terms of the details of the situation (to their own advantage needless to say), and also emotionally, turning up the emotional volume to detract attention away from the facts, and towards their need for support. Those huge innocent eyes are extremely hard to resist when they are full of tears. They tend to attract instant sympathy, irrespective of the underlying situation. Consequently, many Phosphorus individuals 'get away with murder', especially in their youth. Since they do not look back, they do not suffer much guilt when they cause inconvenience to others, although they may be shocked and remorseful for a fleeting moment if they are confronted with the pain they have caused. Then it is a thing of the past, and their mercurial mind is off somewhere else. Since Phosphorus is open to so many disparate feelings and impressions, this ability to let go of the preceding instant is a kind of protection, which helps to prevent an experiential overload.

I recently came across an amusing example of Phosphorus' ability to excuse herself. A few years back I loaned a Phosphorus friend (she had responded well to Phosphorus for a serious disorder) a considerable sum of money, which she undertook to repay speedily. Needless to say, she did not, and I gave up any hope of receiving it. A few years later I met her unexpectedly, having not seen her in the interim. She came up to me, and after exchanging a hug, she looked at me seriously and said she had something to say to me. She then explained that she had been aware all this time that she owed me the money, and wanted me to know that she had not forgotten her debt. I waited for her offer to repay it, and when this did not come, I asked her when she planned to return the money. She smiled sheepishly, and said she would buy me dinner some time. I was too surprised and amused to be angry.

Escapism is a cornerstone of Phosphorus' defence mechanisms. When reality gets unpleasant, he is even more likely than Sulphur and Lycopodium to slip out of the door, either physically or in his head, and seek more attractive surroundings. His flight from reality is helped by the use of alcohol, marijuana and other sedatives, and also by immersion in fantasy films and novels. Phosphorus may not live much in the past or the future, but he is not 'present' half the time either, since he is off somewhere in his imagination

(Kent: 'Exaltation of fancy'). He has little staying power, and even in the absence of 'trouble', he is liable to get restless if he has to apply himself for long, either physically or mentally. He is a sprinter rather than a jogger, and he gets both bored and tired quickly. Like Sulphur and Lycopodium he wants to play much of the time, and can get petulant when he is not allowed to. He may even lose his temper, but this is generally short-lived, and is seldom violent (Kent: 'Mildness').

Gambling is one way that Phosphorus may seek both excitement and escape from financial difficulties. Phosphorus has an addictive tendency, and he is particularly vulnerable to the addiction of gambling, whether it be through the football pools, the horses or the roulette wheel. When he loses he can convince himself more effectively than most other types that he will win next time, and so he can quickly bet his way into desperation, and thence to crime in some cases. As I have implied, it is the male Phosphorus who is more prone to both addictive behaviour and deliberate deception. The female Phosphorus more often finds her escape in the form of a man, or at least in her fantasies about him. She is prone to falling in love with a passing stranger when she is in difficulty, who becomes her Knight in Shining Armour. He usually finds her very attractive, and may even be a party to her victim/saviour delusion, but he usually realises eventually that he has bitten off more than he can chew, and then leaves her. The Phosphorus woman is the original damsel in distress (along with Pulsatilla). She is so innocent, so helpless, and so beautiful, that there is no shortage of willing knights to rush to her aid. However, in these situations it is only the wounded knight who is willing to stick around for long, and he is as much a liability as a saviour!

When the Phosphorus damsel does find her knight, she is liable to respond in one of two ways to him. Sometimes she is utterly devoted, and surrenders her life to him. This is not that difficult for Phosphorus, since she has a very open heart, and a relatively weak sense of her own identity. He then becomes the focus for her whole life, and as long as he is loving, she remains utterly contented in her dependence (Pulsatilla, Natrum, Ignatia and Staphysagria). However, since he is everything to her, she is liable to fall to pieces if his affections begin to waver. At this point she will either strike out angrily in a desperate attempt to keep him (Kent: 'Hysteria, Rage'), or else she will dissolve in tears, and be unable to eat, speak or even move for days (Kent: 'Ailments from disappointed love, with silent grief').

Phosphorus' avoidance of the harsher realities of life is accompanied in many cases by a love of glamour. Like a magpie, she is attracted to shiny, colourful objects, and to other charismatic individuals. The Phosphorus woman usually has a natural grace (which is why so many leading ballerinas are Phosphorus), and loves to wear stylish clothes which accentuate her lithe figure. She is also often an expert at turning on the charm. Like Natrum

Muriaticum and Ignatia, she can be very seductive when it suits her. I shall always remember the photo I saw of a Phosphoric friend of mine. She was looking over her shoulder and blowing cigarette smoke towards the camera, her eyelids half-closed, in quite the most sensuous pose I have ever seen.

Many Phosphorous people lead glamorous lives, and they usually enjoy recounting the glamorous parts. Like Ignatia, their beauty and their charm tends to attract more glamour to it, in the form of prestigious social contacts, and glamourous job opportunities. Furthermore, Phosphorus is often very gifted artistically, and is also often promising as an actor or actress, or as a public relations officer. I once met a Phosphoric young woman who was of Russian origin, and worked as a translator for Russian diplomats in America. I am sure that she got the job not only because she was skilled at translation, but also because of her natural charm, and her striking beauty. She lived a high powered life in the top echelons of society, but when I took her case it became apparent that she was confused inside, because like so many Phosphorus individuals, she was not sure who she was. This sense of confusion made her appear evasive and vulnerable when talk centred on her innermost thoughts and feelings, and hence she appeared quieter than most Phosphorus women. However, she did have the radiant charm that is so characteristic of Phosphorus, as well as the typical impressionability. After a dose of Phosphorus 10M she seemed far clearer about who she was and what she wanted, and she said that she had realised how dependent she had always been upon the guidance and approval of others, a dependence she was now determined to overcome.

### The Shining Star

It is no coincidence that the word 'Phosphorus' means 'the bearer of light'. In nature the brilliant phosphorescence of glow worms and certain deep sea creatures derives from their phosphorus content, and the sea itself glows at night with a million sparks from the phosphorus-containing medusae and tiny crustacea that swarm together at certain localities and in certain seasons of the year. The pure phosphorus metal is so unstable that it bursts into flames when exposed to the air, a further expression of its extraordinary reactivity and its light-giving properties. There is always a meaningful correspondence between the original remedy substance and the individual who resonates to it homeopathically. Like phosphorus, the Phosphoric individual has a high metabolism and a tendency to 'burn up' quickly. His colouring is light or reddish, and he is subject to sudden inflammations and burning sensations. Similarly, the Phosphoric personality has much in common with its volatile physical similimum. It is very excitable, and tends to radiate joy and love unreservedly when it is happy. No other type can compete with a happy Phosphorus individual in terms of sheer radiance of joy. Phosphorus' radiance is almost tangible. A joyous Phosphorus face is probably more moving and more uplifting than any other sight I can think of. For those of you who are unsure of what a happy Phosphorus looks like, consider the screen actresses Julia Roberts and Geena Davis. When they smile, the effect is quite electric and irresistible. (I have found that actors and actresses nearly always play characters of the same constitutional type as themselves.) Male Phosphorus actors are a little harder to spot, but the comedian Martin Short is a good candidate. His smile is almost as endearing as the ladies'.

It seems that most Phosphorus individuals have been blessed with a sunny temperament, and an easy access to the kind of ecstasy that mystics strive for years to attain. Few Phosphorus individuals bother learning to meditate, since they are naturally attuned to the joy within, at least when life is running smoothly (they are probably also put off by the fact that it sounds like work). Many would benefit, however, from the kind of meditation which stills the mind, since Phosphorus is very excitable, and her joy is easily threatened. Being so impressionable, there is a tendency for Phosphorus' mood to fluctuate with the tide of external events to a greater degree than normal. One moment she is deliciously happy, and the next she is despairing (Kent: 'Laughing alternating with sadness'), because somebody said something that upset her, or she saw a tragic occurrence on the news. This emotional seesaw effect is also seen in Ignatia, but the moods of the latter tend to be more dramatic, and the negative emotions in particular tend to be much deeper and more lasting. Unless Phosphorus has had a long run of difficulties that have worn her down, she tends to be pretty resilient to life's blows, and bounces back enthusiastically after a brief period of depression or anxiety. Of all the constitutional types, Phosphorus is the lightest emotionally. Others like Lycopodium and Tuberculinum are relaxed and unemotional much of the time, but they do not have the same buoyancy of spirit of Phosphorus. Like Peter Pan and Shakespeare's Puck, Phosphorus is an airy sprite (it is no accident that these three begin with 'P', a very top-heavy letter, like the triangular face of Phosphorus, which touches the earthly pole so tentatively, and expands as it opens up to the heavens - you see how the subject matter of Phosphorus affects the author, and begins to make him wax lyrical!). She has no time or liking for heaviness, and just as you think she is pinned down by some pressing matter, she is up and away, flying beyond it, whether it be resolved or no.

Phosphorus is a very social animal. No other type enjoys company and depends upon it quite so much (Kent: 'Desires company'). When Phosphorus is alone she tends to get restless and lonely, but in company she shines (unless the company is threatening), since she loves to share herself with others, and to share in their thoughts and feelings. Her natural joy is infectious, and her simple 'live for today' philosophy is refreshing to more sober types, who brighten up a little in her company. She is just as open when she is unhappy, but unlike Natrum or Ignatia who tend to make a meal of it when they share their suffering, the very act of sharing it tends to bring Phosphorus rapid relief. Furthermore, Phosphorus is so impressionable that a little reassurance is all she needs to dispel her anxieties, and a little encouragement suffices to dispel her gloom.

When she is happy, Phosphorus tends to be very playful. Even at work she will be bouncy and chatty, and since her work very often involves service to the public, she is likely to have plenty of playmates to share her sense of fun with. A Phosphorus nurse is like a breath of fresh air in a hospital ward. She will dance through the bedpan duties as if in a musical production, making the sorriest of patients laugh with her mischievous sense of humour (Kent: 'Mirth, hilarity'). Some of the other nurses may actually resent her cheerfulness and popularity, and may take advantage of her innocence and openness. I have come across several young Phosphorus women who complained of bitchiness from their female colleagues. This may in part be an expression of Phosphorus' oversensitivity, which sometimes verges on paranoia, but it is also in part the result of jealousy. Very often Phosphorus appears like a golden child, sent from the heaven to add a little magic to a lacklustre world. Because of her charm, she tends to be very popular, and may, for instance, attract a very handsome boyfriend. Furthermore, she is rather dramatic in her expressiveness, and does nothing to hide her joy in the blessings she receives. Consequently, she tends to alienate some less fortunate mortals, who tire of being constantly reminded of how wonderful her life is.

Like Medorrhinum and Lachesis, Phosphorus functions predominantly from her right brain, being more attracted to harmony than to logic. The majority of Phosphorus individuals are gifted artistically, and many become poets, painters or dancers, in their spare time if not professionally. Phosphorus reflects her lightness of spirit through her art, and is attracted to art which is light, wispy and gentle. She is liable to prefer watercolours to oils, and amongst the oils to prefer light and dreamy styles such as that of Monet, to heavier and more realistic ones. Similarly, her taste in music is likely to favour the romantic, such as ballads, and also light lively music such as jazz. She may be very moved by heavier pieces, such as opera and Beethoven, but they tend to make her too morose. Phosphorus avoids anything which will weigh her down. Her art is an extension of her self, which resonates with the beauty within her soul, and stirs in her awe and ecstasy.

Phosphorus men have the same lightness and sensitivity as the women. They may have little stomach for routine and responsibility, but as long as they are able to find a niche in life which permits them to be their brilliant selves, they are just as beautiful as the women (Phosphorus men are beautiful rather than handsome, just as some of the more cerebral Ignatia women are handsome rather than beautiful. Nat King Cole was a good example of a male Phosphorus artist. His beauty and his innocence endeared him to a whole nation, and enabled him to become the first black performer in America to have his own television show. Like no other performer of his time, Cole visibly enjoyed his public performances, in a most natural and unselfconscious way.) The greatest male ballet dancers are usually Phosphorus. It is said of Nijinsky that when he was in ecstasy he could float momentarily at the height of his leap, as if his body were as light as air. All Phosphorus people have an ethereal quality, which makes one almost expect them to float. They are usually very pleased with their own elfin quality, and make the most of it, unlike China, who is even more ethereal in many cases, but far too lacking in confidence to make a show of herself.

Phosphorus' own self-love tends to add to rather than subtract from his beauty, unlike the pride of Lycopodium and Nux, which is more insistent. Like these other types, Phosphorus tends to be vain and self-indulgent, with the difference that he does not separate himself from others in the process. Although he is pleased with himself, he tends not to judge others (unless they fall into a particular category of people which he is prejudiced against). Indeed, he is generally very accepting and tolerant, and quick to praise another's virtues. Unlike Natrum, who deep down rejects himself, but on the surface may reject everyone else, Phosphorus loves and accepts himself, as he loves and accepts most people he knows. Like Sulphur, his love may not be reliable in a practical sense, but it is real enough to the Phosphorus individual who feels it.

One of the most refreshing things about Phosphorus is that he says exactly what he is thinking or feeling. He may remain silent if he doesn't like you, but he will seldom put on a polite front like most other types. Similarly, he is not shy when it comes to expressing his friendship and affection. Phosphorus is beautifully transparent in all but the most slippery of cases, and is generally too open for his own good. Privacy is a term that he seldom considers. He has nothing to hide, whether he is walking around naked in front of his children, or telling a stranger his life-story. When he does reveal the most intimate details of his life, he expects his listener to be interested, but if they are not, he will shrug his shoulders and think to himself that they are the loser, unlike Natrum and Ignatia, who are mortified by such 'betrayal'.

## *Woolly Thinking and Confusion of Identity*
The weak sense of personal ego that enables Phosphorus to experience the world with such childlike intensity also gives him a rather vague and delicate sense of his own identity. Phosphorus is like a psychic sponge, which absorbs the sensory, emotional and intellectual input from the environment more indiscriminately than most, and struggles to find a stable centre psychologi-

cally amidst the shifting currents of feeling and impression. This impression-ability of Phosphorus has both immediate and longterm consequences. In the moment he can be overwhelmed by a new and startling idea (especially one which is either very beautiful, or very threatening), or by an intense but fleeting emotion. At such times he has no past, and no identity of his own; he becomes the emotion, or the idea, and loses all sense of perspective. It may take a minute for him to come back to his senses, or it may take much longer. When Phosphorus falls in love, for example, he is in a perpetual state of intoxication which tends to dissolve concrete impressions, or to cast ev-erything in a pink, shimmering light, even the tax assessment, and the boil on his beloved's nose. Similarly, a threat to his personal security, or to a loved one, can induce in him a state of free-floating anxiety that makes even a kitten appear menacing to him. Such immediate swamping of Phosphorus' tenu-ous grip on his own identity is generally short lived, and either subsides to be followed by a period of relative stability, in which he can think straight, or is replaced by a different but equally intense impression which has been stimulated by new circumstances. Little wonder that Phosphorus has a ten-dency to become mentally and emotionally exhausted from time to time (Kent: 'Prostration of mind'), and to fall into a kind of apathetic zombie state, in which he either does nothing at all, or acts as if in a dream, func-tioning on 'auto-pilot' until he has had time to recuperate and recollect himself (Kent: 'As if in a dream').

The long-term consequence of Phosphorus' impressionability is that he tends to borrow his identity from those around him. We all grow up with a considerable degree of conditioning inside of us, and tend to adopt many of the attitudes of our parents, both intellectually and socially, but Phospho-rus is even more malleable than most. The Phosphorus adolescent, for ex-ample, may accept all of his parents' attitudes and beliefs without question, long after most of his peers have begun to wake up to the deficiencies and excesses of their own parents. A good example is the Phosphorus child brought up in a religious family. Irrespective of the actual nature of the re-ligion, it will be followed faithfully by the Phosphorus individual, and ques-tioned less than it would be by any other constitutional type (except perhaps Pulsatilla). Similarly, the Phosphorus child is liable to grow up with politi-cal and moral opinions that are carbon-copies of his parents. If his parents were moralistic, he is moralistic. If they were criminals, he will condone crime, and since his parents, like most parents, tended to think and to in-sist that they were right about most things, the Phosphorus child grows up thinking that his parents are always right. The dawning of that awful realisation that one's parents are fallible occurs far later in the average Phos-phorus than in most other types, and this realisation may be too frighten-ing and unsettling to be fully accepted by Phosphorus, who tends to cling to trusted attitudes as he would to a tree in a hurricane. This is not to say that all Phosphorus people are rigid and narrow-minded. If their parents were flexible and open-minded, then so will they be. If his parents were rigid and strict, however, Phosphorus grows up in something of a quandary. He will adopt many of his parents' strict attitudes, but he will be uneasy with them, since he is such a warm, spontaneous type by nature, and his human warmth will constantly be at loggerheads with his adopted severity. In the end he is likely to soften many of his parents' more rigid attitudes and practices (such as a refusal to ever borrow or lend), whilst still maintaining some in theory, and others in practice.

An excellent portrayal of a Phosphorus man who is caught between his rigid moralistic upbringing and his natural, spontaneous self can be seen in the figure of Oscar Hopkins in Peter Carey's tragicomic novel 'Oscar and Lucinda'. Oscar is the son of an evangelical preacher of a particularly rigid kind, and grows up in Cornwall in the nineteenth century. His father once caught the young Oscar tasting a Christmas pudding, a delicacy so decadent that it amounted to an abomination in the eyes of the preacher, who struck the child a mighty blow to the head, forcing him to expel the tasty mouthful. Oscar grew up with his father's puritanical spirit, believing that he must deny his own pleasure in order to win his heavenly father's approval. He lived the life of an ascetic at Oxford, where he studied Divinity in preparation for joining the priesthood, and kept to himself, since he could not relate to the worldly interests of his fellow students. Despite Oscar's impeccable morality, he was disowned by his rigid father for abandoning the latter's Plymouth Brethren faith, and becoming an Anglican. Oscar did this at the tender age of eleven or so, since he could not believe that his father's severity could be pleasing to God. In typical Phosphorus fashion the young Oscar relied on 'signs from above' to guide him to the correct faith. He did this by throwing a stone over his shoulder, onto a grid of squares in the shape of a cross. Each square represented a different Christian denomination, and the stone repeatedly fell on the Anglican square. Now convinced that his father was 'in error', Oscar suffered terrible visions of the Hell that awaited his father, and left home to seek refuge in the home of the local Anglican priest, a man who had always appeared pathetic, even to Oscar. Although he rejected his father's religion on account of its severity, Oscar never lost his puritanical attitudes. Unlike his Sulphur father, however, he never tried to impose these upon others, whom he always saw in the best possible light.

At Oxford, Oscar had no means to pay for his tuition. He waited for several weeks for a solution to reveal itself (Phosphorus will often just hope for the best when difficulties arise), and eventually it did, in the form of a colleague who took him to the races. Oscar knew nothing about betting, except that it was not considered morally sound. Nevertheless, he was suddenly convinced that God had guided him to the races to show him how he might earn his living whilst studying to be a priest. He felt an overwhelming conviction that a certain horse would win, put all his money on it, and his intuition was richly rewarded. This is a good example of Phosphorus' opportunistic thinking. Oscar retained all of his high principles, but reasoned that it was the purpose for which he gambled that mattered, not that gambling was immoral in itself. Since he was still a very pious man, he never once spent his winnings on anything other than his board, tuition fees and meagre rations, and he gave away the excess to charities. His actions, though extreme, are in keeping with the great faith in Life or in God that reassures most Phosphorus people, who tend to be both careless and unselfish with money, since they are more concerned with emotional and spirituals goals, or with just 'going with the flow', and trust that God will provide for the morrow.

The figure of Oscar Hopkins is so faithfully and intricately portrayed by the author that it reveals a hundred and one typical Phosphorus peculiarities. Although Oscar gambles initially merely to pay his bills, he becomes intoxicated with the thrill of it, and it eventually is his undoing. Many Phosphorus people have an addictive personality, not because they are hiding from pain like the Natrum addict (although there is some element of this in every addict), but because they cannot resist the ecstasy that their addiction brings them. Oscar is extremely kind and gentle, and also rather timid. He is one of the more introverted Phosphorus individuals, whose upbringing generated a lot of fear. Phosphorus can appear either boisterous and extroverted, or timid and quiet, depending upon the amount of fear he experienced as a child, and the amount of fear he is experiencing in the moment. Even the quietest Phosphorus like Oscar has moments of wild abandon, when nothing can contain his joy, nor inhibit its expression. I was fascinated to observe that a whole chapter of the book is dedicated to Oscar's enthusiastic description of the phenomenon of phosphorescence at sea. Did the author know his homeopathy, or was this merely a beautiful example of 'synchronicity'? The book should be read by all student homeopaths, not only for its detailed portrayal of a Phosphorus personality, but also for its equally consistent portrayal of proud and timid Silica, in the form of Lucinda Leplastrier.

One reason why Phosphorus individuals have a poor sense of their own identity is that they identify so strongly with other people, especially their parents and their partners. Phosphorus has a tendency to exaggerate, and if he loves somebody, (or some principle), he is liable to put them on a pedestal, and to resist fiercely any attempts by others to knock them off. His identification with the other leads him to adopt the same opinions, the same mannerisms and even the same habits as the one he admires and respects. He may identify not with an individual but with an organisation or a religion, in which case he is likely to be the most devout and trusting member of that group, and will not examine evidence that may be critical of the faith's dogma, or the party line.

Just as Phosphorus idolises, or at least, idealises those he loves, so he exaggerates the negative qualities of those he dislikes. For example, if his father was strict and cruel, the young Phosphorus may at first seek his approval, and love him unconditionally, but eventually even Phosphorus will close his heart in the face of constant abuse, and when he does this, he may turn his father into an image of all that is evil, choosing to forget the latter's many good qualities. Even then, he may maintain the hope for decades that his father will return to his mother, and that she will miraculously reform him into the loving father he never had. Phosphorus cannot bear disharmony, and often plays the role of peacemaker, even to the point of sacrificing his own interests to avoid a family upset.

Phosphorus has a great tendency to generalise. He finds it hard to take in the myriad aspects of the river of life in which he floats (like a boat without a rudder at times), and rather than consider them piecemeal, he will make sweeping generalisations to make his image of the world more manageable. He starts with his own personal experience, and then tries to make new information fit the same patterns, without exercising very much discrimination. For example, ask a Phosphorus girl what she thinks about Russians, and she might reply, "Oh, they're lovely people! I met one once and he had such a nice smile!" In contrast, Natrum might reply realistically, "I don't know, I've only met one", whilst Lycopodium is quite liable to disguise his personal inexperience of Russians by launching into an intellectual discourse on the Slavic character, using information he has gleaned from books.

The 'woolly thinking' that is so characteristic of Phosphorus (as opposed to the erratic, disjointed thinking of Argentum) results from his general lack of focus. Like the phosphoric Russian translator, he may develop sufficient discrimination in certain areas to function effectively, but vast areas of his life may be left floating in a kind of no-man's-land. For example, he may be oblivious of his state of health, his bank balance and his wife's birthday, yet be able to function reasonably as a school-teacher. Like Sulphur, his mind tends to neglect details (though unlike Phosphorus, Sulphur may be extremely knowledgeable about the details of those subjects that interest him) and also unpleasant practical necessities. Phosphorus is less intellectual than Sulphur, being more concerned with leading a carefree or a glamorous existence than with intellectual ideas. (The difference is like that between Einstein and Peter Pan.)

Because he is open to so many things, Phosphorus often becomes scattered mentally. Whereas Sulphur will ignore practical necessities in favour of a single obsessive interest, Phosphorus will flit like a butterfly from one passing interest to another, without ever developing more than a superficial understanding of each. He may have quite a sharp mind, and be gifted, for instance, at mental arithmetic, but he has very little mental discipline (Kent: 'Irresolute'), and he usually makes a restless and impatient student (unless he is studying something which appeals to his ethereal nature, such as painting or ballet).

Scattered thinking tends to make Phosphorus appear vague or muddled at times. Although the Phosphorus nurse is conscientious, she may have difficulty following instructions to the letter, and she may mix up one patient's temperature with another's pulse whilst filling in the observation sheets. Generally, Phosphorus has enough mental clarity to get by at work, but not without numerous minor slips and oversights. I have seen Phosphorus individuals make use of their vagueness deliberately to excuse their omissions. One Phosphorus patient of mine would 'smudge over' the details when he wanted to hide something he was ashamed of, and a Phosphorus friend of mine had a similar habit of confusing the issue with a smokescreen of unrelated observations when she was trying to avoid an unpleasant fact.

Phosphorus is oversensitive to many influences, and it is when she is under stress that she appears most muddled. At these times she may do silly things like putting the clothes into the dishwasher, and the dishes into the washing machine, and when she realises her mistake, she is just as liable to laugh as to cry.

### Fear and Anxiety

The degree to which a person is fearful as he grows up depends both on his constitution and the degree to which he feels threatened by his environment. Phosphorus is more sensitive to his environment than most, and during his childhood any disharmony within the home will generate anxiety, which becomes part of his personality if it continues for long.

It is Phosphorus' extreme openness to external impressions which makes him vulnerable, combined with his relatively weak sense of identity. Because he is constantly bombarded from all directions with a barrage of sensory impressions, and the heady mix of emotions which they trigger, he tends to panic sometimes when it all gets too much for him, and he can no longer process the kaleidoscope of feelings and thoughts swirling around inside. Thus Phosphorus is particularly prone to anxiety when he is under pressure, and also when he is excited or in new surroundings. Unlike Pulsatilla and Calcarea, he is adventurous by nature, and is quite liable to leap at any opportunity to experience something new, but when does, his delight may be followed by anxiety. This is particularly the case in Phosphorus children. Like Ignatia children they are very excitable, and in their excitement they sometimes overstep the limits of what they can cope with experientially. For example, a Phosphorus child may meet a lot of new children at a birthday party. At first he is stimulated and keen to interact with his new playmates. In his excitement he shouts, dances about, and plays tricks on the other children. Having become intoxicated with excitement (Kent: 'Excitability even to ecstasy'), he is then presented with a change of circumstances, which overloads his ability to cope. It may be that a clown is brought in to entertain the children, and the clown's appearance scares rather than amuses him. Had he not been so excited, he would not have been scared, but his mind cannot cope with something new to digest, and he responds by panicking and crying for his mother.

The Phosphorus adult is also prone to anxiety when life gets too hectic. At such times he is liable to invent problems which do not exist. For example, a young Phosphorus man on the eve of his wedding day may develop the fear that he is going to have a car accident, or imagine that his bride no longer loves him, (Kent: 'Fear of imaginary things'). The next day his fear may appear foolish or be forgotten, but at the time it generated a great deal of anxiety.

Similarly, in times of stress Phosphorus will often magnify a small problem or threat out of all proportion. His imagination runs riot, unrestrained by common sense. A Phosphorus woman feeling pressured by difficulties at work may become afraid that her indigestion is a sign of cancer (Kent: 'Fear of impending disease'), and this fear may trouble her until the difficulties at work subside, at which point it suddenly disappears. A Phosphorus man who is struggling with a difficult relationship may become convinced, when his girlfriend postpones a date, that she is seeing another man, and this fear obsesses him until he sees her again, and she assures him that it isn't so. Although generally an optimist (often hopelessly so), under stress Phosphorus tends to imagine the worst, and to suffer a great deal of anxiety as a result. Fortunately, his fears are more easily dispelled than most by a little reassurance. Lacking boundaries himself, he needs someone else to protect him at times, and to say that everything is alright. Such reassurance has as great a positive effect on him as minor threats may have a negative effect. Thus his innocence and impressionability are as much a blessing as a curse.

Phosphorus is more fearful when alone. The presence of people (even unfamiliar people), helps to anchor his awareness in the here and now, and prevents it from flitting off into imaginary terrors. Being alone at night, or in the dark, is particularly likely to make Phosphorus anxious (Kent: 'Fear of being alone', 'Fear of the dark'). Female Phosphorus individuals are even more prone to anxiety than their male counterparts, particularly at night. Their fertile imagination will work overtime in the dark, conjuring up spooks out of every shadow and every noise (Kent: 'Sees faces wherever he turns his eyes'). Phosphorus, like Medorrhinum, has a fear of ghosts and spirits, and is far more likely to believe in them than most people, but then she has more reason to, since like Medorrhinum, she is relatively clairvoyant.

Hypochondriasis is a common cause of concern for the Phosphorus individual. Any little symptom or blemish may evoke the fear of deadly disease, especially when Phosphorus is going through an anxious period generally. At other times she tends to be blissfully unaware of her body, or aware of the bliss running through it (whereas Arsenicum is seldom very far from the fear of illness and death, even in the good times). Again, this anxiety can usually be dispelled fairly quickly by the physician when it is misplaced, unlike that of Arsenicum, which resists reassurance.

One of the most characteristic fears of Phosphorus is an inexplicable dread that something terrible is about to happen. This is presumably a result of fearful imagination combining with a memory of accurate past intuition. Because she has been right about her intuitions before, she reacts all the more strongly to any feelings of dread which she experiences. (The fact that the majority of her premonitions were inaccurate never occurs to her.) At such times it is hard to reassure her, because she feels she knows more about the future than others, and she may be sure that her premonition of disaster is reliable. Nevertheless, once she has relaxed and the other causes of stress in her life have subsided, her dread will dissolve, (unless it is a true intuition, in which case it is liable to persist).

Because she is so vulnerable, so open to the violence of the world, a Phosphorus person who has known quite a lot of suffering sometimes develops a suspicious, paranoid attitude. If, for example, her mother was cruel to her when she was little, she may grow up expecting harm from almost anyone, especially from women who remind her of her mother (Kent: 'Suspicious'). The Natrum woman who has suffered and become somewhat paranoid tends to have a prickly, defensive persona. Phosphorus, by contrast, becomes timid. If she feels under attack she will not fight back like Natrum, but withdraws to a place of safety, or at least remains silent, in an attempt to avoid aggression. If she feels that there is nobody that she can turn to for support at such times, she can become quite panicky, and may withdraw into herself. In her isolation, there is nobody to counter her paranoid fears, which may thus intensify rather than abate. However, Phosphorus seldom develops true paranoid insanity.

When Phosphorus feels threatened she is liable to resort to 'magical thinking' to ward off danger, much as a child does. If she is religious she will pray intensely for protection, but if she is not, she may perform her own mental ritual to protect herself. For example, in times of perceived danger she may close her eyes and count backwards from ten to one, as if the danger will magically disappear by the end of the count, or she may collect lucky charms and wear them religiously. These charms may be manufactured commercially for the purpose, such as miniature horse-shoes, or they may take the form of any object that the Phosphorus individual has decided is lucky for her. Thus she may collect coloured shells, or carry around with her a locket of hair from an old lover, for the purpose of protecting her from evil. Phosphorus is not listed in Kent's repertory under the rubric 'Superstitious', but it should be added in black type. Peter Carey, in his faithful portrait of the phosphoric Oscar in his novel 'Oscar and Lucinda' depicts Oscar on a boat holding onto his caul (a membrane which occasionally covers an infant's head at birth, which was kept for him by his father) for grim death in an attempt to ward off his phobia of the sea.

Although Phosphorus is prone to many fears, his adventurous spirit, extroversion and 'joi de vivre' often predominate as far as external impressions go, giving the impression of a care-free happy-go-lucky personality. This impression is generally true, since Phosphorus is so 'transparent' emotionally. The majority of Phosphorus individuals are prone to frequent but transient bouts of anxiety, which do not overshadow their buoyant spirits for long. A few who have known greater hardship than the others may become anxious much of the time, but even these more damaged Phosphorus spirits are liable to respond remarkably quickly to a safe loving environment, in comparison to more introverted types like Natrum and Ignatia.

### *Physical Appearance*

In keeping with the charismatic nature of the Phosphorus personality, the appearance of the Phosphorus individual is often very beautiful. The body is generally tall, slim and very lithe, being more flexible than most, to the point of being double-jointed. The limbs tend to be long and graceful, like those of a dancer, but not as fragile as those of Silica. The body is generally held in a very loose, relaxed manner, and tends to move with effortless grace. (There is a variant of Phosphorus, however, which is tall, lanky and awkward in movement, rather like a new-born foal.)

The Phosphorus physique is very similar to that of Tuberculinum, a very closely related type. Both types are often freckled, and both are prone to Pectus Excavatum, or sunken breast bone. However, the Phosphorus physique is more graceful than that of Tuberculinum, which is more wiry.

The facial features of Phosphorus are usually highly characteristic. The most prominent features are the eyes, which are unusually large, and bordered by very long eyelashes, giving a most attractive appearance of innocence. The complexion is usually very soft and smooth, even in the men, and the skin is silky to the touch. The face is angular in outline rather than rounded, and tends to be triangular in shape, with a pointed chin and a broad forehead.

Phosphorus generally has a wide mouth (reflecting an open nature) with delicately curved lips. The teeth are usually large and prominent, and the upper front teeth are sometimes 'bucked', that is inclining forwards.

Most Phosphorus people have an impish quality, and the men are often rather androgynous in appearance.

The hair is usually straight and silky, and is frequently light brown or reddish, although blonde and even black do occur.

Famous Phosphorus personalities include the actresses Michelle Pfeiffer and Julia Roberts, and the actor Martin Short. The Australian super-model Elle McPherson is also likely to be a Phosphorus, as is Julia Robert's ex-husband Lyle Lovett, who has the typical ulta-wide mouth, as well as a kind of 'gawky' look that is common in Phosphorus individuals.

# *Platina*

*Keynotes:* Hysteria, pride, nymphomania

Platina is a rare constitutional type, known in homeopathic circles principally for its sexual obsession. I have seen only a handful of Platina individuals, hence the following description is necessarily brief.

Platina individuals can be divided into those who are more or less sane and stable, and those who are insane or on the borderline of insanity. They have many features in common psychologically, characteristics which become distorted and exaggerated as Platina becomes less healthy psychologically. As far as I know, Platina is an exclusively female remedy-type.

## The Sane Platina

The sane Platina woman is a sensitive, emotional person, not unlike Ignatia in many ways. Like Ignatia, she is passionate, not just sexually, but about many things. However, it is her intense sexual desire which she is most likely to complain about to the homeopath. The sexual desire of Platina is more intense and more persistent than that of any other type. Although it may bring pleasure when it is indulged, it is so demanding that it usually causes distress as well. This otherwise sensible woman complains that from time to time she cannot escape from sexual thoughts (Kent: 'Sexual thoughts intrude'), which interrupt her normal thinking with sudden intensity, as if they were not her thoughts at all, and are accompanied by tremendous sexual desire. Because she is a sane, sensitive woman, she knows that this is abnormal, but she may be too ashamed to seek help, or she may think that there is nothing that can be done about her sudden sexual impulses. Either way, it is likely that her 'problem' will remain hidden from the vast majority of people.

In order to cope with their sexual urges, some Platina women resort to frequent masturbation. Others simply resist the urges, and yet others become promiscuous. Those who do act out their sexual obsession are generally less healthy psychologically, partly because they have 'given in' to their abnormal impulses, and hence are no longer in control of themselves, and partly because their promiscuity deprives them of the stability of a one-to-one relationship, and exposes them to the unpredictable influences of their many partners.

From the outside, the first impression one may get of a relatively sane Platina woman is a certain haughtiness. She will tend to treat others a little dismissively, as if they were not worth her time (Kent: 'Haughty', 'Indifferent while in company'). I once worked in a community along with a young woman who seemed to keep to herself, apart from mixing with a select few friends. When our paths crossed, she always seemed very aloof to me, and at first I thought that she didn't like me for some reason. One day she was suffering from a bad bout of 'flu, and a friend of hers asked me if I would treat her homeopathically. I called in at her room, and offered to take her case. Rather than thank me, she went straight into describing her symptoms, and at the end of the interview she thanked me in a terse, unconvincing manner, as if to say, "That will be all thank you. Be off with you." She later told me that the remedy had helped her, and again thanked me in a perfunctory way, as if it were her duty to do so. I noticed that she never smiled at me when we passed each other, and I wondered why. Eventually this woman came to me one day and asked me for some Platina. I asked her why she wanted it, and she said that she "had a sexual problem." She seemed too embarrassed to elaborate, but said that a homeopath had given her Platina 200 and it had helped for a while. Although she wouldn't describe her sexual problem to me, she smiled when she alluded to it, as if she were either flirting with me, or was pleased when she thought of her sexuality. This impression was combined with the contradictory embarrassment. Clearly Platina women such as her are pulled two ways by their sexual obsession, seeking help for it whilst at the same time enjoying the stimulation it brings. Having witnessed the haughty way in which she had behaved towards me, I was inclined to trust the prescription of Platina made by the other homeopath, and I gave her a dose of Platina 10M. A couple of weeks later she told me that her sexual problem had become much more manageable. Although she did not want me to take a full history, she did admit to one other Platina characteristic. She was divorced, and told me that she had been prone whilst married to sudden impulses to stab her husband with a knife (Kent: 'Sudden impulse to kill').

Platina's pride is accompanied by a sensitivity to rejection which is ironic in view of her own attitude towards other people. Like Natrum and Ignatia, she easily feels slighted, ignored or abandoned (Kent: 'Ailments from scorn', 'Oversensitive', 'Delusions—deserted, forsaken'). Like Natrum she is often averse to conversation and company, feels worse for consolation, and better for crying. Again, like Natrum and Ignatia, when she does get close to somebody, she may be devastated when she loses them (Kent: 'Ailments from grief'), which goes to show that Platina's emotional depth should not be judged by her sexual desire.

Alternating states are highly characteristic of Platina individuals. Even the sane Platina woman is subject to alternations of mood (Kent: 'Mood alternating'), but these alternations become extreme in the less healthy Platina.

One day she may be morose, and the next she is euphoric. One day she is calm, and the next she is extremely irritable and tense. It is not just that her mood is variable. It actually alternates between two distinct moods. Similarly, Platina is subject to alternations between physical symptoms and psychological states. One Platina patient complained of sexual excitement alternating with depression, and another of headaches alternating with anxiety. The periodicity of the alternation may be anything from a day to over a week.

### The Insane Platina

A sane Platina woman may, as a result of life's difficulties (especially if they involve grief or a shock of some kind) gradually deteriorate mentally towards insanity. I treated one such lady before she completely lost touch with reality, with the result that she was able to revert to a reasonably normal existence. When I first saw her she complained principally of various rather bizarre physical symptoms, such as shifting numbness, and a sense that her head was being squeezed in a vice. At first I did not see Platina in her history, but on the third visit she trusted me enough to tell me about some of her more unusual mental and physical symptoms. She began rather shyly to tell me that she was subject to powerful sexual urges. She was married and religious, and felt a little guilty about these urges, which she did not act upon. I asked her if she had any sexual fantasies, and she said that she did. Her fantasies were actually more like hallucinations or delusions. She said that she felt at times that she had the body of Jesus, and she was very angry with Jesus for taking over her body, since it gave her the sexual feelings of a man, which she described as 'brutish'. She said that at these times she wanted to make love with women (Kent: 'Love sick with one of her own sex'), or that Jesus was making love with her. She was aware that these feelings were 'crazy', and was able to talk sensibly with me, but she also treated these delusions as more real than imaginary, and felt that she was being made love to or possessed by Jesus. It is typical of the more insane Platina woman to be subject to religious delusions, whether or not they become mixed with her sexual fantasy (Kent: 'Religious—alternates with sexual excitement', 'Religious affections'). This patient of mine also described the inflation of the ego that is so characteristic of Platina, and which becomes more and more extreme as the pathology progresses. She said that she felt as if she was sent to bring light to the people and that she was looking down from a great height on suffering humanity. Although she took these delusions seriously, she also commented "It's ego, isn't it?," indicating that she still had considerable insight into her condition.

Sometimes we can learn more about a person from their family than from them. A young woman once told me a harrowing tale of her upbringing with her insane mother, who was almost certainly a Platina constitutionally. Her mother was a religious fanatic, and sometimes described herself as 'the Bride of Christ'. She would talk about demons in the house, (Kent: 'Fear of evil'), and would sometimes talk to thin air, telling her children not to bother her whilst she did this. One day she emptied all the furniture out of the house in order to find a demon who she said was lurking inside the house somewhere. (She ordered her terrified children to assist her.) My patient told me that her mother acted as if she were a queen, expecting those around her to do all of her chores, whilst she went out and had a good time. In particular, she treated her daughters like slaves, whereas her sons could do no wrong, presumably because she found them attractive, and used them as surrogate husbands (her husband had committed suicide when my patient was four years old). Nothing her daughters did was good enough for her, and they lived in constant fear of punishment. My patient also lived in constant fear of being killed by her mother. She had a vague, very early memory of having a pillow held over her face by her mother (Kent: 'Propensity to kill'), and two of her baby sisters had died of 'cot-deaths'. She also had a feeling that her mother had sexually molested her when she was very young. Her mother gave the impression publicly of being very chaste after becoming a widow, but in fact had several affairs with men from her religious community. Unfortunately, I never had the opportunity to treat my patient's mother, but I was grateful for such a graphic account of life with an insane Platina woman.

The alternation of mood seen in the sane Platina can become an alternation between sanity and insanity as the pathology progresses, or between two markedly abnormal mental states, such as intense sexual arousal with rampant fantasising, and religiousness, with either delusions of grandeur or fear of damnation (Kent: 'Imagines being doomed'). Violent thoughts may become persistent as sanity recedes, particularly the thought of stabbing somebody at the sight of a knife. (Alumina has the same compulsion, but is fairly easy to distinguish from Platina in most cases.) I have not seen it, but there is presumably a danger of the delusions of grandeur and divine mission combining with the impulse to kill, and hence making it more likely that they will hurt someone.

One symptom that is highly characteristic of Platina as she becomes more unhealthy psychologically is the tendency to laugh inappropriately (Kent: 'Laughing over serious matters'). Hyoscyamus also laughs inappropriately, and is often sexually obsessed, but the laughter of Hyoscyamus is more generalised, in that she will laugh at anything and nothing, whereas Platina laughs specifically at the most serious things that are said or that she thinks. She will finally get up the courage to tell her homeopath about her sexual fantasy, and immediately after describing it she will laugh. Or she will laugh during the interview when she considers talking about a serious matter, such as her fear that she is going insane (Kent: 'Fear of loss of reason'). She does not find these matters amusing. She simply cannot stop herself from laughing. The other type who laughs at serious matters is Natrum Muriaticum. Here too there is no amusement, but simply a reflex response with which the person attempts to avoid the fear implicit in the situation.

The delusions that Platina experiences about being a great person, looking down from a great height, are accompanied in many cases by an illusion that her body is very large (Kent: 'Delusions as to the greatness of the body'). The only other type who commonly describes this is Cannabis Indica. In contrast, Platina may experience other people as very small - a visual hallucination which is consistent with her pride. Along with these hallucinations come strange and highly characteristic bodily sensations, the commonest of which are the feeling that her body is dead (Kent: 'Death—sensation of'), and generalised or localised numbness. Another common sensation is that of a constriction or ring around a bodily part (which is also seen in Plumbum cases).

Like all exclusively female remedy-types, Platina tends to suffer from gynaecological and hormonal problems. The alternation of mood is particularly marked perimenstrually, and also after childbirth (Kent: 'Mania-puerperal', 'Anguish during menses'). One Platina patient said that she was torn between her great love for her husband, and 'insane anger', particularly before her period. Her love was as passionate as her anger, and she found another outlet for her fiery emotions through singing. She not only sang a lot at home, but also sang in a choir. As her mental state deteriorated, she found that she could no longer sing publicly, because she began to feel panicky (Kent: 'Fear of crowds, excitement'), and she greatly missed this outlet for her feelings. This particular patient also had a fetish, which I have not seen in other Platinas, but which is not surprising, in view of the intense sexuality, and distorted mentality of the unhealthy Platina. Her fetish involved chairs. She felt a compulsion to sit wherever someone else was sitting, or had just sat, and when she sat in a chair that had just been vacated, she felt a sensuous thrill and a sense of contentment.

### Fear and Panic

Virtually all 'hysterical' types are prone to feelings of anxiety and panic, and Platina is no exception. As with Alumina and more psychotic types like Hyoscyamus, anxiety increases as Platina's grip on reality becomes more tenuous. Fear of people, particularly large groups of people, is a common complaint, as is the justifiable fear of going insane. Other fears reported by Platina individuals include fear of immanent death (Kent: 'Presentiment of death'), fear of ghosts (which may result from hallucinations of spirits) and the fear that they will kill someone. Free-floating anxiety is also common in the more insane Platina, alternating with feelings of power and superiority.

Platina is a very sensitive individual, and like Ignatia she can be frightened by the intensity of her own feelings. Hence she is liable to feel anxiety after anger, or after intense sexual arousal. She is very excitable, and this may be one reason why she tends to keep to herself. She knows that she can only take so much stimulation before she feels panicky and out of control.

### Physical Appearance

I have seen too few Platinas to gather much information about their physical appearance. One impression that I am left with is the fullness of their lips in most cases, which is consistent with their passionate nature. I have seen both thin and fat Platinas, blondes and brunettes.

# Pulsatilla

*Keynote:* The feminine principle

Pulsatilla is often thought by homeopaths to be a common and easily recognisable type. In my experience neither of these assumptions is correct. In adults Pulsatilla is both uncommon and easily confused with other remedy-types, especially with Silica, Phosphorus, Staphysagria, Lycopodium, Calcarea and Natrum Muriaticum. All of these types can be emotional and passive, but homeopathic students tend to be given the impression that Pulsatilla is the emotional, passive type, and hence the remedy is over-prescribed.

### The Pulsatilla Child

No type is as universally feminine as Pulsatilla. There are a few Pulsatilla men, but the vast majority of adult Pulsatillas are female. At risk of attracting the indignation of feminist readers, I would venture to suggest that Pulsatilla is the most feminine of types because she lives almost entirely through her emotions, and does not suppress them. She has an intellect, but it is used exclusively in the service of her emotional needs and desires. This is why her ideas can appear so changeable. Emotions are very changeable things, especially when they are given free reign and not suppressed, and since Pulsatilla's thoughts are generally concerned with emotional satisfaction, they tend to be flighty and unpredictable.

Young children of both sexes are often Pulsatilla constitutionally. As they grow up, the majority of Pulsatilla children change into other constitutional types, leaving surprisingly few adult Pulsatillas (this is one reason why many blonde children become darker as they get older). Between the ages of two and five children are functioning primarily from their emotions. (Before this their focus is principally physical, and after this the intellect becomes increasingly dominant.) It is precisely this age-group of children which contains a large proportion of Pulsatillas. Once the intellect begins to take over and 'edit' the child's emotional life, the Pulsatilla state has gone.

Pulsatilla children of both sexes are highly emotional. They are generally devoted, affectionate and mild providing their emotional needs are met by their parents, but they tend to demand instant gratification, and if they feel deprived they will cry and be petulant until their needs are met. Pulsatilla is such a natural type. If the Pulsatilla child hurts, she cries, whether the hurt is emotional or physical. There is no attempt to disguise her pain, and once it is over, it is forgotten immediately. This is very much like the Phosphorus child, who is often confused with Pulsatilla. The difference is in the degree of emotionality. Pulsatilla is always emotional (though her emotions may be soft and gentle much of the time), and hence personal in her interests and her responses, whereas Phosphorus is more detached and impersonal. To be sure, Phosphorus children can be highly emotional at times, but their principal focus is more active, curious and adventurous than Pulsatilla, who is more concerned with being loved than with exploration. This pre-occupation with personal emotional satisfaction is the cornerstone of the Pulsatilla personality, around which all other attributes revolve.

Little children are very often selfish in their attitudes. This is especially true of Pulsatilla. In the playground Pulsatilla will jealously guard her hoard of sweets (Kent: 'Avarice'), and perhaps deign to give one to her most special friend (as both a reward and an incentive to be nice), whereas the Phosphorus child will share her sweets freely with her playmates. Like Natrum, Pulsatilla is always looking for emotional security, and very easily feels rejected (Kent: 'Forsaken feeling'), whereas other sensitive children like Silica and Phosphorus are actually more robust emotionally. They may require stimulation and attention, as well as a reasonable amount of affection to be happy, but they do not need the constant reassurance that they are loved that is so characteristic of both Pulsatilla and Ignatia. It is this emotional insecurity that makes Pulsatilla selfish. She tends to put her own emotional needs before all else, and will create a scene if necessary to be noticed and taken care of. Alternately, she may whine and moan continually if she is unhappy, in an attempt to attract loving attention (Kent: 'Moaning, groaning'). As soon as she receives the love she is looking for, she is blissfully happy, and as long as it is forthcoming, and obvious, she does not have a care, at least not for long. Like Calcarea, Pulsatilla is very simple in her needs. She simply wants to be loved, and as long as she has this, she is soft, mild and contented. She will then languish in her contentment, making the most of all of her pleasant personal contacts, and also of her sensual appetites.

As one would expect, the Pulsatilla child is extremely dependent upon her parents. She will become anxious if they are out of her sight for more than a few moments, and in public she will tend to stay very close to them, often holding a parent's hand, or even clinging to her mother's dress. As long as she feels loved, she will take great delight from the little playful interactions that make up much of her communication with her parents, and she is particularly fond of physical contact. All Pulsatillas have a great need for physical warmth and contact, whether they be children or adults. They will languish blissfully in the arms of a loving father, utterly devoted and at peace, and will jump at any opportunity for physical affection. Favourite aunts and uncles will also be enjoyed enormously by the Pulsatilla child, particularly if they indulge her, and are physically affectionate. When Pulsatilla is feeling happy and secure, she has a very characteristic 'coyness' which is extremely charming, and attracts a great deal of affection. Her wide, innocent eyes are at once shy and playful, and her smile is both tentative and a little pleased with itself, as if to say, "Be nice to me—look how lovely I am!" Adult Pulsatillas lose none of this coy charm, and they know how to use it to their advantage.

Away from home, the Pulsatilla child is timid with strangers. Like Silica, she will hold back from them at first, whilst she assesses whether they are safe and friendly or not (Kent: 'Bashful, timid). If they appear hostile, she will become frightened very easily, and will not speak to them at all, but instead hides behind her parent. When she has established, however, that the stranger is 'nice', she will lose her reticence far more quickly than will Silica, and very quickly she will be flirting with them, showing them her favourite toy, and telling them her most prized secrets (such as the name of the boy at school she is in love with).

Although she is very trusting with those she loves, Pulsatilla can be very suspicious of strangers, and will not necessarily be won over by a show of friendliness (Kent: 'Suspicious'). The doctor who murmurs reassuring words as he attempts to insert an auroscope into little Pulsatilla's ear may be met by screams of objection long before he touches her. Whom Pulsatilla likes and whom she dislikes is a highly personal and idiosyncratic matter, and once they have been decided, her preferences are very black and white, though they may be short-lived. Although she cannot bear the nasty doctor, and will cringe when she sees him, one day he suddenly redeems himself, and she flashes her winning smile at him, her seal of approval.

After personal interaction with loving intimates, Pulsatilla's next love is the enjoyment of the senses. As well as being highly tactile, she loves visual beauty, and also the taste of her favourite food. Once again, she is highly personal and 'fussy' about her preferences, whether she be five or fifty years of age. The young Pulsatilla will adamantly refuse to wear a dress if she doesn't like the colour, and her palate is often extremely fickle. It is this tendency towards highly personal and specific preferences which resulted in Pulsatilla being included in Kent's Repertory under the rubric 'Fastidious'. She is not fastidious in the sense of tidy and orderly like Arsenicum and Natrum. She is simply fussy, like a spoilt child who has to have her own way. Naturally, the more the Pulsatilla child succeeds in manipulating her parents with her sudden outbursts of emotion, the more spoilt she will become. Many Natrum and Ignatia children are equally fussy, and manipulate their parents into spoiling them. These three types have a lot in common, the principal difference with Pulsatilla being her relative absence of emotional suppression. Like Natrum and Ignatia, Pulsatilla will tend to get very jealous of other children if they are favoured by her parent. In fact, she will get jealous of anyone who takes up her parent's time, or the time of her best friend (Kent: 'Jealousy'). In her jealousy, she is apt to behave petulantly, taking her spite out on her competitor, as well as on her loved one. Thus she may break her brother's new toy if she thinks it is nicer than hers, and refuse to eat her lunch if he is the centre of attention on his birthday.

Pulsatilla is one of the more fearful types. Pulsatilla children in particular are prone to all manner of fears, especially when they are feeling insecure as a result of inadequate parental attention, or a change of circumstances. Like Calcarea and Natrum, Pulsatilla is fearful of change, and reacts anxiously to relatively minor threats to personal security. Most Pulsatilla children are afraid of the dark to some extent. They usually say that they are afraid of ghosts (Kent: 'Fear of ghosts at night'), whereas half of the Natrum children who admit to being afraid of the dark say that they are afraid of 'men', like their adult counterparts. Being alone usually makes Pulsatilla anxious, especially in childhood. Even adult Pulsatillas tend to be very dependent on company.

Aggression is especially threatening to Pulsatilla. She buckles and cries at the slightest hint of aggression, whether verbal or physical, and in families she will usually give way silently rather than face the wrath of an angry parent, and as an adult will often play the role of peace-maker. In this role she relies more on appeals to the heart than on reason. Pulsatilla cannot bear disharmony, especially between her loved ones, and she will beg them to be nice to each other, for her sake if nothing else.

### The Adult Pulsatilla-Personal Concerns

Pulsatilla is more personal in her interests than any other type. Her principal concerns revolve around her loved ones, and her life is devoted to a search for and then a celebration of personal love. Pulsatilla nearly always has someone to whom she is devoted. As a child it was usually her parents. Later on her devotion is transferred to her boyfriend, and then to her husband and her children. As long as she is with her loved ones, and their love for her is evident, she is happy, and is relatively free from ambition. Feminists tend to see red when they are confronted with Pulsatilla. She is quite happy to stay at home and look after her husband and her children. In fact this is what she lives for. She is extremely nurturing, and indulges her loved ones as much as she likes to be indulged herself. She couldn't care less about politics or philosophy, or the state of the economy (Kent: 'Cares about domestic affairs). As long as her home life is going smoothly, she lives in blissful ignorance of much of the world's drama. In this she resembles Calcarea (who is also very similar in physical appearance, and can easily be mistaken for Pulsatilla). However, even homely Calcarea tends to have more interests than Pulsatilla that do not revolve around her loved ones, such as a career, or a creative hobby. Pulsatilla generally chooses her pastimes according to the preferences and the availability of her mate or her children. If her husband plays chess, she will learn to play chess. If he is away for a few weeks, and the children have left home, she will feel lost, and will be forced to do something solely for herself. One Pulsatilla patient of mine, an attractive and sophisticated lady in her late forties, had lived a life of domestic contentment until her husband died. After this she felt entirely at sea for a year or so, having done everything with him up till then. She had to begin to learn how to live in the world, without the protection of, and the preoccupation with her husband. At first she was very afraid of meeting new people on her own, and practical tasks like selling her house sent her into a panic. Eventually she learned new skills as a masseuse and reflexologist and became quite proficient at promoting herself in a very business-like way. In order to expand her interests and her profits, she studied as a nutritionist, and was extremely serious and dedicated to her studies. Like her, many Pulsatilla women do not even consider their individuality until they are left suddenly without their loved ones. Then they wonder who they are, and what their life is about, before finding another mate to devote themselves to, or alternatively, pursuing some worldly activity to give their life some direction and stability.

Adolescence can be a very difficult time for Pulsatilla. Her usual emotional changeability is exacerbated by hormonal instability, and by the pressures of developing sexuality. It is a time when Pulsatilla's attachment to and dependence on her parents must be released to some extent, usually before any stable relationship has been established to take its place. Pulsatilla does tend to hold onto her parents and rely on them for a longer period than most other adolescents. When she does finally leave home, she can enter into a very unstable, distressing period if she does not have a stable romantic relationship. I came across one such Pulsatilla woman in her early twenties. She was attending art college, and sharing a house with a friend whom I also knew. Her flatmate complained to me that her Pulsatilla friend was constantly asking her advice on how to live her life, and then complaining when her advice was ignored and things turned out badly. In particular, the Pulsatilla woman was constantly jumping in and out of unsuitable romantic or sexual liaisons, and then complaining to her flatmate about how miserable she was without a partner, or how miserable she was with a particular boyfriend. Many Pulsatillas enter into relationships impulsively, in a desperate attempt to find the emotional security they crave. This particular young woman (the term 'girl' seems more appropriate, despite her age) suffered from a great sense of being 'lost', since she had no strong relationship to steady her. In order to attract approval she immersed herself in various fashionable interests, including environmentalism, which she would debate with her fellow students, but which she felt little real passion for. Her appearance was usually very dishevelled, in a rather 'punk' way which was fashionable amongst art students, but which succeeded in reflecting the confusion inside her. Those Pulsatillas who are fortunate enough to step from the parental home into a loving, stable romantic relationship cope more easily with adolescence and early adulthood, and avoid much of the confusion and homesickness of the others.

### Emotional Instability

I was about to write that of all the common constitutional types, Pulsatilla is the most emotionally unstable, after Ignatia, when I reflected that Pulsatilla is really rather uncommon. I have come across considerably more Ignatias than adult Pulsatillas, and Ignatia is not a very common type either. The principal difference between Ignatia and Pulsatilla is the degree of emotional intensity. Both have very changeable moods (Kent: 'Mood alternating'), but Ignatia's emotions are far more intense, since they are deeper, and they have the volatile power of suppressed emotions behind them.

When things are going well for Pulsatilla, and she is in a loving and stable relationship, her negative moods may be relatively infrequent. When they do occur, they are likely to be triggered by a perceived threat to her emotional security. Even 'healthy' relationships tend to have their ups and downs, and Pulsatilla is very sensitive to any withdrawal of affection. If her husband is more aloof than usual because he is tired after work, she may worry that he doesn't love her anymore, and in her worry she may exaggerate his aloofness out of all proportion, working herself up into an emotional state, so that when he says that he doesn't like her new perfume, she bursts into tears and runs to her bedroom. Pulsatilla is prone to all manner of emotional states, (Kent: 'Mood - timid, sullen, suspicious, tearful, sad, restless, obscene' etc), the majority of which are brought about by a threat to her relationships with loved ones, or by a lack of a loving relationship. As long as she feels loved, she will tend to be mild and cooperative, but once this is threatened, she has none of the disciplined, automatic defences of Natrum Muriaticum. Rather than suppressing her sadness, she will cry. Rather than suppressing her anger, she will shout or smash dinner plates. When things are not quite so bad, but there is some disturbance in her relationship, Pulsatilla may be edgy or constantly irritable (Kent: 'Discontented with everything'). In this state she may not say what the problem is, and she may not even know, but she will take out her frustration and tension upon her family, complaining about this, or weeping about that (Kent: 'Causeless weeping'). Pulsatilla is listed in Kent's Repertory in black type or italics under no less than fifteen rubrics beginning with 'weeping'. Crying is her most frequent response to emotional pain. In most cases it is gentle crying, rather than heavy sobbing (Ignatia, Natrum Muriaticum), which responds well to reassurance and affection.

However, Pulsatilla tends to become very attached to people (and pets), and after a bereavement or separation, she may break down in hysterical weeping , and feel like committing suicide (Kent: 'Grief'—black type, 'Mood—hysterical', 'Inconsolable').

Pulsatilla is just as prone to positive emotions as negative ones. She gets excited easily, particularly when she is in love, or is sharing some anticipated good fortune with a loved one. At such times she may be so excitable that she exhausts herself, and then cries without knowing why, or develops a headache (Kent: 'Ailments from excessive joy'). She is generally very fun-loving, and extremely sociable. Apart from 'larking about', and flirting with attractive men (Pulsatilla is a great flirter, especially if she is unattached), she will tend in company to talk about personal issues, and to be interested in the personal side of other people's lives, rather than wanting to talk about theoretical or global matters. In this she resembles Calcarea, and also many Natrum women. She may try her hand at an intellectual debate, but her opinions are likely to be borrowed from her husband, and she will argue emotionally, and without the benefit of facts to back her up, unless she has been forced to make her own way in the world for some time. Otherwise, many of attitudes are likely to be grafted from those of her partner or parents. If her husband is a communist, she will become a communist. If he is a Catholic, she will convert without question, and because she does not question she will probably believe in her new faith. It is not that she is stupid. It is just that her mind takes second place to her heart, a long way behind the latter.

Like other predominantly female types, Pulsatilla is very prone to hormonal disturbances, and the psychological upsets that accompany them. She tends to be at her most unstable premenstrually, at which time she may feel slighted very easily, and cry at the drop of a hat (Kent: 'Weeping before menses'). She is also prone to anger and irritability premenstrually, although crying tends to predominate. Menopausal and post-natal hormonal changes can also upset Pulsatilla's delicate emotional balance. She is listed in Kent's repertory under the rubrics 'Insanity—menopausal', and 'Insanity—puerperal', but I am sure that emotional lability at these times is far more common than insanity in Pulsatilla women.

### Passivity, Simplicity, and Sensuality

Pulsatilla is not a very dynamic type. Like Calcarea, she likes a stable, sensuous life of ease, in which she derives her main satisfaction from loving and supporting her family. Like Calcarea and Phosphorus she is natural; uncomplicated by intellectual defences. She feels no compulsion to make her house immaculate, or to be doing something 'useful' in her free time. She is quite happy to be lazy when she can (Kent: 'Indolence'), unless her mate demands of her that she be productive. Even then, she will tend to resist his demands passively, doing what she wants when he is not around, (unless he is aggressive enough to intimidate her, or makes her think that he may leave). When she is in her element, Pulsatilla is like a vine, pregnant with luscious grapes, indolent but full of the Earth's vitality, generously, but almost nonchalantly supplying those around her with succour. In her role as mother and wife/lover she is natural and spontaneous, but rather than being the solid and dependable mother hen like Calcarea, she is the Earth Goddess, passionate and sensuous with her mate, bountiful and relaxed with her brood. The difference between Pulsatilla and Calcarea at home is really one of degree rather than kind. Calcarea is more down-to-earth, matter-of-fact and practical, while still being somewhat sensuous and idle. Pulsatilla is basically sensuous, nurturing and delicate in her feelings, more emotional than Calcarea, more feminine, and less pragmatic.

The similarities between Pulsatilla and Calcarea are numerous, and a comparison of the two types helps to clarify the nature of each, since it reveals the subtle differences, which reflect different essences. One could say that the essence of Calcarea is structure, inertia, and 'materiality'. She is concerned with permanence, practicality and common-sense. The essence of the adult Pulsatilla is fecundity, sensuality and nurturing. She is the epitome of all that is purely feminine. Nevertheless, each type contains the other's essence as a secondary 'theme'. Calcarea is sensuous and nurturing, and Pulsatilla is 'concerned with domestic affairs', and usually makes a capable cook and housewife, as well as a loving mother and passionate lover.

An excellent (if somewhat extreme) example of a Pulsatilla woman in her element can be seen in the character of Emma Badgery in Peter Carey's hilarious novel 'Illywhacker'. Emma is first depicted as a shy and proper school mistress in the Australian outback. She rapidly falls in love with the young Charles Badgery, after he rushes to her aid and removes a large goanna (a huge lizard) that has been sitting on her back for an hour, whilst she is too terrified to move. The couple move to Sydney, where they open a pet shop, and Emma, in true Pulsatilla style, lives a life of total unquestioning devotion towards her husband, happy to work with him, doing all manner of menial and dirty tasks without a care, and making passionate love with him when the work is done. The two innocents live blissfully like this until Charles, a patriotic and unwittingly insensitive Sulphur, goes off to enlist in the army without telling his wife, it being the middle the Second World War. Whilst he is out, Emma hears where he has gone and why. In a panic she rushes across to the barracks, but she is too late—he is no longer there. It turns out that Charles was not accepted by the Army for medical reasons, but his silent abandonment of Emma left a lasting scar on their relationship. She became a caricature of a Pulsatilla. When Charles arrived back at the pet shop where they lived, he found her huddled on a bed of straw inside a large cage, cuddling her youngest child. She seemed half awake, and would not respond to Charles' entreaties to come out from the cage, except to make little whimpers like an injured animal (Kent: 'Delirium with sleepiness', 'Moaning during sleep'). Although she gradually regained something like normal consciousness, and she frequently ventured from the cage to play with her children, or to have tea with her girlfriend, she spent every night in her cage, which her husband furnished for her with silk cushions, expensive curtains, and a mattress. He waited on her like a devoted slave, bringing her meals, and cups of tea, and imploring her to forgive him. She talked little with him (Kent: 'Indisposed to talk'), and punished him with her sulky, petulant moods, whilst at the same time she languished in the concern he showed her, lapped up the luxury she enjoyed in her safe little cage, and slept snugly there with her two youngest children. I have never seen a Pulsatilla woman behave this hysterically, but Emma's hysteria is very much in keeping with Pulsatilla. It was a reaction to a sudden withdrawal of love (Kent: 'Ailments from mortification' ), a very passive reaction, which resembles the kind of hysteria attributed to Pulsatilla in Kent's 'Materia Medica' ('Insanity in woman who was mild, gentle and tearful…she sits in her chair all day answering nothing or merely nodding her head for "Yes" and "No"). Pulsatilla women (and also children) often punish their loved one with a kind of emotional hysteria, which usually vanishes magically once they feel reassured of the latter's love. Emma's hysteria is interesting, because it not only ties her husband to her in an utterly devoted way, but also supplies her with a snug, cosy nest and the kind of sensual luxury which Pulsatilla enjoys. Although she is somewhat insane, she is sane enough to converse normally with her friend (as long as her unusual behaviour is not discussed), and to be a mother to her children. This kind of highly selective hysteria is a characteristic of Pulsatilla. If she is feeling insecure in a relationship, she may behave normally with others, but demand absolute devotion from her mate, and dissolve into hysterical tears, or withdraw into silence if she does not get it.

Pulsatilla is a creature of whim, hard to fathom from a logical point of view, full of contradictions (a man's idea of a typical woman). Her attitude to sexuality is particularly unpredictable. The old materia medicas are full of references to Pulsatilla's aversion to members of the opposite sex, or to sex itself, and yet Pulsatilla is a very sensual, passionate type, and is generally devoted to her man. The aversion referred to in the old texts is probably due to a combination of two factors. Firstly, when Pulsatilla is insecure she will act petulantly, and say she hates those she loves, and will withdraw from sex to punish her mate. Secondly, Pulsatilla is very impressionable, and she will take any religious teachings in her upbringing very seriously and literally, hence the aversion to sexuality described by the homeopaths of the last century, a time when religious teachings on sexuality were stricter and more widely adhered to than today (Kent: 'Religious aversion to the opposite sex'). Pulsatilla is a very sensitive and vulnerable type, who is passionate, but more interested in love than sex per se. One can easily imagine her developing a repugnance to sexual matters in general, if she is exposed to coarse sexuality when young. She is an intensely romantic person, who may be awoken rudely from her fantasies of Price Charming by the lecherous attitudes of ordinary men. On the other hand, Pulsatilla is also listed in Kent's repertory under the rubrics 'Lascivious' and 'Nymphomania'. Emma Badgery would entertain strange men in her cage whilst her husband was at work, and her youngest son did not resemble his father, having oriental features which nobody dared comment upon. I have not come across the lasciviousness attributed to Pulsatilla, (Kent: 'Erotic insanity'), presumably because it is a feature of Pulsatilla's hysteria, which is not often seen these days.

## Confusion and Partiality

Because Pulsatilla lives so much in her emotions, her thinking tends to be somewhat 'woolly'. It lacks precision and clarity much of the time. Pulsatilla women are liable to give up easily when rational analysis is required, including the analysis required for practical tasks like changing an electric plug. She will most likely, if she attempts such a task at all, attach the wires any old way. (A good example of this is the Pulsatilla character Eva in the American comedy series 'Green Acres'). The resultant failure of the plug to work will then confirm to her that she can't do such tasks, and she will avoid them in future. In actual fact she only needs a little patient instruction, but very often she would prefer to leave it to the men, not only because she is afraid she can't do it, but also because she is not very interested in logical, rational things, whether they be practical or theoretical. Her mind is lazy rather than unintelligent, and it is often rather 'rusty', since she tends to leave the thinking to others. However, when she is forced to study, she will gradually acquire proficiency in intellectual discrimination.

Pulsatilla is very prone to indecision. This is presumably because she listens to her emotions, which react both positively and negatively to every possibility. For example, if she tries to decide between two men who have asked her out on a date, she may reason thus; 'Harold is so good looking (heart skips a beat), but rather uncouth (imagines that he might treat her roughly), whereas Jimmy is sweet (reassured but wonders if she will get bored), but his mother is so dominating (fears her herself now). On the other hand...' This is rather like the thinking of a four year old child, which is very partial and lacking in objectivity, revolving as it does around likes and dislikes. A more distinct example of emotional preference determining opinion was given to me by a Pulsatilla woman who came to me for treatment of premenstrual tension. She was a widow, who was in the process of investigating meditation techniques and esoteric philosophy, which she found fascinating, when her two sisters, who were both born-again Christians, declared that she was dabbling in Satanism, and that they would have nothing to do with her if she continued along her present path. She asked me if I thought that such practices were evil, having more or less convinced herself that they were, in order to justify to herself abandoning them, and hence keeping her sisters' love. I could sense that she was ambivalent about the matter, and was both pleased and disturbed when I said that I did not think that her interest was unhealthy. She was an intelligent woman, but she was in the process of abandoning her own reason to keep the love that she needed.

Like other highly emotional types, Pulsatilla can get into a mental fluster when she is upset. If she has had a row with her husband, she will not be able to think straight, and will forget what she has gone shopping for (Kent: 'Vanishing of thoughts'), get on the wrong bus, panic and then burst into tears. Like Phosphorus, she is likely to attract instant sympathy when upset, and will probably find someone kind to drive her home, where her husband will be contrite, and will step around her on tiptoes until she is more herself again. She does not mean to be so confused, but when she is upset she will fall back upon trusted methods of getting by, such as prolonging her crying until sympathy and help arrive. If such help is not available, she will cry until her upset is exhausted, and then she will be able to collect her thoughts again and work out what to do.

### Innocence

Along with Baryta, Graphites, and Phosphorus, Pulsatilla is the most innocent of constitutional types. Like a child she will tend to say what she feels and thinks, without any cleverness. I have a Pulsatilla friend, a young woman who is very concerned about the environment, who was appalled to hear that local forests were being logged. She immediately wrote a letter to the Minister for the Environment, which she showed to me. It was touching in its childlike candour, and said something like 'Dear Minister, please stop the logging of the trees as there won't be any left soon, and the animals will have nowhere to live'.

The Pulsatilla wife will most likely be her usual innocent self when her husband brings the boss home for dinner. She will have no airs and graces, and when she needs to relieve her bladder she is liable to announce unselfconsciously "I'm just going for a wee," as if her husband's boss were her sister. Whether such innocence is considered charming, foolish or impolite by the latter depends entirely upon his personality. Thus exactly the same innocent demeanour can win Pulsatilla instant approval, from both her husband and his boss, or disdain from the latter, and rage from the former, who imagines that his prospects of promotion have just gone out the window!

The Pulsatilla friend who wrote the letter had, not surprisingly, a Pulsatilla mother. The latter used to embarrass her daughter in public by proudly announcing to all and sundry (including strangers at the bus-stop) her daughter's every achievement, including the fact that the latter had qualified as a nurse. She was so proud of her daughter that she couldn't understand the latter's embarrassment at such public praise. This is another example of Pulsatilla's innocence and lack of interest in the norms of social behaviour.

Every manner in which a child expresses innocence can be seen in the adult Pulsatilla woman. She is just as thrilled as a child when her mate surprises her with a present. She is as excited as a child at the prospect of a day-trip to the country (particularly if it doesn't happen very often). And she is as perplexed as a child when she is punished and doesn't know what she has done wrong. Such innocence in an adult is also seen in Phosphorus and Baryta Carbonica. The latter is usually fairly easy to distinguish from Pulsatilla, since there is generally a degree of backwardness or mental retardation that is not characteristic of Pulsatilla. Phosphorus can be more difficult to differentiate from Pulsatilla on the mentals alone. However, there is a difference in the 'flavour' of the innocence of each type, rather as there is a difference in the 'flavour' of the emotionality of Pulsatilla and Ignatia. The innocence of Phosphorus contains within it an impish, ethereal quality, such as that of Puck in Shakespeare's 'A Mid-Summer Night's Dream'. It is an androgynous quality, reminiscent of the joi de vivre of youth. The innocence of Pulsatilla is more feminine and more vulnerable, and is reminiscent of the innocence of a much younger child, between the ages of, say, three and five. Whereas the innocence of Phosphorus seems to shout 'Ha! You can't catch me!', that of Pulsatilla sings gently of roses and butterflies. It is the difference between Peter Pan and Alice of Wonderland. Both are very loving and very open, but Pulsatilla is softer, more personal and more emotional.

### The Pulsatilla Man

Although Pulsatilla is a common type amongst young boys, it is rarely seen in men as a constitutional type. The Pulsatilla men I have seen were very soft men, who were shy of strangers, and very loving towards their family. One of them complained of indecision. He was always agonising over choices, whether they were important or trivial (Kent: 'Irresolution'). As one would expect, the Pulsatilla man is lacking in both positive and negative masculine qualities. He finds it difficult to assert himself, and will tend to give way to keep the peace, like Lycopodium and Staphysagria. However, he is far more emotional and sensitive than Lycopodium, and also more nurturing. He does not have the emotional evasiveness of Staphysagria. Unlike the latter, he knows what he feels, and is able to express it, once he has gained your trust.

It would not be surprising to find a Pulsatilla man staying at home whilst his wife went out to work. Some degree of role-reversal is almost inevitable, given the femininity of the type. The Pulsatilla men I have treated were all married, and all were more concerned with family life than with their careers (a refreshing change from what one generally finds). One said that he was insecure, and needed frequent reassurance from his wife that she still loved him, but the others seemed more secure in their relationships. None were 'effeminate' or homosexual. In fact they all had a fairly objective, masculine exterior, but were quick to admit their more delicate feelings when asked.

Shyness can be a major problem for the Pulsatilla man, especially with the opposite sex. Since our society generally expects the men to do the wooing, shyness affects male Pulsatillas romantically more than their female counterparts. One of my male Pulsatilla patients had endured years of loneliness without a girlfriend before meeting his wife, because he was too shy to get to know girls. Kent lists Pulsatilla in his repertory under the rubric 'Aversion to women'. I suspect that the aversion he refers to is really fear, which arises out of shyness.

The Pulsatilla man may easily be confused with Phosphorus men, who are far more common. Both are sensitive, and Phosphorus men are often nurturing, but Phosphorus is less shy, more spirited and more extrovert.

### Physical Appearance

Pulsatilla has a characteristic appearance in the majority of cases, at least in Caucasians. The hair is usually blonde or light brown, the eyes blue or green, and the lashes naturally curved outwards. The face tends to be rounded (unlike Phosphorus and Silica), and the skin is pale, often with a blonde down on it like Calcarea. The figure is generally full, with rounded hips and well-developed breasts, resembling that of Aphrodite, the goddess of Love. The lips tend to be full and well curved like cupid's bow, reflecting both sensuality and sensitivity.

### Postscript

Adult Pulsatillas are surprisingly uncommon in my experience, considering the frequency with which one comes across Pulsatilla children. The vast majority of Pulsatilla children grow up into other constitutional types (principally Natrum Muriaticum), with only a few growing up into Pulsatilla women, and exceedingly few into Pulsatilla men. Pulsatilla embodies 'the feminine principle' more purely than any other type, and the relative scarcity of adult Pulsatillas is presumably a reflection of the patriarchal society in which we live, which undervalues the feminine, and systematically abuses it, until it becomes something suppressed and twisted, resulting in either slavish or masculinised women. There is a very close resemblance between Pulsatilla and Natrum Muriaticum, the former being more natural, the latter a more 'artificial' type that I believe has been created over thousands of years by the suppression of emotion. Homeopaths often give relatively open, expressive Natrum women Pulsatilla, which fails to act. The difference between a Pulsatilla woman and a relatively open Natrum woman appears subtle at first, and requires a lot of sensitivity on the part of the homeopath to recognise. Basically, Pulsatilla is always herself - pure emotion, whereas Natrum learns to disguise herself with cloaks of efficiency, rationality and acceptable mock-emotion. The more one strips away a Natrum woman's artificial defences, the more she resembles Pulsatilla. (However, it is important to realise that she does not turn into a Pulsatilla. In my experience, it is rare for a person to change their constitutional type, whereas it is common for people to grow into more healthy versions of their type.)

# Sepia

*Keynote:* The independent woman

Sepia is a predominantly female type, and like Ignatia, Pulsatilla and Natrum Muriaticum, it constitutes its own unique 'version' of woman. One could say that each of these types represents a different 'archetype' (literally, ancient impression) of the feminine, and when combined their collective attributes and essences constitute the whole realm of Woman.

Sepia's natural independence sets her apart from other women. She seeks to be herself, unfettered by the expectations of others, especially those of men. In this she differs from Natrum women, who generally seek independence as a reaction against the hurt they have received, a protective mechanism. Sepia is naturally independent. She is not running away from anything like Natrum—she is just being herself, and refusing to let other people mould her personality to their own ends. This independence of Sepia sometimes gives her a certain masculine appearance to others, since we expect men to be more independent than women, but it is not really masculinity. The hardened exterior of a defensive Ignatia or Natrum woman is masculine—an efficient, aggressive front which protects the sensitivity beneath. The average Sepia woman has less of a front, and her independence results from her celebration of her own uniqueness, and the sense of power she receives from her own connection with her body and the Earth. This sense of power is feminine, since it depends upon being sensitive to one's body, and centred in it, and upon a natural wisdom which has little to do with the intellect. Masculine power, in contrast, is more dependent upon aggression, brute force, and intellect. The difference is like that between Karate, which is an extremely offensive, 'cutting' martial art, which can cause a great deal of harm to an opponent, and Aikido, the 'soft' martial art which is entirely defensive, and depends upon flexibility and the ability of the practitioner to 'go with the flow' of his opponent's movements.

I have chosen five sub-types to represent the different attributes of the Sepia woman. Three of these are traditional roles of independent women throughout history. The other two, the Drudge and the Shrew, represent what happens to Sepia when she surrenders her identity to others, particularly her family.

## The Witch

The Witch, or the Wise Woman, has always been around, and has always attracted a mixture of fear, respect and fascination from ordinary mortals. Whether she be a witch of the Middle Ages, mixing potions and making spells, or a priestess in Ancient Greece or India, initiating neophytes into the Mysteries, the Wise Woman has always dedicated herself to her 'craft', her wisdom, rather than to husband and family. Most witches are Sepia, and most Sepia women have something of the witch in them. They are naturally somewhat clairvoyant, and are usually fascinated in things psychic or mystical. Furthermore, they have a sound, detached intellect, which is subtle, and can easily grasp hidden mysteries which cannot be seen by purely deductive, masculine reasoning. Sepia loves to delve into hidden mysteries, whether of the personal psyche, or of a more philosophical nature (Kent: 'Theorising'), and like Phosphorus and China, she has the sensitivity in many cases to intuit what she cannot deduce intellectually. For example, a Sepia woman will usually be able to tell if her husband is being dishonest, even though he has left no tangible clues. She can simply feel it. Similarly, she will get the feeling that she shouldn't have anything to do with the nice man at work, and subsequently she finds out that he is a dangerous psychopath, who had succeeded in fooling everyone else with his pleasant, normal exterior. Unlike Phosphorus, she usually has enough internal clarity to separate her intuition from her fears and her wishes, though this difference disappears as Sepia becomes more anxious. Sepia is like a cross between Phosphorus and Natrum Muriaticum—as intuitive and as natural as the former, and as deep as the latter. She is usually more 'grounded' than Phosphorus; more down to earth and sensible, and hence she is able to make more use of her intuitive faculties. Natrum is also sometimes highly intuitive, but her intuition is liable to become mixed with personal unconscious fears, and also with wishful thinking. Sepia is more able to be impersonal when it comes to intuiting information, and does not suffer from the compulsion of Natrum to make things appear either positive or dramatic. She is a natural seer, who is not only intuitive, but also grounded in her body, and impersonal in her perception. In contrast, Phosphorus tends to get carried away by flights of fancy, and Natrum often distorts her intuition with highly personal bias, and pursues it as a means of appearing 'special'. Like true Wise Women, Sepia is liable to keep quiet about her intuitive faculties, not only to avoid scorn (and persecution in the past), but also because she is not egotistical about her abilities, and her wisdom tells her that those who need it will be guided to her.

Witches can be either black or white, and like the majority of ordinary people, most are somewhere in-between. Your 'average grey witch' will use her intuitive abilities both for selfish ends, and to help others. Similarly, the average Sepia woman is neither saintly nor Satanic. She is liable to favour people she likes, and to ignore those she dislikes, or sometimes to punish them. I once got to know a Sepia woman who lived next door to me. She was very refined and intelligent, and also tremendously self-possessed. When she spoke, she spoke with a natural authority which was both relaxed and free from pride. She was studying Traditional Chinese Medicine, working as a Shiatsu practitioner, and also pursuing creative writing, which came to her spontaneously as if from the Muse, and was of publishable quality. Like many Sepia women, she had an air of mystery about her; not the seductive mystery of an Ignatia or Natrum vamp, but a more quiet, self-possessed depth, which gave the impression of great wisdom. We made a date for dinner at her place, and the next day I phoned and cancelled it, explaining that I had remembered a prior engagement. I saw nothing of the woman for several weeks, and eventually when we met again, she said in a matter of fact way that she had been so angry with me for cancelling after she had prepared the food in advance, that she had put a 'hex' (a bad spell) on me. She said this in all seriousness, and later in conversation she related how she had once been involved with a man who practised magic (the witchcraft kind, not the theatrical), and had been plagued by him telepathically after she left him. Eventually, she let out such a scream at him psychically that he was driven close to madness, and stopped harassing her. When one hears stories like this from impressionable Phosphorus women one is inclined to take them with a pinch of salt, as one is when they are told by emotionally effusive Natrum women seeking the limelight, but this Sepia woman was highly intelligent, very sober and powerful in an understated manner, and I had no difficulty in believing her.

Because Sepia is naturally attuned to both psychic and bodily energy, many Sepia women become healers of one sort or another. My witchy neighbour was not the only Sepia woman I have known who dedicated herself to the healing arts. I have known several such Sepia healers, and each of them had a characteristic quiet poise, was physically graceful, and entirely free from pride. The majority of healers I have known have been Natrum women. Some of these were relatively natural and unselfconscious, but even these Natrums tended to over-intellectualise their art, and to use a great deal of 'New Age' jargon, as well as making an effort to be positive. Sepia, in contrast, simply does what she is good at, and generally has no need of elaborate intellectual constructs to justify what she is doing, nor any need to emphasise the positive.

Sepia embodies feminine wisdom, or intuition, whereas Pulsatilla embodies the nurturing and sensuous side of Woman. She generally has a sharp intellect, but is not interested in mechanical or dry intellectual knowledge, which she leaves to men, and to more masculinised women. Instead she focuses on knowledge which is directly about life itself (like the healthy Ignatia woman). Thus Sepia women are likely to become horticulturalists, vets, nutritionists, doctors and nurses, but not company directors or statisticians. I have come across many Sepia women in the nursing profession. Like the natural healers, they have a love of life, and an empathy with people, but their intellect is generally stronger than their intuition, and hence they choose a more conventional and practical form of service.

In the old days, many people were very afraid of witches. With the help of both ignorance, and the teachings of a male-dominated Church, witches were seen as almost universally evil, and were hounded and burned at the stake. Today men are still afraid of the power of an independent Sepia woman, whose wisdom and subtle intellect is often more than a match for merely deductive reasoning. Because she tends to be herself, rather than try to conform or please (like Pulsatilla and Natrum), Sepia is often a puzzle to men, who are either fascinated by her mystery, or leave her well alone. Healthy Sepia women stand their ground with men in our society, but they do not usually try to compete with men like Natrum and Ignatia women, since they honour their feminine wisdom, and prefer to explore it quietly. They may fear the brutality of men, but they seldom allow their fear to coerce them into conforming to men's expectations.

This self-possession and independence from men that is so characteristic of Sepia is beautifully portrayed by Jenny, the principal female role in the novel 'The World According to Garp'. Jenny has a fiercely independent disposition, which eschews conventional morality, without trying to be different. Since she wants a child, but does not want a husband, Jenny makes love to a dying soldier, whose injuries have left him mute, and virtually unconscious, and with a permanent erection. There was no malice or perversion in her action, simply a pragmatism that ignored conventional mores without hurting anyone (in the book the soldier thoroughly enjoyed it). Jenny brings up her son Garp single-handedly without much trouble, since she possesses all the qualities of worldliness and authority that the father usually provides, as well as the nurturing instinct, which she uses to good effect in her work as a nurse. When her son has grown to manhood, she writes a book about the sexual exploitation of women that becomes a best-seller, and enables her to found a centre for the rehabilitation of abused women. Although her centre is full of women who hate all things masculine, Jenny herself has a balanced view, abhorring the exploitation of women by men, without rejecting men as individuals. Her fearless intellectual championing of women's rights is accompanied by a tender heart, and an ability to relate impartially to people of both sexes, and from all walks of life. Like other Sepia women, she is able to stand up to the Patriarchal leaders of society, whilst still retaining her own deeply felt connection with nature, and with the feminine in general.

## *The Dancer*

Every homeopath knows that Sepia women love to dance, and feel better in general for vigorous exercise. These isolated details tell us something more general about Sepia as a type, namely, that she is usually 'well connected' to her body. Unlike the majority of people in modern times, healthy Sepia women are still aware of the energy inside their body, its natural flow, and the discomfort that results when it is blocked. Most people have retreated from their body into their intellect, and are no longer aware of their body energy. Children are aware of their bodies, but this awareness is rapidly knocked out of them by an over-analytical world, which has forgotten how to feel, not only emotionally, but also physically. The analytical types, such as Lycopodium, Kali and Natrum, are the most out of touch with their bodies. More spontaneous types like Phosphorus, Sepia and Medorrhinum retain body-awareness to some degree, and this is especially true of Sepia, so long as she stays emotionally healthy. (Being aware of the body does not mean being fit. It is much more subtle than that. A sportsman may have tremendous stamina, but be unaware of his bodily energy, whereas a delicate Silica woman may be totally in tune with her body.) It is because she can feel the pleasure of her physical energy that Sepia is often attracted to dance, and also to yoga, Tai Chi and other physical activities which involve the experience of physical harmony. Through these activities she maintains contact with her life-force, whereas when she ceases to be physically active, she begins to feel deadened inside. This happens to all inactive people, but Sepia feels the deadening effect of inactivity more than most. This is partly because she has had the experience of physical vitality to compare it to, but also, I believe, because her nervous system is more finely tuned than most, and hence more easily 'clogged up' by both physical abuse, and the numbing effects of monotony and inactivity. A draw-horse will take any opportunity to be lazy, whereas a race-horse will fret when it is forced to be idle. Similarly, Calcarea enjoys inactivity, whereas Sepia needs activity, preferably rhythmic harmonious activity, to feel alive.

Some people have 'natural rhythm', and Sepia usually does. You can tell the people with natural rhythm on the dance floor. Their movements are effortlessly graceful, whether the activity is a slow waltz or a frantic jive. Kali is generally the stiffest of all, whilst Phosphorus and Sepia are generally 'as loose as a goose', and Natrum lies in between, with some stiff and some loose. Sepia's natural rhythm lends itself to musical ability as well as dance (Kent: Sensitive to music'). There are many gifted Sepia musicians, and also a good many Sepia artists. Sepia may be a little less visionary than Phosphorus and Lachesis, but she often has great sensitivity when it comes to the five senses (Kent: 'Sensitive to sensual impressions'), making her naturally adept not only with music and dance, but also the visual arts, and physical healing arts like massage and Shiatsu. Generally her art is quieter and more subtle than that of more extroverted types like Phosphorus and Lachesis, except her dancing and music, which may be just as wild as any other's.

Sepia's natural connectedness to her body is accompanied in many cases by an attunement to the Earth, and to natural cycles. In olden times it would have been Sepia in particular who danced to celebrate the harvest, or the coming of Spring, and whilst these dances eventually became ritualised, they would have began as spontaneous offerings which welled up in the bodies of sensitive Sepia women. Witches have always had a close connection with Mother Earth and her cycles, and have used the products of the earth to make healing potions, aphrodisiacs and also poisons. Today's Sepia woman may not go in for 'the craft', but like her witchy ancestors, she has a feeling for the earth, for its beauty and its hidden wisdom, and she is liable to go into a meditative state when she takes time to be surrounded by nature (unless she has lost herself, as so many Sepia women do, as they succumb to society's dictates, and drift into the worlds of the Drudge and the Shrew).

Because she is an 'earthy' person, in touch with her body and the earth, Sepia tends to have a lot of common sense. As long as she is not undergoing emotional upheavals, she tends to be practical, and also gifted at practical crafts, such as weaving and basket-making. In this she resembles Arsenicum, who is also very much at home with the material world. Sepia's 'down to earth' quality, together with her usually sharp intellect, gives her in many cases a wry, understated wit, and also an ability to accept the ways of the world. Although she may be acutely aware of the madness of the consumer-culture, deforestation, political corruption and other manifestations of a Patriarchal culture out of control, she is rarely utopian like Phosphorus and Natrum, whose idealism can blind them to practical reality. She is more likely to take the view that her own individual pursuit of health, truth and service on a local level will do more for humanity than any drum beating, which she is not cut out for anyhow. I am reminded of a charming Sepia lady I once treated who was once a ballet teacher, and at the age of fifty or so was still lithe and grace-ful. Her dark complexion, greying hair, high cheek-bones and dark eyes in deep hollow sockets gave her a look that was not only sophisticated, but also subtle, serious and wise. After the death of her husband she had struggled with intestinal cancer for some time, before embarking upon a new explo-ration of life. She travelled from Australia to California, where she got her-self adopted by a San Franciscan mission church which served the poor black community. She revelled in her new role as a coordinator for charitable services to these people, not only because she enjoyed helping, but also because her self-possessed Bohemian temperament loved learning all the street slang, the black handshakes, and mixing with a culture that was raw and vibrant in comparison with middle-class white America (or Australia).

Like the middle-aged housewife who comes alive on the dance-floor, she came alive amid the hustle and bustle of down-town San Francisco.

A good many Sepia women have an untamed, Bohemian quality. I am sure that there are a lot of Sepia gipsies, with their dark looks, their clairvoyance, and their refusal to conform. The witch and the dancer combine to some extent in the woman. She is totally feminine, but neither submissive nor passive, and she will strike out like a wild cat if she is threatened or abused. The more Bohemian Sepia women I have met were generally healthier emotionally than the others, and I believe this is because Sepia is naturally a free-spirit, not a conforming house-wife. Pulsatilla and Natrum women can be themselves as housewives, and many can find all the fulfilment they need through their roles as wife and mother. Sepia, on the other hand, needs some degree of freedom and independence to be happy, and this is why so many Sepia women become either bitter or depressed when they sacrifice their individuality to the service of the family.

Any type can appear Bohemian, but some are naturally that way, whilst others jump on the band-wagon and try to imitate them. Natrum and Phosphorus are great imitators, and Natrum in particular will sometimes adopt the role of the wild, untamed woman. This may be real to some extent, and in some cases, but it is often an attempt to appear 'cool', and therefore desirable. In contrast, Sepia women who appear Bohemian are usually being themselves, rather than looking for approval. They wear their hair long, their clothes loose and often home-spun in appearance, because it resonates with their sense of freedom, not because it is fashionable.

Other types who may be naturally Bohemian include Phosphorus, Medorrhinum, Tuberculinum and Ignatia. All of these types tend to be spontaneous and artistic, attributes that are an integral part of the Bohemian type. They function more from the visionary right side of the brain than other types, and are thus less conventional in outlook. Of all these types, Sepia is probably the most sensible and quietly 'centred'. She is not looking for wild experience, or that is not her main goal. Rather, she seeks to explore the mysteries of her own psyche, of the earth, and of her fate. She may be a dancer, and an artist, but as Bohemians go she is subtle and keeps her own counsel, when compared to the wildness of Tuberculinum and Medorrhinum. It is Sepia's lack of attraction to glamour, thrills and utopian ideals that enables her to function within conventional families as well as on the fringes of society. Tuberculinum and Medorrhinum must have their stimulation to be happy, and this stimulation generally requires more than being a wife and mother. Sepia's needs are more subtle, and because of this, they can easily be neglected, in favour of the normal, sensible, expected roles of a housewife. She needs to feel independent and also creative, and may choose an unconventional, Bohemian lifestyle because of this. On the other hand, because her needs are more internal and self-reliant than other spontaneous types, she may feel that she can create the space to meditate, dance or write whilst enjoying conventional family life. Many Sepias do manage to do this, but many others gradually lose sight of themselves in their attempts to please their husband and children.

Whereas a healthy Phosphorus or Tuberculinum is basically an extrovert, a healthy Sepia tends to be a mixture of introvert and extrovert, like Medorrhinum. She is generally sociable, and able to mix with all types of people, because she is herself. On the other hand, she needs time to herself to go within, and then to come out and be creative. Her introversion is not that of the depressive, who dwells upon unpleasant thoughts and feelings from the past (though the unhealthy Sepia may do just that), but rather a meditative focus within, which is richly rewarding rather than depressing.

### The Courtesan

Some readers will be surprised to see the courtesan as one of Sepia's subtypes, since homeopaths tend to think of Sepia as being sexually uninterested. This is because homeopathic literature and teaching has concentrated almost exclusively upon the pathology of Sepia, which results in the main from her giving herself up to man. The emotionally healthy Sepia woman, who is her own independent self, generally has a high but well-controlled sex drive, and as long as she honours herself in her relations with men, and does not simply 'submit' to the personality of the other, she gets a great deal of pleasure from her sexuality.

In keeping with her natural independence, the healthy Sepia woman likes to remain in control of her body. She cannot bear the thought of being a man's 'sexual spittoon', and hence she will refrain from sexual relations until she either finds a man who will not try to possess her, or she will have very brief or intermittent affairs. In between times, she is generally more able than most women to switch off her sexual urges, or to sublimate them into other activities, such as social, artistic or sporting pursuits.

Those Sepia women who are not married, and are not misanthropists, tend to honour their body by withholding it from men until they feel moved by a special attraction (this celibacy may have moral or religious overtones to it, but this is not usually the case). Very often, Sepia will be attracted to a man by a kind of magnetism that is part sexual, and part psychic or spiritual, but not the kind of 'falling in love' that overtakes other people. She feels a special chemistry between herself and this man, who is often either a man of considerable personal power, or one who shares her subtle understanding of life. In fact, Sepia is often attracted by a meeting of minds or spirits more than a meeting of hearts. She is quite capable of personal love, but this is not her main mode of inter-relating, which is either physical, mental or spiritual, rather than emotional. As a result, Sepia women can appear rather cold and aloof compared with warmer types (Kent: 'Indifferent to loved ones'). Certainly the emotionally unhealthy Sepia shrew is very cold, and the apathetic Sepia drudge has no feelings left in her, but even the healthy Sepia woman has a certain separateness from others. This is not due to self-protection as in the case of Natrum, but rather, like the Arsenicum woman, she loves gently without surrendering herself to the other, and without losing her independence, or she loves passionately in the moment (Kent: 'Lascivious'), and then goes about her own business. (I cannot imagine a witch who is devoted to another man, but I can imagine a partnership of equals between a witch and a warlock, which may involve affection, respect and sexual passion.)

The courtesan is perhaps an extreme representation of Sepia's sexual independence, but it is nevertheless quite consistent. In contrast to ordinary prostitutes, courtesans used to be awarded considerable respect in society. They were proud women, who slept only with the noble, the wealthy or those men they found attractive. I once knew a Sepia woman who had done just that. She was a highly intelligent and refined artist, who had studied Japanese, and had lived in Japan for some time. (Sepia women are often attracted to Japanese arts, since the latter tend to emphasise poise, subtlety and physical harmony.) Whilst she was studying in Japan, she became short of money, and since she had always wanted to explore her sexuality more, she decided to become a high-class prostitute. She arranged to sleep with wealthy men, and men she liked, for very high fees, and enjoyed doing so for a while. As soon as the fascination faded, she stopped doing it. She told me this about herself with no sign of embarrassment or shame. To her, sexuality was something to explore like any other subject, and if she could make money at the same time, so much the better.

Not many Sepia women become courtesans, but many have the detached, amoral passion of the courtesan; a passion which is not compelling like that of Platina (except in the moment), but which can rise instantly in the presence of the right partner. At other times it is dormant, rather than suppressed. Many Sepia women can tolerate celibacy so easily that one would assume they have no sexual drive, but this is not the case. If they are healthy, their life is their passion, and this may or may not include sexual passion, depending upon whom they are with.

There is a connection historically between the courtesan and the 'wise woman'. Sexuality has always been used in occult traditions to harness and direct subtle energies. Witchcraft and magic in the Middle Ages had a reputation for indulging in orgies, as part of the 'Black Mass'. This is hardly a very high form of wisdom, and was presumably a reaction to the oppressive sexuality of the Catholic Church at the time (and also was undoubtedly exaggerated by the Church for its own ends). Nevertheless, ritual sex of this kind can be seen as a means by which the participants 'felt their power', albeit in a degenerate form. It involved no conquest of woman by man, but was rather a meeting of equals, that was characterised by lust and possibly also a certain mystical or Dionysian state of mind, but not affectionate love. In this sense it is consistent with the sexual practices of many Sepia women. Higher forms of 'sexual magic' have also been practised in the past, and still are to this day. In Ancient Greece and Ancient India, the Priestess was almost certainly a Sepia woman. She was a seer, who was revered and answerable to no-one but the Gods. Part of her sacred duties included the initiation of neophytes through sexual union. Provided they had been prepared through extensive practice of meditation, this initiation was mystical rather than lustful, opening up new vistas in the neophyte's awareness. The Priestess knew when the neophyte was ready for initiation, and did not make her choice on the grounds of sexual attraction. In Eastern spiritual traditions tantra is still practised today, and is gaining popularity in the West. True tantra involves no lust at all, and can only be practised successfully by spiritually advanced people. Through sexual union, the tantric lovers raise the energy in their bodies, until it illumines their minds, producing an expanded state of consciousness. This and other forms of 'sexual magic' are especially attractive to Sepia, because she has such a subtle awareness of her own bodily energy, and tends to regard sex as either a natural function like eating and drinking, which is neither moral nor immoral, or as a sacred activity. She is as liable to reach ecstasy through dancing or meditation as she is through making love with the right partner, and more liable than most other types.

Sepia's independence, both sexual and otherwise, is often surrendered at the feet of male domination, and when this happens, the result is the bitterness of the shrew, and the apathy of the drudge.

### The Shrew

When my Sepia neighbour put a hex on me, she was acting as the shrew. When she is crossed, particularly by men, Sepia can get very angry, and this anger becomes chronic when she has been put down often enough, resulting in a permanent state of bitterness. Few Sepia girls grow up truly healthy emotionally. They are at a disadvantage from the start, since their independent, meditative nature is often either missed by their family, and hence is not catered for and nurtured, or it is seen as unhealthy in a woman, and deliberately opposed. When Sepia is allowed to be herself in childhood, she will develop sufficient self-assurance to avoid abusive conditions and relationships later on, and will be able to honour her own interests, which usually include either artistic or metaphysical pursuits or both. On the other hand, if her father expects her to show him respect when he behaves disrespectfully or foolishly, she will react in a 'spirited' manner, at first opposing his attitude quietly, and then more vehemently as he begins to try and crush her 'rebellion'. Sepia adolescents are renowned for their temper, which can be fierce and explosive. It is generally assumed that they are both spirited, which they are, and also that they are naturally irritable or volatile. Sepia adolescents only become irritable when they are not understood, and not allowed to be their independent, subtle-minded selves. Whereas other types, like Natrum and Lycopodium, may buckle under and acquiesce to the dictates of parental pressures to be normal, obedient and dependent, Sepia will resist such pressure for a long time, with outbursts of temper, and floods of tears which totally bemuse her well-meaning parents. Eventually her own mind and body become a battle-ground, as the pressure of conditioning threatens to overwhelm her own identity, and she wonders who she is, what is right, and why she is so sensitive and irritable much of the time. From this point on, she becomes oversensitive to criticism and opposition of any kind (Kent: 'Anger from contradiction', 'Offended easily'), particularly when it comes from men, whom she has learned to fear and resent, since they so often try to tame her. The tension that results from this battle between Sepia's independent, sensitive nature and society's insensitive attempts to mould her into something more pliable often reaches such intensity that she wants to scream (Kent: 'Feels as though she must shriek'), or to smash crockery. (When she does resort to such measures, they do break the tension inside, and help to restore her sanity.)

Sepia is often said to suffer from a loss of her femininity, as indicated by her aversion to men, her indifference to her children, and her aggressiveness. All of these do occur, but they occur not so much because Sepia has lost her femininity, but rather, because she has surrendered her independence. Sepia is naturally very feminine, but her femininity is of a special kind, being intuitive, and sensitive to life and the body. She represents one pole of Womanhood, whereas Pulsatilla represents the other, more nurturing, passive pole. It is when Sepia is pressured by her upbringing and her society to deny her own form of femininity that she becomes aggressive, and ultimately may come to hate men (Kent: 'Aversion to members of the opposite sex').

Like all other predominantly female types, Sepia is prone to mood changes during times of hormonal flux. As a practitioner of deep psychotherapy I have found that such hormonally related moods are always the result of suppressed anger or sadness from childhood, as well as from present conditions, and they disappear when the patient has been able to bring the suppressed emotions to consciousness in their original context (e.g. anger towards her father, not anger projected onto her husband), and to feel them fully. Sometimes Sepia does actually develop abnormal levels of sex hormones, but even these are reflections of suppressed emotion, which disappear when the emotion is released (see Arthur Janov's 'The New Primal Scream' for evidence of physiological normalisation resulting from emotional de-repression). More often, Sepia's hormonal levels are normal, but the rapid change in hormonal status which occurs premenstrually, postnatally and at the menopause makes her more unstable emotionally, because it destabilises the normal repression mechanisms which keep suppressed pain at bay (in all of us). Sepia is particularly prone to anger and irritability at these times, because she is naturally a spirited, independent type. Natrum, in contrast, is equally or more prone to sadness at such times, because her need of love, and sensitivity to being unloved, is greater than her need for independence.

When Sepia is upset, she is as likely to be tearful as angry, (Kent: 'Weeping—involuntary', 'Mood—tearful'), and her tears flow very easily in most cases, unless she has become worn out emotionally, in which case apathy and emotional dullness take over. Her tears are usually more the result of exasperation and tension than of sadness. They can be elicited by the slightest thing going wrong, when she is tense before her period, or generally tense because life is not going well for her. Again, it is those Sepias who have surrendered their natural independence that suffer most from hormonally related mood swings, since they are the ones who have had to suppress the most anger.

Several constitutional types are prone to anger and tearfulness premenstrually, including Natrum, Sepia, Lachesis and Alumina. When tears are clearly being suppressed, Natrum is most often the constitutional type, whereas when tears are freely flowing, and the temper is sudden and intense, both Sepia and Lachesis should be considered, and are usually easily differentiated on account of the former being chilly and the latter hot-blooded. However, there are many cases in between, with some tearfulness, some irritability, and occasional temper, where any of the above types and others may be indicated, and other features of the case will be more helpful. Sepia is often indicated when the woman complains of 'becoming another person' for a week or more before her period, during which time she is a veritable fiendess, snapping at anyone and everyone, complaining about the slightest little thing, and smashing glasses in the kitchen. Although her problem is due to suppressed anger, it can often be alleviated or cured by Sepia in high potency. (Presumably the remedy removes some of the tension in the nervous system which resulted from suppressed anger, and also reduces the 'leakage' of emotion through the barrier between subconscious and conscious minds which occurs at times of hormonal flux.)

Bitterness is a quality that can be possessed by any constitutional type, but is characteristic of a few, in particular Arsenicum, Natrum Muriaticum, Sepia and Nux. Sepia is actually less liable to become bitter than Natrum, because she suppresses her anger less. Once she has lost her temper, the tension is eased. She is more likely to enter into transient periods of resentment, which are over relatively quickly when she explodes, especially if she receives an apology from whoever she was resenting. More often than not it is her husband or boyfriend, who has taken her for granted in some way, thus activating the constant tension inside that results from compromising her true nature. In contrast, Natrum is more likely to swallow her resentment for a long time, for fear of losing her partner's love, and when she finally 'flips', she may be resentful for months, during which time no amount of apologising will placate her.

In view of Sepia's tendency to rebel against man's domination, one would expect to find a great many Sepias amongst the feminist movement. This is indeed the case, although they are easily outnumbered by Natrums, since the latter are so much more common generally. Like the Natrum feminist, the Sepia feminist usually has a sharp intellect, with which she whips the defenders of the Patriarchal system. If anything, she is more dispassionate than her Natrum comrades, who are more liable to be governed by hate (Natrum is listed in Kent's Repertory in italics under the rubric 'Hate', whereas Sepia is not listed at all). Like Jenny, the Sepia heroine in 'The World according to Garp', Sepia feminists tend to concentrate on clarifying the wider issues of gender politics, whereas Natrum feminists are more intent upon revenge. (Having said that, there are a good many Natrum feminists who stick to the issues in a reasonably dispassionate manner.)

## *The Drudge—Apathy and Acopia*

Once the Sepia woman has compromised her true nature for long enough, she begins to lose her spirit. As this occurs, she experiences a gradual deadening of her appetite for life. She starts to live life more and more like a robot, going through the motions of her usual activities, with no enthusiasm or motivation inside her. Because she has lost contact with her own 'life-force', she feels sluggish both mentally and physically (Kent: 'Dullness, sluggishness'), and her emotions are also blunted, producing a kind of indifference to everything. This is particularly likely to happen to the Sepia housewife who has no interests outside of her family to stimulate her. When she had children she gave up her sport, and no longer had time to write her poetry, or perhaps the inspiration to write dwindled gradually as she immersed herself more and more in feeding babies, changing nappies, and cooking meals. As she loses herself, Sepia starts to worry about the fact that she feels less and less for her husband and children (Kent: 'Indifference to loved ones'), apart from irritation. She also loses the enjoyment she used to feel from socialising, from eating and drinking, and from making love (Kent: 'Indifferent to pleasure').

As this condition progresses, the Sepia woman feels more and more drained of energy, and finds it harder and harder to face the day's chores (Kent: 'Aversion to business'). She gets up in the morning and dreads the coming day, because she has no energy, and no motivation. (At this stage the improvement she feels when she goes dancing, or engages in vigorous exercise is most noticeable.) She may also have no patience to deal with the children, and finds herself shouting at them for the slightest thing. In the evening she tries to be cheerful for her husband, but the act takes all of her energy, and she cannot keep it up for long. In bed she has no desire to make love, and often shrinks from her husband's touch (Kent: 'Fears touch, contact'). When she does make love, she feels nothing, or she feels weepy or irritable afterwards. Her mind slows down until she makes mistakes with the simplest of tasks (Kent: 'Prostration of mind'). She burns the dinner, puts bleach in the washing instead of fabric conditioner, and forgets appointments. Gradually she begins to feel panicky, because she is going downhill, and she feels she can't cope any longer. She becomes prone to weeping for no apparent reason, and she weeps whenever she tells another person how she is feeling (Kent: 'Weeping when telling symptoms'). Eventually, her inability to cope starts to make her more and more anxious. At first, she is anxious about realistic things; principally that she won't be able to cope with the things she has to do. As she fails to cope with her daily tasks, the anxiety increases, and attaches itself to more and more fears. She begins to fear that something terrible might happen, that she has a fatal disease, or that her husband will leave her. She worries excessively about finances, and she worries that she is going insane (Kent: 'Fear of insanity). In her anxiety she may become very restless, and she may feel that she has to get out of the house (presumably because her housework and her identity as a housewife have robbed her of herself). Alternatively, she may develop agarophobia, and feel terror when she is away from home. This is connected in part with her fear of meeting people and being unable to cope with their social expectations. Even at home she may be very frightened of having visitors, because she is no longer in a fit state to talk to them. She withdraws more and more, and yet she feels more frightened when she is totally alone. She wants someone near to reassure her, but she does not want to have to talk. Eventually, she may feel so hopeless that she considers suicide, although her anxiety and depression are usually tempered before this by antidepressants and sedatives. These will help her to get through the day, but what she really needs is to turn back the clock and find herself, and then to rearrange her life so that she has time for herself.

The above progression varies somewhat from case to case. Sometimes anxiety predominates over apathy, sometimes weeping is the most prominent feature, and sometimes dullness and indifference is the main complaint. The depressed Sepia woman can be quite difficult to differentiate from a depressed Natrum. Generally tears come easily, but sometimes they are suppressed, and sometimes depressed Natrums cry very easily. Furthermore, some depressed Natrums are very apathetic. Some Sepia women enter into deep depressions that are more or less indistinguishable from a deep Natrum depression, with withdrawn brooding, self-recrimination, despair and a tendency to dwell on past unpleasant events. In these cases the generals, the physical features, and the previous personality will help to differentiate a Sepia from a Natrum depression. It can generally be relied upon that Natrum people develop Natrum depressions, and Sepias develop Sepia depressions (i.e. depressions that respond to Sepia), although there is the occasional exception. For example, a Sepia woman may enter into a Natrum state after a bereavement, or a Natrum woman may enter into a Sepia state during pregnancy (though she is more likely to develop Natrum symptoms during pregnancy). In these cases, the generals and physicals will help in the selection of the correct remedy.

Fear is a common finding in Sepia women, but it tends to occur predominantly in those Sepias who have lost their real identity. (This can happen as early as a few years old.) Those Sepia women who retain their independence and creativity, whether they are married or not, tend to be relatively free from fear. I have often come across Sepia women who were somewhere in between. They were seeking to strengthen the independence they knew that they had lost, and were often pulled in two directions, between being themselves, and devoting themselves to a relationship. It is possible for Sepia to do both, but only with a man who does not try to dominate. He does not have to understand Sepia's interests, nor share her subtle sensitivity, but unless he lets her be herself, she will either go under, or leave. A great many Sepia women are dependent upon men for emotional security, and also for support in making decisions, and for practical help. Those who realise that they must regain their lost identity tend to go through periods of great confusion, when they are not sure who they are, or what they want, and during these periods they may be quite anxious, since they are attempting to let go of dependencies which have both imprisoned them and supported them. In particular, such women are often afraid of men, especially aggressive men, since they are trying to stand up for themselves, without the support they have been used to, before they have regained their own sense of power.

These 'in-between Sepias', who are neither independent and confident, nor totally submerged under the pressure to conform, often have a certain 'scatty' quality. They are torn emotionally between the safety of being what others expect a woman to be, and the frustration that it entails. This internal war has a confusing and disorientating effect on many Sepia women (and girls), and as a result they appear a little muddled from time to time. Since they are often still very spirited people, they may simply laugh when they say the wrong thing, or do something silly, such as giving their husband cat food by mistake, whilst Puss gets the paté. The characters portrayed on the screen by the actress Shirley Maclaine often have just this kind of scattiness, as well as a fiercely independent streak, and more often than not, a wry sense of humour. Phosphorus is also scatty quite often, and a good many Sepia women are given Phosphorus by mistake, particularly the more extrovert, effervescent ones. Even the scatty Sepia woman is generally a lot more focussed mentally than Phosphorus, at least most of the time. Furthermore, Sepia is not a dreamer to anything like the same extent as Phosphorus, and whilst she is sometimes very upset by the sufferings of others, she is seldom overwhelmed or affected for long by another's feelings, whereas Phosphorus can be so empathic that she totally loses herself in the other person.

To confuse matters further for the student and inexperienced homeopath, a good many of the 'in-between Sepias' have some of the innocence of Phosphorus. They are often quite naive about worldly things, both because they rely excessively on men to take care of them, and also because they are often uninterested in mundane matters like politics, financial matters and even social etiquette. They would rather get on with their own creative pursuits, and also their friendships, and leave worldly details to the men. The more independent Sepia woman may also take this attitude, not because she cannot understand politics or high finance, but rather because she knows that she would lose her soul if she tried to enter these somewhat inhuman worlds.

Those Sepia women who see the journey of self-discovery (or self-remembrance) through to its conclusion are rewarded with the peace and understanding of the wise woman, the joy of the dancer, and the satisfaction of loving relationships which do not bind and weaken those involved. Sepia is capable of being a loving wife and mother, without giving up her identity. The healthy Sepia mother is less sentimental and less possessive towards her children than most other mothers, but she is not cold. Her own strength of mind tends to rub off on her children, making them more independent and individualistic than other children. She is an equal partner in her marriage, and takes as many decisions and as much responsibility as her mate, but this does not mean that she is unfeminine. On the contrary, her wisdom, her natural connection with her body, and her understated, somewhat mysterious sexuality is most feminine, in a strong, uncompromising way.

### The Sepia Man

I have very little to say about the Sepia man, since I have only treated two, which makes me think that they are very rare. One of these men looked very much like Sepia women look, in the sense that he was of spare build, bony, with a very dark complexion. He was quiet and rather introverted, and also sensitive and nervous. I forget now what his main complaint was, but I remember that he had very little interest in sex, his libido having always been low. Basically, he resembled other Sepias (who happened to have been women) very closely both physically and psychologically, and I had no difficulty in spotting the remedy, which worked, despite the fact that I had never seen a Sepia man before.

The other Sepia man I have treated was a young man who was suffering from chronic hepatitis. He had mousy brown hair, and numerous dark moles on his face and torso, and he had a quiet, shy temperament. He was clearly in awe of his rather insensitive father, who was a butcher, and looked to his father frequently when answering questions. Thus far his description could easily apply to Pulsatilla, and indeed like Pulsatilla he would cry easily when he felt low. However, he was not as emotional as the other Pulsatilla men I have treated. He had a passive 'fay' quality that made one think of the more feminine types, and his physical symptoms fitted Sepia very well. His illness improved remarkably quickly after a few doses of Sepia 200c, and so did the passive feeling of depression to which he was prone. He required a weekly dose of Sepia 200c for a few months to get him over his hepatitis, which made me inclined to think that Sepia was his constitutional remedy long term, and not just a remedy for an acute illness.

Kent states that Sepias of both sexes develop an aversion to the opposite sex. I have not seen it much, but I suspect that both male and female Sepias are more prone to homosexuality than most other types, as a result of this tendency towards aversion to the opposite sex.

### Physical Appearance

Most Sepia women have a very characteristic appearance. Like traditional images of witches, they tend to be very thin, bony, and have long, thin limbs and digits and a long neck. The face is bony and angular, and the nose is usually long and thin, and is often hooked to some extent. The complexion is characteristically sallow, and the hair is usually straight and black, (or sometimes reddish or mousy brown), and is generally worn long. Moles are commonly found, both on the face and the body, and the woman tends to be hirsute, with dark facial and bodily hair. The eye sockets are often deep and hollow looking, giving an intense, mysterious appearance. The waist tends to be very slim, and the hips are often narrow, though a common variant of the Sepia physique has a body reminiscent of the biblical Eve (or at least of medieval portraits of her), with small breasts, narrow waist, full hips and a rounded, relaxed stomach. A great many of the Sepia women who have not found their true identity become overweight with time, since they become sedentary, and use eating to diffuse some of their sense of dissatisfaction.

# *Silica*

Keynote: Delicate and determined

Silica is a relatively uncommon constitutional type. Like all highly refined types, it is seen in only a small proportion of the population, probably one to two percent, and because of its rarity, it is easily missed, and also over-prescribed. Silica has some characteristics in common with Pulsatilla, Calcarea, Nux Vomica, Graphites and Arsenicum, and may be confused with any of these, but the totality of the Silica personality is quite distinct and unique (as is the physical appearance). All the Silicas I have seen were fe-male.

### Intellectual Refinement and Depth

Silica is probably the most refined of all the constitutional types. Almost everything about her is refined, including her intellect, her aesthetic appre-ciation, her moral sensitivity, and her appearance. Only Ignatia and Arsenicum come close to the refinement of Silica, and all three are quite distinct and different types.

Silica is an intellectual in most cases. This alone is enough to differenti-ate her from Pulsatilla, who is sometimes confused with her on account of her timidity. Silica's intellect is refined and subtle, like that of Sepia and Arsenicum, but more so. Providing she has a clear head, Silica can discrimi-nate very acutely, whether she be considering a mathematical problem, the personality of a new acquaintance, or a complex moral or philosophical is-sue. Unlike Arsenicum, who is often orientated primarily towards material concerns, Silica is usually a deep thinker, like many Sepias and Ignatias. She is liable to be attracted to metaphysical poetry for example, and to spiritual or religious issues, as well as to matters of social justice. Kent recognises this depth when he says of Silica (in comparison to Pulsatilla) 'it is a deeper, more profound remedy'. This is true not only of its physical actions, but also of the corresponding personality of the Silica individual. Silica tends to take life fairly seriously, not because she is a depressive, but rather because she wants to plumb its depths, especially intellectually. Far from being frivolous, she tends to be quiet, thoughtful and discerning, and this often puts her in the role of an observer. She will stand back from the hustle and bustle of life and watch with an eye that sees far more than she lets on. She stands back partly out of fear that she is not rugged enough to take the rough blows that life may deal her, and partly because she wants nothing to do with vulgarity. Her delicate sensitivities are appalled by the brutality, unconsciousness and dishonesty she sees in the world, and as a result, she keeps herself somewhat separate from all but the most gentle and genuine of people (rather like China).

All the Silica people I have known have been intelligent, discriminating individuals, who were more interested in the subtleties of the life sciences, such as psychology, medicine and in one case podiatry, and in the arts, than in the cut and thrust of commercial business. Kent notes that Silica is not suitable for the treatment of 'business brain-fog', but rather, for the mental exhaustion of 'professional men, students, lawyers and clergymen'. In other words, she has a subtle and profound mind that tends not to be interested in business purely for the sake of making money, but rather in the pursuit of knowledge, and its application for the betterment of both the Silica individual and society. Silica is not only too delicate for the commercial world. She is also too principled, and too interested in more cerebral and more spiritual aspects of life. All the Silica individuals I have treated, or known personally, have been idealistic people, but like many Sepia women, they are usually practical as well, rather than being dreamers like many Sulphur and Phosphorus individuals, and some Natrums. Silica tends to focus upon one or two skills which are either artistic or which serve humanity in some way, and to then pursue these skills diligently, rather than getting caught up in the enthusiasms of different idealistic movements. She is basically cautious by nature (Silica should be added to both 'Cautious' and 'Carefulness' in Kent's Repertory), and though she is excitable, and may be swept off her feet initially by a pleasant surprise, or a new idea, she soon simmers down and looks at the practical realities.

Silica's mind is highly precise, like that of Arsenicum. She will usually dot all the i's, and cross all the t's, and in general do her work and her research with precision. She tends to be painstaking (Kent: 'Conscientious about trifles'), and thorough, but has less of the obsessive orderliness that is so common in Arsenicum, and does not impose her standards upon others to the same degree as the latter. This is because she is usually more interested in the content than the form of knowledge. For example, a Silica music teacher is likely to have a highly sophisticated understanding of music, but she is more concerned with teaching the spirit of music and its appreciation, and also how to play an instrument, rather than ensuring that each pupil can read music, and correctly identify every chord, which may be the principle focus of an Arsenicum music teacher. Silica's knowledge is often underestimated, since she is seldom didactic like Kali, Arsenicum, Sulphur, and Lycopodium. She tends to keep her light under a bushel, and avoids showing off. She will reveal whatever is appropriate, and retain the rest of her knowledge until she finds those who can appreciate it. Even then, she will usually share her knowledge and opinions in a quiet, even tentative way. She wishes to understand many things, and she will enjoy discussing them with other like-minded people, but there is no egotism in her self-expression. Rather, she is liable to appear earnest, since that is what she is.

## *Timidity, Determination and Obstinacy*

There is an apparent contradiction in the personality of Silica, which is highly characteristic. Though she is one of the most timid of constitutional types, she is also one of the most stubborn and determined. She is timid because she lacks confidence in herself, and because she fears aggression and the unpredictability of life. As a result, she is tentative when it comes to expressing herself, and she holds back from new endeavours for fear that she will fail, or that circumstances will prove too much for her to cope with. Whenever anything is highly refined, it becomes delicate, and Silica's delicacy makes her try to protect herself by holding herself back, by keeping quiet, by retiring. Her delicacy is both physical and mental. On the physical level she is very sensitive to adverse conditions, such as incorrect diet, and strenuous labour, and she easily becomes tired if she over-extends herself. Because she lacks stamina, and is so easily disturbed by unfavourable conditions, becoming either anxious or developing a headache or an upset stomach when she is required to take on too much, Silica is often given a sheltered upbringing by her concerned and protective parents, and this in itself can make her even more timid. Psychologically Silica is usually stronger than she thinks. She underestimates her capabilities, and fears that she will fail when attempting new tasks. As a result, she may delay for a long time before testing herself. I once knew a young Silica woman who was training at a massage school. At the end of her training she passed the final examinations, and then decided to repeat the whole training, in order to feel more confident of her abilities before beginning to practise professionally. Another Silica woman I knew took course after course in various methods of healing, and others in teaching techniques as a musician, because she felt her credentials were not good enough to attract clients, despite the fact that she was very gifted both as a healer and as a music teacher. The results she obtained in her work were pleasing to her, but she always had the fear that business would fall off, or that she would cease to get good results after a while, because she was inadequately qualified.

Another reason why Silica is afraid to dive too energetically into activity is that she knows that her stamina is not great. This is especially true of mental work. After studying for a while her brain will get fuzzy, and she will be unable to concentrate (Kent: 'dullness from mental exertion'). There then ensues a vicious circle, in which confusion produces anxiety, which leads to more confusion. Silica is prone to anticipatory anxiety, and is particularly likely to panic before examinations and public performances. Because she prepares diligently, she is usually quite capable, and generally succeeds despite her nerves, but she may avoid taking on all sorts of tasks and opportunities because she is afraid that she is not up to them. She is liable to become more contented and more adventurous as she gets older, after having seen over the years that she usually succeeds once she finds the courage to embark upon a project.

Silica's timidity extends beyond her belief in her abilities. It also affects her socially. She tends to be shy until she knows someone well, and knows that they are harmless. Even then, she will usually be a little quieter than her friends, although she doesn't lack a sense of humour. She is at her most timid in dealing with persons in authority, and also with aggressive people. I know one Silica woman who used to mumble all the time, so that people had to constantly say 'pardon?'. This tendency was even more marked when she was nervous, especially during interviews, and hence she constantly 'undersold herself', since people equated her hesitant self-expression with lack of ability. This was not the case, since she was both confident and able at her work, but not during interviews.

Despite her timidity, Silica generally knows what she believes and what she wants. She may or may not have the courage to go out and say what she thinks, or do what she wants, but her mind is not easily changed. In fact, it is surprisingly stubborn. To understand this, we must bear in mind that Silica is an intellectual type, and one with a particularly subtle mind. She has faith in her own understanding once she has grasped something, and she is inclined to stick to her guns in the face of opposition. In fact, when it comes to intellectual argument, Silica can sometimes come alive and project herself into the conversation with an assertiveness that takes others by surprise, having sat quietly and a little nervously whilst the conversation interested her less. She has a love of truth, and will often forget her fear and dive to defend the truth when she feels it is being attacked. At these times she will speak with passion and determination, as if her life depended upon it (Kent: 'Fearlessness'), and she will resist fiercely any attempts to contradict her (Kent: 'Intolerant of contradiction').

One example of the apparent contradiction between Silica's timidity and her determination is her proneness to both indecision and firmness of views. Her indecision is most apparent when she is nervous, and when she is mentally or emotionally exhausted. She will then lack the confidence to make decisions for herself, and will try to rely on other people to make them for her. The decision may be as trivial as which film to see at the cinema, or as important as which career choice to make. The more timid she is in general, the more she will suffer from indecision (Kent: 'Irresolution'), and this will depend upon many factors, including her upbringing (and especially the degree to which her parents respected her views), her emotional security at the time, and her financial security. Any of these factors can adversely affect Silica's ability to make up her mind, and this will vary from day to day. When she asks someone to make the decision for her, and they refuse, she is liable to feel anxious, and she may agonise for a long time over it, basically because she is afraid of the consequences if she makes the wrong choice. This is just another consequence of her general lack of faith in herself.

The other side of the coin is Silica's tendency to have fixed views. Although she may be unsure about many things, she is also unusually sure about some. For example, if she is a Christian, she will tend to have absolute faith in her beliefs, although these may not necessarily be the orthodox articles of faith that she was taught as a child. She will think it through for herself, reject what does not stand up to examination, and then stick doggedly to the rest. I remember having a conversation about religion with one such Silica woman, a friend of mine who was responding positively to Silica for treatment of arthritis. She had rather radical Christian views, which rejected much of popular Christian teaching, and incorporated a lot of more contemporary progressive thinking, but she would not entertain any questioning of the few pieces of traditional belief that she retained. It was as though she had put a fence up around the territory of her belief, and fortified it, saying to herself, "I will venture this far, but no further."

One can interpret Silica's intellectual stubbornness in several ways. It could be due to a fear of uncertainty, and consequent defensive reaction of certainty. Alternatively, it could be due to a love of truth, and a refusal to see truth contradicted. Finally, it could be due to an excessive attachment to certain ideas, in the same way as Arsenicum is often attached to the idea of 'paying one's own way', or Kali Carbonicum is attached to the idea of being rational. I suspect that all three are true to varying degrees. Certainly Silica sometimes gets very attached to certain ideas, be they religious, political, moral or 'scientific'. She also tends to get very attached to certain familiar things and favourite habits. I remember a meeting I once attended of a group of practitioners I worked with for a while at a clinic in England. One of them was a herbalist, a young lady with very characteristic Silica features, being of slight build, with a very pale complexion, rather bony features, and a soft yellow down on her upper lip. She kept quiet for most of the meeting, and when she did speak, she was tentative to the point of being apologetic. Her attitude suddenly changed when we came to discuss whether or not newspapers should continue to be left in the waiting room for the patients to read. Some of the therapists thought they should be removed, since they were full of such negative stories which were not good for anyone. At this point my Silica colleague piped up with a spirited defence of the newspapers. Her face was red with emotion as she insisted that we continue to leave out the papers.

When asked why, she replied that she often had free time at the clinic, and enjoyed reading the newspapers. Such idiosyncratic attachments come as a surprise from the normally meek and sober Silica individual. They reveal the passion with which Silica relishes that which she enjoys, and the indignation she feels when they are threatened. This same Silica herbalist who defended her right to her papers so vigorously eventually came to see me for a consultation. Her main complaint was irresolution (yes, cases are sometimes this simple and consistent!), which had dogged her throughout her life. She said she was forever in a quandary, hesitating before a given course of action, or before a choice which had to be made. I gave her Silica 10M, confident that it would help her, and found a week later that she had not taken it. When I asked why, she said that she couldn't decide whether or not it was the right course of action. I told her that the only way she would be able to decide was if she took the remedy!

Silica's stubbornness is often a refusal to give up a familiar or cherished habit or belief. This rigidity can be quite detrimental to her, as the following example demonstrates. I once treated a young Silica woman for a mild form of rheumatoid arthritis. She had a moderate amount of pain in her hands, but refused to take any conventional medication. She told me that her grandmother had eventually become crippled with arthritis, and she was afraid of ending up a cripple herself. I gave her a regular dose of Silica 30c, which clearly helped, and later occasional doses of 200c, again with good effect. After a while I found that the remedy was not acting for very long at all, and I discovered that she was using marijuana against my advice. I told her that the drug would interfere with the treatment, but she said that it was her only vice, and she wouldn't give it up. This surprised me, in view of the fact that she was highly intelligent, used the drug only occasionally, seemed emotionally stable, and was afraid of becoming a cripple. I realised that it was just another example of Silica's attachment to a given circumstance, one which sadly would do her more harm than most.

It is this kind of attachment that presumably led Kent to list Silica in his Repertory under the rubric 'Monomania', an old-fashioned term for obsession. I have not found Silica to be an obsessive type, except in her attachment to certain ideas and certain habits, which she does not try to push onto other people, but is unwilling to give up herself.

Another example of Silica's determination is the way she sometimes reacts to a dominating personality. Although she is timid, she will often stand up to officiousness in others, and resist them with great presence, even though she may be quaking inside. It is quite common for Silica to feel anger and fear at the same time. She is at once angry at the attempted domination, and afraid of confrontation, but whereas others like Lycopodium and Staphysagria would back down, Silica will often stand her ground despite feeling very afraid inside. Lucinda Leplastrier, the wealthy but inexperienced owner of a glassworks in Peter Carey's comic novel 'Oscar and Lucinda' is a perfect example of a Silica woman. One of her principle attachments is gambling, and one evening she is found playing poker with Oscar, the newly arrived vicar, by one of the more pious parishioners (in Sydney at the turn of the century). The parishioner lets it be known that he is outraged by this indecency on the part of both of them, and whilst Oscar tries to placate him politely, Lucinda adopts her most formal expression and berates the interloper for barging in, ordering him to leave immediately via the window, (through which he had climbed in, having spied their game of cards), along with his grossly obese wife.

Silica is surprisingly good at standing up for herself when she feels she is being imposed upon. Suddenly the blood will rise to her cheeks, and she will object most strongly to the way she is being treated. Generally she is not pompous or egotistical, but she will not tolerate disrespect, since she has a great deal of self-respect, despite her lack of faith in herself at times. Similarly, she will often speak up for someone who is the victim of abuse or injustice, even if she hardly knows them. Her own sense of justice and propriety is profound and personal, rather than arbitrary or conventional, and her defence of innocent victims is a natural expression of her strong convictions.

Because of her timidity, Silica can be over-defensive at times, especially when she is faced with a forceful personality. She fears that her fragile independence is being threatened, and may react hastily and inappropriately. I remember suggesting rather confidently to my herbalist colleague that her indecision would be helped by taking Silica, and then finding that my confident, almost nonchalant manner seemed to make her resistant to taking it. It was as though she felt I was pushing her into a corner and leaving her no choice, and that she had to assert herself to defend her freedom. This tendency often appears as wilfulness in Silica children (Kent: 'Obstinate'). They will gladly cooperate with their parents wishes as long as they feel they are being respected, but as soon as they feel they are being ordered, they will dig their heels in and resist, irrespective of whether they actually want to do what was ordered or not. The Silica child is unlikely to throw a tantrum like Sulphur or Tuberculinum, two other wilful types, but she will get her own way just as often by quiet resistance. If her resistance is broken by force, she will not forgive her parent easily, and will tend to withdraw her affection to punish them. Like the Silica adult, the Silica child is proud and stubborn, without being arrogant or aggressive. She expects respect for her views and her preferences, and as long as she gets it, she is willing to compromise and cooperate, but as soon as she feels she has lost it, she will withdraw her trust, and require a lot of coaxing before she will cooperate again.

One result of Silica's obstinacy in the face of pressure is a refusal to be rushed. She likes to take a long time to think things over, and this can be exasperating for more go-ahead types like Nux and Sulphur. In a marriage, Silica will often be the brake upon her husband's enthusiasm, not because she is a kill-joy, but because she wants to think things through and make sure a course of action is safe and affordable before she commits herself to it. This refusal to be rushed even shows itself in Silica's movements. She not only walks with poise, her back generally perfectly straight yet relaxed, she also has a tendency to dawdle at times. I play tennis with a Silica friend who is willing to run to reach a short ball, but in between play she walks at such a slow pace to retrieve a ball that one would think she was exhausted, and she refuses to ready herself in the usual tense alert way to receive a fast first serve, preferring to stand nonchalantly with her racket by her side. This is presumably another example of Silica's tendency to conserve energy, in case she may need it later on. She will not be pushed into losing her cool unless the situation is dire, and then she may be more likely to panic than to speed up.

## *Integrity*

Integrity is a quality that is hard to define, but one which nearly all Silica individuals possess to a high degree. Silica's integrity is not so much an adherence to codes of ethics, which is more typical of Natrum, Arsenicum and the Kalis, but rather an innate sense of what is right and wrong for herself. Lucinda Leplastrier breaks one taboo after another, since she has no time for the stuffy, hypocritical morality of the Victorian upper classes, yet she is acutely sensitive to her own conscience, and cannot rest when she feels she has been unkind to someone (unless she thinks they deserved it). Silica individuals tend to be very principled people, without being rigid or moralistic. They tend to apply their principles more to themselves than to others, and are not particularly critical of another's behaviour, unless it clearly hurts someone else. They live and let live, and though they may keep themselves apart from the masses, this is more out of respect for their own fragility and sensitivity than out of arrogance. Silica knows that she is very refined, but she is seldom if ever contemptuous. More often she is modest, and liable to understate her gifts and her achievements. She considers self-congratulation to be vulgar (although she will allow herself a brief moment of excited indulgence), and seldom tries to make herself the centre of attention, yet she is not prone to self-denigration either. She is measured and sensible in her activities and attitudes for the most part, with a degree of poise and self-control that appears stately rather than rigid. I am inclined to think that the Princess who slept on a dozen mattresses and still felt the pea on the ground was a Silica. She felt the pea because she was unusually sensitive (Kent: 'Senses hyperacute'), and her sensitivity was her proof of being a princess. Like Arsenicum, Silica very often has a dignified air about her that suggests aristocratic origins or royalty, but unlike the former, her dignity is quiet and modest, rather than insistent.

Loyalty is one aspect of integrity, and I have found my Silica friends and patients to be very loyal to their own friends, and to those they have made a commitment to. Occasionally this may be detrimental to them, since they may get dragged down by friends who are less careful, or less scrupulous, but that is a price that Silica is willing to pay to preserve her own self-respect. I once knew a very refined Silica woman who had adopted a drug addict as a friend. She went to great lengths to help him, and was always available for him when he was in need of her, and would not abandon him as his health and sanity deteriorated. The relationship was very much one of carer and cared-for, and involved no sexual or romantic association. This Silica lady's dignity and self-possession contrasted starkly with her friend's roughness, yet she was not troubled by the latter. Neither was she particularly emotional about his suffering. Silica usually has a caring heart, but like other intellectual types, she is often able to avoid sentimentality and over-attachment when it comes to caring for others, without appearing cold. This is very similar to the detached yet sensitive way in which many Sepia nurses look after their patients. Silica has quite a lot in common with Sepia. Both types are naturally sensitive, independent, and have relatively subtle intellects. Apart from the generally obvious difference in complexion, (the most dark and the lightest of constitutional types), other differences include Silica's delicacy—Sepia is generally more robust and less timid—her obstinacy and her mildness.

Although Silica individuals have high principles, I have not found them to be obsessively conscientious like some Arsenicum and Kali people are. All the Silica people I have known and treated were precise when it came to their work or their art, but none of them appeared to agonise about minor matters of propriety.

### Warmth and Spontaneity

Just because Silica has a subtle mind, and a dignified, sensible nature, we mustn't assume that she is a dull or overly serious person. The majority of Silica individuals have a lightness about them, which results from a combination of cheerfulness and a relative lack of heavy suppressed emotion. When Natrum, Sepia and Ignatia become unhealthy emotionally they suppress negative emotions, leading to a kind of brooding heaviness. Being more intellectual and less emotional than these types, Silica tends to be 'lighter', not only in complexion and in body, but also in mood. Other intellectual (or at least, 'mental') types like Lycopodium and Argentum have a certain lightness, but they lack the gentleness and profundity of Silica. Only Silica has this combination of subtlety, lightness and depth, although the most healthy Mercurius, Sepia, and Ignatia individuals come close. In contrast, Arsenicum is subtle and 'deep' in many cases, but lacks 'lightness' (because he worries too much about material concerns), whereas Phosphorus is subtle and light, but lacks depth both emotionally and intellectually.

The lightness of mood that one often encounters in Lycopodium, Phosphorus and some Staphysagrias all too often relies upon a flight from unpleasant truths. Silica's lightness is seldom an evasion. When her life is beset by problems, she tends to worry a lot, and will usually face the problems eventually, when she has mustered up sufficient courage. It is when she has her life in order that Silica relaxes and enjoys life. She is neither escapist nor an opportunist, but once she has dealt with any pressing problems, she will enjoy living with a quiet relish that is no less delicious than the more excited ecstasy of Phosphorus or Tuberculinum. Most Silicas take delight equally in solitary or meditative pursuits such as art, reading and gentle walks, and in more social activities. Although Silica is shy initially, she will soon warm to a pleasant stranger, and she tends to have several friends, rather than being a loner. One of the more attractive aspects of Silica's personality is her ability to get on with all sorts of people. This results in part from her lack of egotism. Although she is very discriminating, she tends not to be very judgmental, and will usually give someone the benefit of the doubt. In company she is liable to be quiet if the gathering is large, but in a small group, especially one to one, she can be both chatty and playful.

Although she is often an intellectual, Silica seldom gets 'stuck' in an analytical mode of thinking, unlike many Sulphur, Kali, Lycopodium and Natrum individuals. (Sulphur and Lycopodium in particular often have difficulty in separating their ego from their intellect, which they use to impress people. Natrum and Kali tend to hide behind their intellects, since they are often afraid of intimacy). Silica is usually able to be herself in company once she feels safe, and can let her hair down without her intellect getting in the way. She is not overly secretive, but in keeping with her natural dignity, she will tend to reveal her private life only to intimate friends whom she can trust, and will respect another's privacy without having to be asked. As a result, she tends to make firm and loyal friendships. Silica's natural dignity and poise frequently endears her to a great many people, and wins their respect. Even when she is having fun, she tends to retain this poise, just as Phosphorus tends to retain her charm even when she is trying to be intimidating. (Even in a pillow-fight, Silica retains a certain dignity, preferring a few strategically placed blows to a rampant, all-out attack.)

Although Silica is more forgiving than most, when she does develop a dislike for somebody she can be stubborn in her enmity, as she can be in other matters. She is unlikely to become aggressive with her enemies, but she will make her dislike apparent with a mixture of avoidance and non-cooperation, in the same way that the Silica child will express her displeasure to her parents. She is sensitive, and will protect herself from unpleasantness in this way, knowing that her constitution would neither relish nor withstand outright aggression very well.

## *Physical Appearance*

Physically Silica has a characteristic appearance. In keeping with her psyche, Silica's body is refined and delicate, like that of Phosphorus, but even slimmer and lighter. The limbs are often so thin that one can imagine them breaking like matchsticks. In Caucasians the hair is blonde (often very blonde), or light brown, and is straight and exceedingly fine in texture. The skin is generally very pale, and fine to the point of looking almost transparent, with fine blue veins showing through, and is often covered in a fine blonde down. The facial features are long, thin, delicate and angular, reflecting the refined intellect, and the eyes are generally blue, grey or green.

# Staphysagria

*Keynote:* Suppressed anger

Staphysagria is often given acutely for the physical effects of suppressed anger. In these cases the patient's anger and resentment is clearly felt, but not expressed. The force of it rebounds upon the body, producing physical symptoms. It is important for the homeopath to realise that acute states of Staphysagria can arise in any constitutional type, and also that the anger of the person who is constitutionally Staphysagria is usually much less apparent than in acute cases. Staphysagria's anger is often so well suppressed that it is not only unexpressed; it is not even felt. (This compares with many Natrums, whose sadness may be completely suppressed much of the time.) This gives most Staphysagrias a certain mellowness or sweetness that belies the time-bomb of anger ticking away beneath the surface of consciousness.

The source of Staphysagria's suppressed anger is usually to be found in his childhood. (In my experience, male Staphysagrias outnumber females by three or four to one.) The parents were often restrictive and authoritarian, and the young child learned that it was not safe to express his displeasure; that only led to stricter punishment. Sometimes the parents were not particularly strict, but they put the child down verbally, telling him that he was 'good for nothing'. Staphysagria responds to this repression in one of four ways, producing four different sub-types, which I have called the Sweet, the Wild, the Subdued and the Smooth Staphysagria. All of these have problems expressing their anger, and due to their suppressed anger, many find it difficult to express themselves in general.

Sometimes one of the child's parents was Staphysagria constitutionally, and the habit of suppressing anger was learned without any overt repression of the child. The child subconsciously senses his parent's fear of aggression, and this fear is infectious.

Each of the four sub-types we are going to consider is capable of displaying the classic smouldering resentment of Staphysagria, but the Sweet type takes extreme provocation to 'mobilise' his suppressed anger.

When Staphysagria does become resentful, the picture is similar for all subtypes. The main point is that the anger is obsessive. It takes over the personality, creating enormous tension in the body and the mind, which feel like they could explode. The commonest cause of this resentment is rejection by a loved one, usually a partner, especially when the rejection is done in an aggressive, hurtful way.

Once Staphysagria's old, subconscious anger has been brought to the fore, it 'attaches itself' to the present circumstances, generating seemingly endless resentment towards the one who rejected him. There may have been genuine cause for anger in the way in which he was treated, but irrespective of the cause, Staphysagria's anger will take more than a few outbursts to defuse, since there is a huge reservoir of past anger feeding it.

The aggrieved Staphysagria person lives, eats and dreams of hurt and revenge. In the consulting room, the homeopath confronted with such a patient will find that he speaks of nothing but his resentment. He cannot be made to focus on other topics for long. His stomach may be in knots from the tension, but he is more concerned with expressing his resentment, in a repetitive, totally unconstructive fashion. I have found that giving psychotherapy to such patients is generally very unrewarding. Even if they can be persuaded to release their pent up anger (and they usually cannot be) the relief they experience is very temporary. It is only in the rare cases where Staphysagria is willing to come back week after week and explore the original causes of his suppressed anger that real progress can be made. Dealing only with the current anger is like lancing a single boil in a body that is utterly septic. No sooner has one vent exhausted itself than another erupts. Fortunately, doses of Staphysagria 10M generally do succeed in defusing the tension remarkably quickly and effectively in most cases. After the remedy is taken there is often a brief 'explosion' as anger that was kept in check pours forth (it is wise to warn the patient so that plans can be made for him to be in a place where the anger can be vented harmlessly), followed by a genuine calm which may last indefinitely. A great deal of suppressed anger can be neutralised by a few doses of Staphysagria 10M, enabling the patient to drop his resentment and get on with his life.

The following analysis of Staphysagria sub-types is based entirely upon my own experience. Although most Staphysagria people fit one of these sub-types in the main, there are always elements of the others present as well. Thus a person may be a mixture of the Sweet type and the Wild type, or of the Subdued type and the Smooth type. Quite often all four sub-types are expressed to some extent in the same individual.

### The Sweet Staphysagria

This type is most often seen in women, but it does occur quite often in men as well. The Sweet Staphysagria is the polar opposite of the popular image of Staphysagria portrayed in the old materia medicas, which is based on the acute picture of boiling anger and simmering resentment. The Sweet Staphysagria is the most repressed of the four types. She learns in childhood to avoid pain by being good, so good that she becomes utterly compliant, incapable of expressing opposition to anything. Staphysagria is a very sensitive type. In particular, she is sensitive to parental aggression and disapproval (Kent: 'Oversensitive', 'Ailments from reproach'). Like Natrum and Aurum, she is mortified by parental anger and criticism, but her response is somewhat different from these. Natrum and Aurum children respond by withdrawing into themselves, hiding their feelings from their parents, but still nurturing a great deal of resentment inside in most cases. With the Sweet Staphysagria the fear is greater, and the response more extreme. Anger and resentment are repressed so completely that they are no longer felt, and their place is taken by a fear of displeasing the parents, and later on everyone else. This makes the Sweet Staphysagria mild and appeasing. She is the mildest, gentlest soul you could imagine, but her mildness is not healthy like that of Silica and Pulsatilla, who are capable of saying no. It results directly from her desperate attempt to avoid aggression, and prevents her from ever really being herself.

The Sweet Staphysagria is most often seen as the devoted wife of a somewhat dominant husband (or the devoted husband of a somewhat dominant wife). In her attempt to gain approval, the Sweet Staphysagria is frequently dominated by, and devoted to her partner. Like Natrum Muriaticum, she will often choose a partner with some form of weakness, such as physical disability, or emotional instability, and by tending to his every need make herself indispensable. In such situations she is naturally open to being abused, and when she is taken for granted, or worse, she will take it without complaint, and will even assume that it must be her fault. When she surrendered her assertiveness in the hope of avoiding aggression, she lost the ability to look after herself, and also the perspective to see when she is being abused. Because the Sweet Staphysagria is so afraid of confrontation, she will blind herself to her partner's unreasonable behaviour, and take the blame herself, in order to avoid the responsibility for changing the situation, and the fear that this would evoke in her. In this way she lives with her head in the sand, forever avoiding the truth of her situation. This refusal to face unpleasant truths is characteristic of all Staphysagria types, and results in an evasiveness that is subtle in some, and obvious in others. The Sweet Staphysagria's principal method of avoiding unpleasant truths is to acquiesce, to agree, or to keep quiet, and to accept the blame herself when things go awry. She is meek to the point of having no personality of her own, so moulded is she by the principal relationships in her life. Her meekness generally is so ingrained that it extends to every aspect of living. If a stranger steps on her foot in a queue, she will apologise. If a manipulative friend asks her for a favour for the thousandth time, she will say yes, even though it will inconvenience her enormously. In this way the Sweet Staphysagria is a veritable prisoner to her fear, living the life of a slave to other people's preferences and expectations.

Like many Natrum and Lycopodium individuals, the Sweet Staphysagria is usually very polite. Even if she hates a certain man's company (because he scares her), she will never be rude to him, and will smile if he makes a joke at her expense. She does come across as very sweet, because she is gentle and considerate, and few of her friends and associates ever realise the extent to which she has repressed her real feelings. She will often function relatively well in society, since she is at pains to fit in, and has often developed a smooth manner in public, knowing the right things to say at the right times. Furthermore, the Sweet Staphysagria is relatively stable emotionally. Her repression of anger is so complete that it seldom if ever erupts, and her fear is generally kept in check by remaining in a safe relationship. Her mood is generally mild, and cheerful providing she is not in the midst of a threatening encounter with somebody, or anticipating one. To all appearances the Sweet Staphysagria who has a relatively stable marriage is contented and at peace, and this may be so as far as the conscious mind is concerned.

Like other Staphysagrias, the Sweet Staphysagria tends to be romantic. In her flight from her own fear and anger, she will imagine the man of her dreams, and work towards turning her present mate into him. To keep the flame of her romantic hopes alive, she may resort to reading Mills and Boon novels, or the romances in women's magazines. If she does find a mate who is loving and attentive, she will return his love and devotion tenfold, and consider herself the luckiest woman in the world. She will still be unable to stand up for herself, but she will not need to, because she will have what she wants, and her mate will help to protect her from life's cruelties. Those who have less agreeable mates will still do all they can to please, but their peace of mind is clouded by the constant fear that they will be rejected.

The Sweet Staphysagria, being so dependent upon her partner in many cases, tends to suffer a great deal when she is parted from him. I once knew a Sweet Staphysagria young doctor, who lived with a highly unstable Ignatia fiancee, who was also a doctor. My Staphysagria friend spoke so softly that he could not be heard above the background noise of street traffic, or the television. He was terribly devoted to catering to his rather histrionic fiancee's whims, and would quietly and apologetically ask his guests to leave if she were in a bad mood. One day I took his case, and he told me that he would get morose and restless whenever his fiancee was away for a few days. He said he missed her terribly, and didn't know what he would do if he ever lost her (Kent: 'Ailments from disappointed love'). Like all Sweet Staphysagrias he was a sensitive soul, and like many he had adopted certain spiritual practices and beliefs. These not only allowed him to explore the spiritual side of existence, but also to justify his acquiescent sweetness. Many Sweet Stapysagrias are attracted to religions and philosophies which advocate unconditional love, pacifism and the turning of the other cheek. Such attitudes come easily to them, but unfortunately this is generally as a result of fear of aggression, rather than genuine spiritual development. (The latter does not entail a flight from aggression, and strengthens a person's will rather than simply reassuring.)

My Staphysagria doctor friend was very idealistic. He winced at stories of cruelty, and had resolved to go to work as a missionary doctor in Africa. During medical school he stood apart from the other students, since he was too delicate to enjoy their ribald humour, and he was not interested in their more materialistic and hedonistic pursuits. His prime interests were spiritual, and he spent a lot of time reading complicated esoteric books, and playing the violin. He was always ready to help someone in need, and to listen to another's point of view, and in most people's eyes he would be seen as the perfect Christian. This may be true if one considers that 'Christian children all should be, mild obedient, good as he', but it does not mean that he was psychologically healthy. Underneath the Sweet Staphysagria's sweetness is a great deal of fear, and underneath that is anger, but this anger can only be reached by the deepest of psychotherapies. The Sweet Staphysagria may admire the indignant power with which Jesus chased the money-lenders from the temple, but he is unlikely to find sufficient courage to emulate him. In the face of aggressive opposition he is likely to either back down, or to reason politely, and if this does not placate his adversary, he is liable to tremble with fear, and to be physically sick after the encounter. Few of us are relaxed and confident in the midst of aggression from a stranger, but the Sweet Staphysagria is more upset than most by direct aggression, and it will leave him feeling nervous for hours or days afterwards (Kent: 'Timid').

One consequence of abandoning one's sense of power is a certain lack of mental clarity. Nothing clouds the mind like fear, and fear of upsetting other people very often sends the Sweet Staphysagria into paroxysms of indecision, particularly when he is trying to accommodate the wishes of more than one person. Should he listen to his mother or his girlfriend, and if he listens to his girlfriend, will his aggrieved mother ever forgive him? Such quandaries are common when one lives one's life through other people, and this is usually the case for the Sweet Staphysagria.

Staphysagria individuals often have a fine intellect, and the Sweet type is no exception. The men in particular are very often professionals of some kind, and are married as much to their jobs as to their wives, but whereas other workaholics are motivated by greed or by a need to prove their worthiness, the Sweet Staphysagria workaholic works out of duty, to serve his fellow man. I once treated a paediatric surgeon for chronic dyspepsia. He was very prominent in his field, having won many accolades in his profession, and he was confident when he talked about his work (without any trace of pride). One might expect a high-flying surgeon to be a Nux Vomica or an Arsenicum, or perhaps a perfectionist Natrum, but it soon became clear to me that this was a very shy man (Kent: 'Bashful'), who cared very deeply for his little patients, and savoured the way they looked up to him as a loving father-figure. Like all Sweet Staphysagrias, he spoke very softly, and appeared modest even when he was describing his greatest career achievements (which included setting up a paediatric surgical unit in a town which had never had one before). When I asked him what he enjoyed doing most now that he was retired, he told me that he loved to play croquet, and was something of an authority on the game, but that he found very little time to play, since he was always being asked to umpire at croquet tournaments all over the country. I asked him why he didn't say no since he preferred playing croquet to umpiring, and he sighed and said, 'I never could say no'. As well as umpiring croquet games, he spent much of his time working on various charitable and medical committees, again because he was made to feel that he was needed, and could not say no. Of course, subconsciously he wanted to feel needed, just as the Sweet Staphysagria housewife likes to make herself indispensable to her husband, but he also felt the frustration of not being able to relax and play in his free time. Like most Sweet Staphysagrias, he was a mild man, who seldom displayed strong emotions, and who looked at the world through the lens of a fine intellectual mind, which was pervaded by an emotional desire for harmony and acceptance.

### The Wild Staphysagria

This sub-type is a little closer to the traditional, angry version of Staphysagria, but even more complex than his Sweet brothers and sisters. The vast majority of Wild Staphysagrias are male (I have never seen a female one). Unlike the Sweet Staphysagria, who copes with anger by completely suppressing it (Kent: 'Suppressed anger'), the Wild type experiences the force of his anger tangentially through the thrills of dangerous adventure and wild sexual exploits. He is the most reckless of constitutional types, taking risks just for fun that would terrify even the most adventurous Nux or Sulphur individual. In fact, he is reckless because his predilection for wild and dangerous adventure is actually an addiction. If his life begins to feel safe and 'normal' he will get very agitated, because the tension of his suppressed anger is rising, and requires another release through another wild adventure. Tuberculinum also gets very restless when he is one place for long, but his addiction is to variety and excitement rather than danger. It is Aurum who shares the Wild Staphysagria's appetite for death-defying activities, but for a slightly different reason. Aurum is comforted by coming close to death, because he feels free from the burden of life at these times. The Wild Staphysagria is not a depressive like Aurum. He needs the thrill of reckless and dangerous antics to purge the tension that resulted from suppressing his anger, which originated primarily in his childhood. If he does not have this release, he is liable to lose his temper, particularly if he feels scorned (Kent: 'Offended easily').

I once treated a young man in California whose passion was mountaineering. He complained of rather non-specific uneasiness in the stomach after eating, and of a very variable bowel habit, and he also wanted help in giving up recreational drugs. He was very animated and enthusiastic when he was talking about his climbing expeditions, boasting about the times when his safety harness broke, or about the thrills of negotiating deadly overhangs. When I tried to find out more about his personality he became more and more vague, his face took on a confused expression, and he started fidgeting in his chair. He didn't seem to have much idea about what he felt inside, and described his feelings as a vague, confusing mixture of emotions, except for those highs of excitement which he felt from climbing, drugs and sex. His whole life appeared to be an escape from the confusing emotions that were there whenever he was not distracted by excitement.

He had had a variety of jobs all over the State, but his favourite, apart from the climbing tours he conducted, was as a caretaker for a few acres of wilderness in the coastal mountains of California. He loved the freedom of the job, and the fact that he was answerable to nobody, and saw people only when he wanted to. Like the Subdued Staphysagria, the Wild type must have the freedom to travel and escape the confines of normal everyday living. He is usually a wanderer, looking for peace of mind, but seldom finding it, since he looks outside, and when he does look inside, he finds a violent chaos which frightens him. Only by re-experiencing the childhood which he has blocked out (through deep psychotherapy) and releasing his suppressed anger can the Wild Staphysagria find peace of mind. Instead he goes outwards and literally loses himself in the thrill of dangerous adventures.

The Wild Staphysagria pays little heed to the dangers he is taking in his pursuit of excitement. The climber lost his girlfriend in one expedition when her harness line broke and she fell to her death, but this did nothing to inhibit his risk taking. Whilst I was treating him he led an impromptu climbing expedition in the coastal mountain ranges. The weather was bad, visibility was poor, and he was warned not to go, but he shrugged off these warnings and persuaded four other inexperienced climbers that it would be alright. It turned out that the group got into difficultires from the start, and one new climber was slightly injured. Thankfully no lives were lost on this occasion. My patient discussed these events afterwards as if he were in a dream. He tried to gloss over both the dangers involved, and the trauma that his terrified charges had experienced, and seemed genuinely confused as to what went wrong. He was keen to make amends by taking out another expedition, 'in safer conditions'. The Wild Staphysagria is very prone to confusion, of a dreamy, absent kind (Kent: 'Concentration difficult, 'vacant feeling'). His emotions are so much more active than the Sweet type's, and their suppression is only partial. The result is a kind of stale-mate, in which the mind goes blank in order to avoid facing the confusion, and the rage that lies beneath it. After a dose of Staphysagria 10M the wild climber became distinctly more stable, less excitable, and he even developed a desire to settle down with his new girlfriend.

In their search for distraction, Wild Staphysagrias will often turn to mind altering drugs. The two I have known best both used drugs liberally, and one not only took a cocktail of 'uppers' and 'downers' himself, but also made a little money by selling them. Like most Staphysagrias, he was a sensitive soul, and he justified his drug-peddling by extolling the mind-expanding (and hence liberating) effects of his merchandise. The cynical, hard drug-pusher who knows he is instrumental in killing his clients and doesn't care a fig is unlikely to be a Wild Staphysagria. It is the habitual user and small time pusher of cannabis who is most likely to be a Staphysagria. I have treated many such people, and all of them had a lost quality, and a tendency to jump at simple solutions to their malaise, such as taking off and having a new adventure somewhere, rather than stopping the drugs and trying some introspection, and finding a regular job. (An excellent portrayal of a Wild Staphysagria can be seen in the recent film 'Point Break', in the character of Bodhi, played by Patrick Swayze. Bodhi is a fanatical surfer, who rides the biggest waves, snorts cocaine at parties, charms and then dumps one woman after another, and espouses a sixties' philosophy of mind-expansion, freedom and Zen. His charisma attracts a group of followers who are willing to take risks, and willing to interpret his total lack of responsibility as 'personal freedom'. Bodhi weds his idealism to his thirst for thrills by staging a spree of bank robberies. He is motivated more by a desire to embarrass the authorities than to make money, and even more by the thrills he gets from doing it. When things go wrong he is determined enough to kill to escape, and crazed enough to feel little remorse, yet he is generally kind-hearted, and will always help out a friend. Like all Wild Staphysagrias, he is full of contradictions, not least of which is his sensitivity and his irresponsibility.)

The Wild Straphysagria is apt to use his idealism at times to justify his dangerous activities. I once treated a man in his late thirties for indigestion. He had a boyish appearance, and a mild, gentle manner. He was very sociable, and spoke in a relaxed and humorous way which put others at ease. At the time I met him he was in between assignments in his work as a journalistic photographer. He had lived a very varied and wandering life, and did not seem very interested in settling down. He told me that he felt most alive when he was covering war stories, and he was in the thick of it, with bullets and missiles flying overhead. The next time I saw him he was in tears. Another regional conflict had broken out, and he did not have the money to fly down and cover it. I asked him why he was so upset, and he said he just wanted to be there where the action was. He then said that he wanted to help the peasants who were in the midst of the conflict, the ones who suffered the most. He really did seem to be beside himself with frustration and sorrow, but I got the impression that his real need was not so much to help the needy, but rather to feel the exhilaration of being where the action was. I gave him Staphysagria 10M, and his indigestion improved rapidly, but I did not see him for much longer, and do not know if he was able or willing to refrain from coffee and drugs long enough to allow the remedy to help balance his personality.

Staphysagria is a very sexual type (Kent: 'Lascivious', 'Libertinism', 'Nymphomania'), and this is especially true of the Wild type. There is a very close connection between lust and aggression (the male hormone testosterone has been shown to promote both), and the poorly suppressed anger of the Wild Staphysagria tends to fuel his libido. Given the type's taste for and addiction to excitement, it is not hard to see why the Wild Staphysagria has a tendency to be promiscuous, and to dive impulsively and passionately into sexual affairs. Whilst I was in California I stayed in two communities, which gave me the opportunity of observing my patients more intimately than is usually the case. One evening I was at a dance, when I was 'accosted' by a man I knew to be a Wild Staphysagria. He had drunk too much alcohol, and had been propositioning a number of women. When they refused him, he asked me for a wrestle, and proceeded half playfully, half aggressively to grapple with me. I could feel tremendous force in his arms, and also a certain sexual excitement which he was trying to diffuse by wrestling with me. The Wild Staphysagria is liable to be both aggressive and sexual when he is disinhibited by alcohol. The same can be said of Natrum men and a few other types, but the Wild Staphysagria is especially sexual, and his sober state is so mild and gentle in comparison.

Staphysagrias in general are very sensitive to being rebuked, and the Wild Staphysagria is particularly sensitive to sexual rejection. I was once a witness to the wrath of a rejected Wild Staphysagria. I knew him as a reckless but mild and gentle man. One day I saw him turn on a young woman who had rejected his advances, hurling abuse at her in a frenzy of indignation which reduced her to tears. I have since seen similar reactions by other Wild Strapysagria individuals, and have come to regard them as typical of the type (Kent: 'Jealousy', 'Anger with indignation').

Like other Staphysagrias, the Wild type is predisposed to vivid and intense sexual fantasies (Kent: 'Sexual thoughts intrude'). These fantasies will often drive him to masturbate frequently (Kent: 'Masturbation, disposition'—black type), and also to engage in wild sexual encounters, including homosexual ones. On the other hand, the Wild Staphysagria is also romantic. He usually yearns for the intimacy and sweetness of an intimate relationship, but his evasiveness and his wildness generally prevent him from finding one that will last. One of my Wild Staphysagria patients had tears in his eyes when he told me of a love-affair that didn't work out. Another stopped taking drugs and appeared to settle down and find a stable relationship after taking the remedy. In almost every case the homeopath will find Staphysagria to be a sensitive, romantic type, irrespective of his anger and his irresponsibility. The Wild Staphysagria often appears like a lost boy, confused, excitable and impulsive, and very sad when he stops and feels his loneliness. His charm and his recklessness will attract a great many fun-loving women, and others who want to mother him, but he is usually unable to sustain a relationship for long, because he cannot face painful home-truths. He prefers to forget his problems by getting 'high', and then leaving when things get ugly.

Unlike the Subdued Staphysagria, the Wild type tends to be emotionally open. He is usually willing to talk frankly about his feelings, especially when he is sad, in a manner that attracts sympathy, since it reveals his vulnerability. He will cry easily when upset, without being ashamed, and he is generally affectionate with his loved ones. His evasiveness lies not so much in his refusal to discuss his feelings, but rather in his inability to face them himself. He is often very confused about the mixture of emotions he is experiencing, and tends to escape from them by pursuing adventure and excitement. When he does try to describe what he is feeling, he will often stop and look perplexed, and then say 'It's kind of hard to say'.

Like the press photographer who identified with the peasants in the wars he covered, the Wild Staphysagria will usually have a dislike of authority. In most cases his anger derives principally from strict parents who punished him as a child, hence it is natural that he enjoys seeing authority figures discomforted, since in this way he tangentially rebels against his parents. Bodhi, the Wild Staphysagria character in the film 'Point Break', robbed banks specifically in order to embarrass the establishment, rather than to make money. His gang wore masks resembling the previous Presidents of the United States, in order to rub in the message that he had nothing but contempt for the authorities. His contempt for authorities is one reason why the Wild Staphysagria tends to be a wanderer. He knows that if he stays in one place or one job for too long, he will come into conflict with authority. It is easier to move on and avoid commitments and responsibilities. Eventually, some Wild Staphysagrias may become burnt out and suspicious loners, having unwittingly rebuffed any love and stability that was offered to them. They then come to resemble the Subdued Staphysagria.

### The Subdued Staphysagria
Whilst the Sweet Staphysagria learns to avoid conflict by appeasement, the

Subdued type does so by avoiding social interaction. This is a very introverted type, a fugitive, who runs away from people in order to avoid a repetition of his past, a childhood in which he was made to feel helpless or worthless, with anger that could not be expressed, because fear of punishment was even stronger. Talking to a Subdued Staphysagria, one gets the feeling that one is talking to a shadow of a man. There is little expression of life - little interest or emotion shown. The voice is dry and monotone, and as few words as possible are spoken. The eyes are reticent and suspicious, and do not make good contact. He appears tense and restless in conversation, and his face never relaxes. One gets the feeling that a smile would crack his face, so set are its muscles in a protective neutral expression. This rigid neutrality or lack of expression is reminiscent of Kali and Aurum, but there are clear differences between these three. Aurum is far more prone to depression and suicidal thoughts than the Subdued Staphysagria, and is generally assertive in the world. Kali is also frequently assertive professionally, is anything but a wanderer, and is generally far more socially interactive than the Subdued Staphysagria.

The Subdued Staphysagria learned in childhood to avoid punishment by laying low, by keeping out of sight. He continues this habit into adult life, and in doing so he seriously restricts his emotional satisfaction. As a child he most likely had few friends, and was overly serious with those he did mix with. He cannot let his guard down, since he may get hurt again. Unlike Natrum, who usually becomes a good actor, the Subdued Staphysagria never develops confident social skills. His expression is almost always sombre, and when he does attempt a smile, it usually appears nervous and tense. I suspect that the reason why the Subdued Staphysagria differs from Natrum in not developing a smooth social exterior lies in the fact that he is both too afraid and too bitter to do so. Natrum is primarily concerned with avoiding emotional pain. I have the impression that Staphysagria (especially the Subdued type), like Arsenicum, tends to be more concerned deep down with survival, and the avoidance of physical abuse. Most of the Subdued Staphysagrias I have treated were beaten frequently by their fathers in childhood. As a result, they feared almost any human contact, and they usually became wanderers in their attempt to avoid being noticed. The popular Western movie image of the high plains drifter is an excellent caricature of the Subdued Staphysagria. He is depicted as a loner who is running away from a terrible secret, which often involves him having been violently and deliberately tortured almost to the point of death. He hides his eyes under the shade of his hat, utters only the bare essentials he needs to order whisky or hire a room, and moves on before anyone develops an interest in him. Typically, the movie's climax sees our anti-hero wreaking revenge upon his oppressors, and thereby restoring some sense of inner peace to his soul. The Subdued

Staphysagria does need to get in touch with his anger and express it, but it is only when he confronts his original oppressor (usually his father) internally and releases his anger towards its original cause, that he can be free of both the anger, and the fear that cripples him so. Projecting his anger onto others may help him to feel more confident, but it will not remove either the anger or the fear permanently.

Not surprisingly, the Subdued Staphysagria tends to be very distrusting (Kent: 'Suspicious'). He will be reluctant to reveal too much about himself to the homeopath, and will tend to cloak his fear with a very rational way of speaking. Staphysagria is a relatively mental or intellectual type, and many Subdued Staphysagrias will devote their time to reading and studying, in place of mixing with other people. Others become very practical, since they move around a lot, and hide from human contact in the wilderness, where they learn to fend for themselves. Natrum Muriaticum may also withdraw to isolated areas, and suspiciously avoid human contact, and the differentiation of Natrum and a Subdued Staphysagria can be very difficult. Generally Natrum is better able to express himself, and his feelings are clearer, even though he seldom expresses them. All Staphysagrias tend to appear confused when talking about their feelings, and to suffer more from intellectual impairment than depression. There is a constant subconscious battle inside between their fear and their rage, and the mental effort required to suppress this from consciousness can sometimes leave the mind blank or confused, especially when present circumstances trigger off the old feelings. The facial features may help in distinguishing between Natrum and the Subdued Staphysagria. Most Staphysagrias develop fine wrinkles radiating out from the corners of the eyes, and their faces tend to remain relatively free otherwise from wrinkles, producing a boyish appearance, like that of Lycopodium, but more so.

On giving a Subdued Staphysagria a high potency of the remedy, the effect can be dramatic. I have seen such people change within a week or so from being withdrawn and 'haunted' to becoming increasingly open and spontaneous. One can actually see the life-force returning to those grey, weary faces, as they soften, and begin to smile naturally for the first time in decades. In the process they may experience some of the anger which they suppressed in childhood, and express it impulsively by losing their temper, or in the safe environment of a therapy session (I advise my angry patients to release their anger by hitting at cushions and yelling), or by working it out through heavy physical exercise. They may never fully reconnect with and release their anger and their fear, but may, with the help of the remedy, find sufficient courage and sense of self to expand their lives emotionally and professionally, to put down some roots, and abandon the old tactic of running away.

## The Smooth Staphysagria

The Smooth Staphysagria possesses many of the characteristics of the other three types, with a few more of its own. It is the most successful of the Staphysagrias from the point of view of social adjustment, and its very 'normality' can make it difficult to spot. Furthermore, none of the four types is very common, and hence the fledgeling homeopath cannot learn about them very quickly from experience, and must rely on accurate descriptions.

The Smooth Staphysagria resembles the Sweet type quite closely, but is able to be more assertive when the situation demands. Like the Sweet type he has a soft, gentle quality which is feminine without being effeminate, and which endears him to a great many people (the softness of the English comedian/singer Des O'Conner is a good example of this kind of manner). In comparison Lycopodium, who is easily confused with the Smooth Staphysagria, is more neutral or masculine, and appears more emotionless. Whereas the Sweet type avoids unpleasantness by giving way, the Smooth Staphysagria is more subtle and slippery. He is generally very diplomatic, and skilled at avoiding situations which might make him feel uncomfortable, whether they involve another person's aggression, or the risk that he will have to talk intimately about his emotions. He generally has a sharp intellect, which he uses not only to explore his world, but also to deflect attention away from his own feelings. He is especially good at using humour to gloss over his personal life, and to lighten the subject of conversation. Unlike the Sweet Staphysagria, the Smooth type will not give way endlessly when he is put upon, and will get annoyed eventually. When he is annoyed he will seldom express his anger directly, but will become increasingly terse in his speech, and he will tend to avoid the object of his anger as much as possible.

The Smooth Staphysagria, as his name suggests, has a casual, 'laid-back' manner which suggests that he is emotionally relaxed and healthy. He is very flexible, and can adapt himself to a wide variety of situations without appearing flustered. His principal weakness is his emotional evasiveness, which is not easy for the homeopath to spot initially, unless the latter probes his patient quite deeply, or asks his patient's partner. Furthermore, the homeopath must learn to distinguish between the Smooth Staphysagria and other suave, emotionally evasive types like Lycopodium and Natrum. Generally, The Smooth Staphysagria appears even softer and 'lighter' than Lycopodium, and does not have the latter's tendency to rationalise everything, and to show off with his knowledge. Like all Staphysagrias, the Smooth type appears modest, although he is often confident socially. He appears lighter and more boyish than Natrum men, and is not so easily embarrassed or threatened by intimacy. (Compare the softness of the naturalist David Attenborough with that of Des O'Conner.) Natrum is a 'deeper' type than Staphysagria, in the sense that he is more able to feel deep emotions, and is more likely to be attracted to profound concerns like the plight of the home-less, or to religious issues. The Smooth Staphysagria just wants an easy life, and whilst he is generally kind by nature, he does not have the need of many Natrums to 'fix' other people's lives.

Although constitutional types are determined more by heredity than by environmental factors, there does seem to be a remarkable 'resonance' between constitutional types and the upbringing they receive. For example, it is common for Ignatia to experience the loss of a loved one in childhood, or for Natrum to be made to perform by his parents. In the case of Staphysagria the child is often either physically mistreated, or made to feel that he is no good. This conditioning then plays a major role in the devel-opment of future illnesses.

I once saw a vivid example of this in the case of a Smooth Staphysagria patient who came to see me for the treatment of a crippling generalised arthritis, which he developed suddenly at the age of eighteen. (It is typical of Staphysagria to develop conditions rapidly, in response to emotional stimuli.) He was very polite and suave, and yet modest at the same time. He appeared open and friendly, and highly intelligent. When I asked him about what was happening in his life at the time the arthritis developed, he said that he had just sat his final exams at school, and was waiting for the results. He had thought he had done badly in these exams, and was very worried what his parents, who expected him to go to law school, would think of him. On further questioning he confirmed that his parents were forever criticising his performance, and his person in general. I asked him how this had made him feel, and he said 'Like I can't do anything'. I then asked what the effect of his arthritis had been on his life, and he said 'I can't do what I want to'. It was clear to me that he had subconsciously chosen to develop his arthritis having anticipated failure in those crucial exams, as a means of justifying his inability in his parents' eyes. It was acceptable to be incapable if he was a cripple, but not otherwise. Ironically he did well in his exams and went on to become a proficient lawyer. I gave him a regular dose of Staphysagria 30c, and his joint pains improved markedly. His condition was diagnosed as Reiter's Disease, an arthritis which follows either gastroenteritis or a sexu-ally transmitted urethritis.

It is interesting to note that Staphysagria's weakest points physically in-clude his digestive system and his reproductive system, and I have found several cases of Reiter's Disease which responded to the remedy. Exactly the same family dynamics can often be seen in the Lycopodium person's child-hood, but the result is somewhat different, because the constitution is dif-ferent from birth. The principal effect of discouragement upon Lycopodium is a lack of confidence in his abilities, with its concomitant anticipatory anxi-ety, and often a compensatory bravado. The Smooth Staphysagria lawyer with arthritis did not suffer from a lack of confidence in his abilities. Neither was he bothered by anticipatory anxiety, nor was he prone to showing off. His parents' expectations left him feeling angry, and also afraid of punishment, and it was to avoid these feelings inside himself that he subconsciously chose to develop a crippling illness.

Staphysagria is far more prone than Lycopodium to develop sudden and serious illnesses in response to emotional stress. Whereas Lycopodium may develop an aggravation of his eczema or his dyspepsia during times of stress, Staphysagria is more likely to develop severe stomach pains, or a sudden and severe eczema. The Smooth Staphysagria lawyer appeared very stable emotionally, as do all Smooth Staphysagrias, but he had paid a terrible price for that stability. His alternatives had been either to express his fear and anger to his parents, or to suffer a mental breakdown, and he chose the least threatening of the three options.

Smooth Staphysagrias are generally very sociable people. Their emotional 'lightness', combined with their easy charm and their wit make them very popular, with both sexes. Lycopodium men are generally more popular with women than men, because their competitive nature tends to make them treat other men as rivals. In contrast, the Smooth Staphysagria appears modest and charming to both sexes, because he is not trying to prove anything. What he is trying to do, like all Staphysagrias, is to avoid his deeper feelings, and it is his very success that makes him seem so likeable.

Some famous entertainers have a light air that is reminiscent of the Smooth Staphysagria. (They also have the light physique that is typical of Staphysagria in general.) I am thinking not only of the afore-mentioned Des O'connor, but also of Fred Astaire, Bing Crosby and the English actor Nigel Havers. (It is perhaps no coincidence that the last two television dramas I have seen involving Nigel Havers portrayed him as a fugitive, whose subtle charms could no longer hide the awful secret he was running from.) Note the somewhat impish features of each of these, which are almost feminine in appearance.

Naturally, since he is hiding from his deeper feelings, the Smooth Staphysagria is liable to be less successful in his private life than he is socially. His partner is liable to find his evasiveness frustrating, since she can never be truly close to a man who is hiding from himself. She is also liable to become angry when he glosses over serious problems, be they practical or emotional. Many Smooth Staphysagrias compromise by learning to take their partner's concerns seriously, and by learning to talk more about their feelings, and this does make for more satisfying relationships, though it may still leave the majority of the husband's emotions suppressed, and hence a threat to future stability. If future events wake up some of those sleeping elephants, a stampede could ensue, in the form of unexplained anger and irritability, irrational nervousness leading to alcoholism, or the development of a serious physical disease. Like all Staphysagrias, the Smooth type is sitting on a reservoir of turbulent emotions. He generally manages to keep the lid screwed down tight, but occasionally circumstances prise it open, and he is suddenly astonished at the intensity of his own feelings.

### Physical Appearance

In my experience, women are somewhat more common than men amongst the Sweet Staphysagrias, but in the other three types they are rare or non-existent. The Sweet, Wild and Smooth types tend to resemble each other physically, and I will deal with these first. Generally the physique is slight, being both shorter and slimmer than average. The face looks younger than its years, with smooth skin and very fine wrinkles, and a characteristic radiation of fine wrinkles from the corners of the eyes. The face is frequently impish in appearance, being thin and somewhat triangular, with the point downwards at the chin. The hair is usually fine, and may be any colour, though a light or medium brown is commonest. The eyes are often 'bright and beady', like those of the cartoon character Jimminy Cricket, whose whole appearance is suggestive of Staphysagria. Some Staphysagrias, particularly those who 'drop out' and become addicted to cannabis, are tall and extremely thin, with bony angular faces and sharp bony noses. They usually have a pale sickly look to them, and a characteristic stoop of the shoulders. When walking this type often keeps both arms stiffly by his side, which looks very incongruous, since his gait is usually a languid lope. The effect is like that of an orang-outang walking. This 'washed out' effete version of Staphysagria is generally a combination of the Sweet, Wild and Subdued types psychologically.

The Subdued Staphysagria often looks very similar to the above, but his features have stiffened into a mask, which is rigid and reveals little emotion. He is generally grey-haired, even when young, and his eyes are very reticent. I have seen one Subdued Staphysagria who had a large frame, the others being small but generally muscular, as a result of pursuing a physical way of life. Most Subdued Staphysagrias have thin or non-existent lips, as a result of their extreme suppression of emotion.

# Stramonium

*Keynote:* Light and dark

Stramonium is perhaps the most dramatic and famous of the remedies which correspond to states of insanity. It is a constitutional type, and it bears close resemblences to Hyoscyamus, Belladonna, Anacardium and Veratrum Album. Like these other types, it is rare, and its mental picture is generally so extreme that the majority of Stramonium individuals are likely to reside in mental institutions. It is interesting that most of the children I have seen who responded to Stramonium were boys, whereas all of my adult Stramonium patients have been women. I conclude from this that Stramonium is more common in males, but that female Stramonium individuals are more liable to remain in the community rather than be institutionalised.

## The Darkness

One of ther helpful differentiating features between Stramonium and his cousins is the intense fear of darkness of Stramonium. Stramonium individuals are subject to all manner of terrors, delusions and hallucinations, and they usualy dread the night, because it is then that they become haunted by the horrors of their own subconscious mind. They will tell you that they hate sunset, because it heralds the beginning of the dark time. Stramonium children often have an extreme fear of the dark, and will not go into an unlit room. They sleep with a light on, and if they wake in a darkened room, they will see monsters in the dark (far more vividly than the wispy shadows seen by other children), and will scream and scream long after their parents have arrived and tried to soothe them. Stramonium has terrible night terrors—nightmares which continue after the child has awakened, whilst the child stares manically and screams like its life was about to be terminated.

Adult Stramoniums are more prone than any other constitutional type to see faces, creatures and illusory people (Kent: 'He sees animals, ghosts, angels, departed spirits'). One Stramonium patient who was diagnosed as a case of multiple personality said that she was forever seeing little men, or strange creatures, that nobody else could see. Stramonium will see these hallucinations more often and more vividly in the dark. They may frighten her because they appear demonic or dangerous, or she may take little notice of them.

It is curious that Stramonium is not only terrified of darkness and evil, but also fascinated by it. This is especially true of Stramonium boys, and presumably of Stramonium men as well. Stramonium boys will be terrified after watching a children's horror story on television, and will be kept awake by horrible visions emanating from the impressions they have seen on the TV, yet they will also admit to being fascinated by ghosts, monsters and by violence. A Stramonium child can easily take on the persona of some terror figure he has seen or heard about, and after he has beheaded his hamster with the kitchen knife he will explain calmly that it was not he but the Executioner from the video film that did it. It is this sudden switch from being a victim of terrifying visions to being controlled by them that makes Stramonium so dangerous, and gives the type its violent reputation.

### Rage and Sexuality

There is no more violent type than Stramonium. The Stramonium child has tantrums that are of an entirely different order to aggressive types like Tuberculinum and Nux. The latter will scream and hit, but Stramonium children will bite, gauge and stab. There is no holding back when Stramonium 'loses it'. The rage is quite insane, and accompanied by a definite desire to maim or kill in many cases. Those Stramonium patients who are brought to see the homeopath are usually calm most of the time, and will talk in a strangely detached manner about how they want to kill when they are angry, and how they have no control at such times. There is an eeriness about this detachment, especially when it is seen in a young child. Young Stramonium children will look at you in the consulting room with a stare that is unnerving and totally devoid of fear. They will speak intelligently and often precociously about their fears and their hates, as if they are talking about a laboratory specimen. Although they will admit to stabbing their mother with a scissors, they appear to feel no remorse afterwards. They simply switch from rage mode to normal mode, as if nothing has happened.

The adult Stramonium women I have treated were all prone to bouts of intense rage, but were able to resist acting it out for the most part. That is why they were able to consult a homeoapth. They presumably lie at the more sane end of the Stramonium spectrum, whilst the majority of the type have less control, and spend their lives in institutions. It is generally true that male members of a potentially insane constitutional type exibit more anger and sexuality than their female counterparts, and this is probably the reason why I have not seen adult male Stramoniums. A trip to a long-term psychiatric ward would no doubt reveal many Stramonium patients, and they would be especially common in high security psychiatric wings of prisons.

The rage that the Stramonium individual feels is often unfocussed; that is, the anger is not directed at anyone in particular. It appears as if they are 'possessed' by a force that is entirely impersonal. The same can be said of the terror that they feel, which is often unrelated to any specific fear, and the sexual desire, which will usually be unrelated to any attraction to anybody in particular.

The Stramonium people I have treated were not angry most of the time. Rather they would suddenly be prone to bouts of rage with which they would struggle for a few hours, and then be calm again, or enter a different emotion, such as lust or terror. Often they would seek help when these waves of emotion were becoming too strong to resist, and usually a few doses of Stramonium 10M would lessen the force of the attack immediately, and repeated doses would gradually reduce the intensity and frequency of all the psychotic phenomena. During an acute episode of rage or terror the remedy may have to be repeated every hour or two. It can then be tailed off gradually, but will often be needed in a maintenance dose of once a week or so, since it is a constitutional remedy for a highly unstable personality.

Most psychotic remedy types are prone to intense sexual desire, and this is especially true of Stramonium. The intensity of desire is as great or greater than that seen in Hyoscyamus individuals, but whereas Hyoscyamus tends to have 'perverse' sexual impulses, with an exhibitionist element, Stramonium either has a feeling of pure overwhelming lust, or else lust mixed with rage. The latter may give rise to violent sexual fantasies. One highly intelligent Stramonium patient was tormented by such intense sexual desire that she signed up with a brothel. After treatment she was able to resist doing this, but only with the help of frequent doses of Stramonium 10M during crises. Another could not get enough sex from her relationship, and was sorely tempted to be promiscuous, but resisted because of her religious beliefs. Religiosity is almost as common as intense lust amongst psychotic types, and frequently the two are seen together.

It must be remembered that psychotic patients often have a psychotic parent, and hence received a very abnormal upbringing. One of the consequences of this is that they are more liable to have been sexually abused as children. Two of my Stramonium patients had been sexually abused in childhood, and both tended to go into psychotic states after the trigger of potential or actual sexual contact.

### The Fractured Personality

Stramonium is very prone to hearing voices, and these voices are often quite consistent and have a personality of their own. All the psychotic types can hear voices, but I have only come across multiple voices in Belladonna and Stramonium cases. The voices usually talk to the Stramonium person, sometimes giving orders or advice, other times mocking or abusing. The subject may believe that she is possessed by numerous entities, and tends to have little control over the voices, but may be able to resist their promptings. My Stramonium case of multiple personality was learning with the aid of a therapist to see the voices as different aspects of herself, and to 'integrate' them into her 'normal' personality. This process was slow but did succeed in making the voices less troublesome. Another aspect of her shaky sense of self was her weak 'boundaries'. She believed that she took on the feelings and the ailments of those around her, and this belief persisted after most of her psychotic symptoms had subsided with treatment.

### Delusions and Hallucinations

Delusions are common in Stramonium individuals. Often the person has some insight, knowing that the belief is 'silly' or unlikely, but still it is clung to, at least to some extent. An example is the lady who grew up planning to marry her father. Part of her knew that this was impossible, yet the thought was a source of security for her. As she grew up and abandoned this thought, she replaced it with the delusion that she was married to her brother. These delusions appeared to be an attempt by the patient to compensate for a terrible sense of abandonment (Kent:' Forsaken feeling'). Another Stramonium patient told me that as a child she felt whilst in the bath that her thoughts would go down the plughole, and thence someone would be able to get hold of them and analyse them. Many of Stramonium's delusions relate to being under attack in some way.

Stramonium's hallucinations are as varied and as bizarre as her delusions. One patient said that as a child she saw worms inside her head after being touched by a child she thought was dirty. The same patient was prone to smelling imaginary odours, and to seeing cats and insects that were not there. Often they would dissapear as she watched them. Such stories confirm that Stramonium is a long-term constitutional state, not just a temporary one.

### Fears and Phobias

We have already mentioned Stramonium's fear of the dark. Another common phobia is tunnels. many Stramonium people dread going through tunnels, and feel panicky when they do so. Some will not travel in a train in case it goes through a tunnel. This fear appears to be closely related to the fear of darkness. Another highly characteristic Stramonium fear is a fear of shining objects or of flickering light. Stramonium patients will report that they feel panicky in a moving car if sunlight is flickering in between a row of trees, or through a fence. One woman said she hated to look at sunlight upon water. When I asked why, she said it was "one of those horrible shiny things." Another common fear is a fear of the colours red and black. These obviously suggest blood and violence and also darkness and evil, things that Stramonium individuals are often both terrified of and fascinated with. I once asked a patient I suspected of being Stramonium if there were any colours she didn't like. She immediately said "Black and red," and I then pointed out that these were the very colours she was wearing. She could not explain the contradiction. It appears she was irresistably drawn to the colours she hated.

Many Stramonium patients have a great fear of being alone. This is especially true when they are feeling anxious to start with. One attractive young lady who later responded to the remedy was so dependent upon her boyfriend's company that she would not leave the house without him. She appeared basically sane, and she talked sensibly, but she was subject to terrible urges to kill her boyfriend, and to overwhelming sexual desire.

### The Light

Just as Stramonium people fear the night and all things evil, and yet are fascinated by them, so they hate bright light, and yet feel better in the daytime, and are soothed by spiritual and religious thoughts. Many Stramonium people cling onto sanity and keep the terror at bay by praying fervently. Another aspect of the light/dark dichotomy is the tendency to feelings of euphoria. At times the Stramonium patient will feel very high, with a rush of energy, and a feeling of closeness to God. One Stramonium patient would run and dance when she was high, whilst another would furiously get all her chores done at top speed. Unfortunately, Stramonium's high spots tend to be less frequent than her downers.

Readers may be confused by the similarity between Stramonium's light/dark dichotomy and that of Anacardium. The main difference is that Anacardium experiences both simoultaneously, and is torn between his two halves, whereas Stramonium experiences them sequencially, and hence is either fearing the darkness or 'being it', without the aweful struggle between the two.

### Obsessive/Compulsive

Like the other psychotic types, Stramonium is prone to obsessive compulsive behaviour. Stramonium children will often have rituals that they must follow in order to avoid anxiety, such as doing up their shoe laces in a particular order, or lining up their toys in a specific way. One Stramonium patient told me that as a child she had to make her bed so that the stripes on her sheets were exactly aligned with her bed, otherwise she felt very threatened. (Stripes appear to be threatening to Stramonium people.) She also said that after a bath she had to have a separate towel to dry her feet, or she felt contaminated. This is reminiscent of Syphilinum, but it was accompanied by many classic Stramonium features, and Stramonium did act very well in her case.

### Hyperactivity

Stramonium children are usually hyperactive. They cannot keep still for long, and in the consulting room they will roam from one object to another, picking it up, putting it down, and going on to the next. Generally their constant behaviour appears more purposeless than that of sane hyperactive types like Tuberculinum and Natrum Muriaticum. The same can be said of the hyperactive Anacardium or Hyoscyamus child. These hyperactive children appear oblivious to the conversation between their parent and the homeopath, and will interrupt whenever they like, and ignore all remonstrations and threats. On the other hand, they will often interrupt to comment on something that has been said about them, either denying it or elaborating, which shows that they are more perceptive than they might appear. In school they will tend to distract other children, and their concentration span is usually very short.

The Stramonium adult is only hyperactive when in a manic phase, which is a minority of the time for those outside institutions.

# Sulphur

*Keynote:* The inspired ego

Elemental Sulphur has always been associated with fire. Sulphur is flammable and burns with a stench, which can be smelt at the site of an erupting volcano, and brimstone (the naturally occurring form of mineral sulphur), is said to fuel the fires of hell. When Sulphur powder is left on the skin it produces a burning irritation, hence its use homeopathically for skin diseases. Even the mineral's yellow hue reminds us of its fiery affinities. The Sulphur individual is fiery in every sense of the word. Fire has always been used to represent the Divine Spirit in mankind, which lights up the clay of the physical body. There is a distinct spiritual element to most Sulphur individuals, which is inspirational rather than merely intellectual. Fire also represents the passions, and there is no more passionate type than Sulphur, whether one is considering the appetites of the flesh, intellectual inspiration, romantic love, or zealous enthusiasm for virtually anything under the sun. Whatever interests Sulphur he pursues passionately. Fire is also anger, and Sulphur's vivacity can easily spill over into irritation and outright rage when his determined will is blocked, or he feels wronged in some way. Finally, fire represents the spark of creativity and genius. Sulphur individuals are generally very creative people, particularly intellectually. I believe that true genius belongs almost exclusively to the Sulphur constitution, and that virtually all of the great scientific and philosophical minds recorded in history were Sulphurs, from Socrates to Einstein, as well as the greatest of the great composers. The world would be a dull place without Sulphur's inspiration, optimism and eccentricity.

## Intellectual Inspiration

The gift of inspiration is possibly the single most characteristic quality amongst Sulphur individuals. (The only Sulphur people who are not inspired are those who were inspired, but have become cynical as a result of disappointment and adversity.) On meeting a Sulphur man one may or may not receive the impression of an inspired soul, depending upon the mood he is in, and what he thinks of you. If you are able to get to know him, however, you will soon witness the infectious enthusiasm with which he shares with you his passions. If he is an intellectual, as a great many Sulphurs are, he will treat you before long to a sample of his theories and opinions. Kali and Lycopodium also love to expound their knowledge, but they do so in a far drier, more sober manner than Sulphur, who visibly delights in sharing his enthusiasms with anyone who will listen. To the intellectual Sulphur ideas possess an inspirational quality, in much the same way that they do to a child when he first conceives of them. Their content may be anything from the structure of the universe to the best way of putting top-spin on a tennis ball. Whatever the idea, if it appeals to the Sulphur individual, it will elevate his spirit, and he will cherish it and attempt to share his prize with others, who very often are quite unable to share his enthusiasm, and wonder what he is so fascinated with.

The Sulphur mind has a tendency to delve deeply into whatever interests it, with a passion that drives the person further and further towards understanding the whole of the subject, with all its ramifications and obscurities. As a result, Sulphur very often displays an astonishingly detailed knowledge of his pet subjects, which is even more surprising in the cases of those Sulphurs who had little formal education and are self-taught, as many are.

Kent gives a beautiful description in his Lecture Notes on Materia Medica of Sulphur's almost fanatical method of enquiry. He wrote, 'Sulphur has cured this consecutive tracing one thing to another as to first cause. It has cured a patient who did nothing but meditate as to what caused this and that and the other thing, finally tracing things back to Divine Providence, and then asking "Who made God?"

In general Sulphur is more interested in understanding 'the big picture', than in focussing upon a single facet of a subject (which is more typical of Kali Carbonicum and Arsenicum). The Genius of Einstein is a good example. Einstein was a failure in the mathematics class at school, presumably because he wasn't interested in doing sums for the sake of it. On the other hand, when he came to consider Time, Space and the structure of the Universe, he was excited enough to pursue his calculations with great determination and accuracy. This reveals another very characteristic Sulphur trait, that of applying oneself passionately to whatever interests one, and not trying at all when not interested. Getting a Sulphur to do something he does not enjoy is virtually impossible, and not worth the effort, since even if he does it he will do it so half-heartedly that it will not be worth doing at all. (Wives and parents of Sulphur individuals know this all too well.)

Sulphurs are intellectual visionaries to a far greater extent than any other type. They relate to the broader implications of new knowledge, and usually do their best to spread their vision, and to make it a reality. The American poet Walt Whitman was a good example of a visionary Sulphur. He wrote about the ordinary people, the workers, the wives and their children, and the commonplace activities that made up their day, and yet at the same time he glorified them. In true Sulphur fashion his expansive and optimistic spirit found great inspiration in the waves of progress sweeping the American continent in the early part of the twentieth century, and prompted him to write 'The Body Electric', a rousing and passionate hymn to the common man, his inexhaustable spirit, and the glorious future that he was fashioning through the tools of industry and technology. Whitman imagined that Man would be liberated from poverty and serfdom by the new technologies that science was creating, but he did not see the dreadful boredom and poverty of spirit that an industrialised, materialistic way of life would bring. Like most Sulphurs, he was caught up in his wonderful vision, and tended to ignore the down side.

It is symptomatic of our times I believe, that Sulphur leaders are no longer seen as often as they were in the last century. The visionary and inspired leadership of men like Abraham Lincoln, like the intellectual liberalism of the Whigs in Britain, struck a cord then with the aspirations of the people, who saw a great future dawning with the advent of the industrialised society, and who still respected the old values of honesty, hard work, and loyalty to the family. Today we live in far more cynical, materialistic times, and those few Sulphur visionaries who do reach the top in government, like Winston Churchill and Jimmy Carter, tend to be toppled very quickly by a political apparatus that serves a society more interested in their pay packet than in nobler concerns. An exception is Ronald Reagan, a very classic Sulphur individual, whose dramatic rhetoric succeeded in restoring national pride to Americans after the shame of the Vietnam war. His unashamed and heartfelt championing of old American values like industry, entrepreneurial spirit and independence won him an extraordinary degree of popularity, which enabled him to survive scandal after scandal, and earned him the title of 'the non-stick president'. He may have been short on detailed policy, but his charisma and his idealistic vision more than made up for it in the eyes of the electorate.

The inspired Sulphur mind can be as original as it is zealous (Kent: 'Ideas abundant, clearness of mind'). Being open to the broader ramifications of an isolated group of observations, many great Sulphur thinkers have synthesised whole systems of thought, and lifted their respective disciplines to new heights of understanding. I am certain, for example, that the majority of the great European philosophers of the last three centuries were Sulphur individuals. Abstract thinking comes easily to Sulphur (Kent: 'Philosophical mania'), and even the Sulphur farmer or physician is likely to have a love of philosophy, usually of a home-spun variety. I once treated a cook who was sacked from his work because he spent more time chatting about the nature of life than he did cooking. He took his misfortune very philosophically, pointing out to me that his colleagues could not be blamed for their inability to appreciate the deeper aspects of life. During the interview he was animated, and he especially enjoyed sharing with me the insights he had gathered about human nature, spirituality, and a great deal more besides. I could easily see why he had been sacked, but I thoroughly enjoyed partaking of his enthusiasms. His minor physical complaints were entirely resolved after a few doses of Sulphur, but I did not see him for long enough to find out whether the remedy helped him hold down a job!

The Sulphur intellectual's fascination with a particular subject leads him to delve ever more deeply into it, and in the process he is apt to discover and record a mountain of information, much of it obscure to all but himself. A good example is the pioneering psychiatrist Carl Jung, who developed a whole new school of analytical psychology. Jung's insights into the human subconscious were as revolutionary and as useful as those of his original mentor, Sigmund Freud, but they were far more abstract and 'spiritual' than Freud's. Freud may well have been an Arsenicum, judging from the way he dispassionately dissected the minds of his patients, and came to a rather rigid and limited view of humanity which saw the human mind basically as that of an animal, which had been forced by society to subjugate and sublimate its baser instincts into more social behaviour. In contrast, the more spiritually inclined Jung saw man as having an inherently Divine core, which he called the Collective Unconscious, which contained both animalistic instincts and far more subtle drives towards 'wholeness'. Jung's intellect was formidable, and in true Sulphur style he was at home both in the world of objective science and in the heady realms of philosophy, myth and legend. Nothing could exemplify more clearly the difference between the reductionist Arsenicum (or Kali) mind and the synthesising Sulphur mind than the theories of Freud and Jung about myth and legend. Freud maintained that ancient legends which had survived for millenia were Man's attempts to represent and make sense of his animal instincts, particularly his aggression and his sexual impulses. In contrast, Jung, who made a lifetime study of mythology, maintained that legends were spontaneous products of the Collective Unconscious, and contained hidden wisdom waiting for the sensitive mind to discover it. Jung's goal was a system of psychotherapy which produced 'self-realised' individuals, that is, people who functioned simultaneously on the mundane level and on the mythic level of the poet and the saint. In contrast, Freud's goal was more modest, being a therapy which produced 'full genitality', or the ability to enjoy sexual love fully with one's partner. The respective attitudes of these two great thinkers towards psychological defense mechanisms are equally instructive. Freud saw neurosis as a weakening of desirable defense mechanisms, and his therapy sought to strengthen the patient's defenses against his subconscious drives. (No one is more defended than an Arsenicum.) In contrast, Jung saw psychological defenses as blocks to the enlightening experience of the Collective Unconscious. He sought to guide the patient beyond his defences and into the unknown. Like most

Sulphurs, Jung was both an explorer and a visionary, and he strived to take his patients with him on a journey of fantastic discovery.

Reading Jung's vast Collected Works is an excellent introduction to the way a Sulphur genius thinks. Jung connects disparate threads of information from every source, and weaves them into a dizzyingly complicated picture of the psyche. His exhaustive and subtle analysis of symbols is enough to keep the dedicated student sweating for years to grasp the enormity of it all, without ever reaching his treatises on 'complexes', personality types and a host of other equally detailed and abstract subjects. Trying to grasp the enormity of the theories of another Sulphur, Albert Einstein, is just as difficult for the average mortal (or even for the average intellectual mortal), and even the mysteries of 'The Organon' and other works by the founder of Homeopathy, Samuel Hahnemann, leave the reader straining to wrap his grey matter around all that abstract theory.

No treatise on Sulphur could be complete without a consideration of Hahnemann himself. The founder of Homeopathy was undoubtedly an intellectual genius, and one who exhibited a host of classic Sulphur personality traits. It is perhaps no accident that Sulphur was the cornerstone of Hahneman's therapeutic arsenal. Homeopaths have long recognised that they tend to see their own constitutional type unusually frequently in their patients.

Hahnemann had a profound knowledge of a great many subjects apart from the conventional medicine of his time. He had studied the writings of ancient physicians like Hippocrates and Paracelsus, and he took a great interest in the more philosophical aspects of disease, as one can see when one reads 'The Organon', and also 'Chronic Disease'. Hahnemann's emphasis upon augmenting the patient's 'Vital Force' is an example of Sulphur's ability to marry abstract and more concrete information into a whole. It was because he was able to see the whole picture when looking at a patient's health that Hahnemann was able to develop such a powerful therapeutic method, one which emphasised the psyche and the general well-being of the patient far more than most other therapies. It is when homeopaths abandon Hahnemann's constitutional approach that they are liable to have less success with their patients.

Many Sulphur intellectuals are gifted at inspiring an audience with their own enthusiasm for their pet subject. A good example is the eccentric astronomer Patrick Moore who has appeared for many years on British television screens. With one eye closed and the other staring with almost manic intensity, he launches into a story about a newly discovered asteroid with all the zeal of a Bible-punching preacher, gesticulating with his hands and raising his bushy eyebrows to the heavens which fascinate him so much. Like many Sulphurs, Patrick Moore speaks very quickly when he is excited (Kent:

'Loquacity'), since there is so much he wants to share with the world. His unruly hair and bow-tie add to the typical Sulphur appearance of the eccentric professor, and endear him to an audience who appreciate his comic persona at least as much as the information he gives them. Another somewhat comical Sulphur scientist who has made scientific matters popular with the general public in Great Britain is Magnus Pyke. His wild gesticulations and dramatic descriptions of physical phenomena have made him a household name. Even his name seems larger than life (the Great Pyke), a quality that makes Sulphur individuals so entertaining, and so frequently seen before the public eye.

### Larger Than Life

Whether they be in the public eye or not, the majority of Sulphur individuals have a tendency to be dramatic, enthusiastic and to think and act on a larger scale than most other people. Some are truly great in stature - visionaries like William Blake and William Wordsworth, thinkers like Albert Einstein and Carl Jung, leaders like Winston Churchill and Abraham Lincoln. Others are inspired by the truly great, and since their spirit resonates with that of their heros, they are able in turn to inspire their fellow man, at least to some degree. Spirit is a quality that is hard to define, and must be felt, and recognised through its outer manifestations. It is Sulphur's spirit that is expansive, and overflows into boundless enthusiasm, dramatism and eccentricity. The majority of Sulphurs are extroverts, and are not shy when it comes to expressing themselves. In fact, there is nothing the average Sulphur enjoys more than an audience. The best raconteurs, for example, are always Sulphurs. Whereas other types, like Lycopodium and Natrum, will adopt a dramatic tone to make a story more interesting, Sulphur need only be himself to bring his story to life. He does not have to learn to be dramatic or passionate; he is dramatic and passionate. Consequently, a great many entertainers are Sulphurs. Furthermore, Sulphur's breadth of interest is generally so great, and his experiences in life so diverse, given his fearlessly adventurous nature, that he usually has a lot of stories to tell. Sir Peter Ustinov is a good example. Like many Sulphurs, he has an international quality that is the result not only of being widely travelled, but also derives, I believe, from Sulphur's naturally broad outlook. (Most Sulphur individuals have more in common with other progressive, 'go ahead' people around the world than they do with their own neighbours). Sir Peter appears to have been everywhere, and met everyone (if one is to believe his stories), and yet when he recounts his adventures he sounds neither arrogant, nor a hanger-on to the rich and famous. Like a great many Sulphurs, he has a naturally regal presence, and remains himself whether he is in a Brooklyn bar or dining with royalty. The title of a Knight rests comfortably on Sulphur's wide shoulders, without appearing either ridiculous or pompous, as it so often does on the shoulders of others.

Most Sulphurs have a great gift for identifying with and relating to people from all walks of life. Their expansive spirit embraces a love for their fellow man and woman which often transcends barriers of class and creed, and allows them to be both garrulous and generous with almost all they come across. Here one must distinguish between Sulphur and the Lycopodium know-all who will speak to anybody because he wants to show off his knowledge. The latter is far more self-conscious, and far more offended when he is spurned or contradicted. Sulphur takes a philosophical approach, enjoying the exchange if his audience disagrees with him, and calmly moving on if they lose interest. He can, however, be just as tiresome as the Lycopodium know-all, since he gets carried away with his pet topic and will speak endlessly, misinterpreting politeness for interest.

Another sociable type who can be confused with Sulphur is the Natrum man who has quite a lot of self-confidence, but wants to be liked by everyone. He is extremely courteous, yet he calls complete strangers by their first names without being invited, including his doctor and his bank manager. He will talk in a polished fashion about virtually anything, but there is no real feeling behind what he says; it is all an act designed to impress. In contrast, most Sulphurs don't care whether or not they impress you, since they are too interested in the subject of conversation, and too involved in the simple pleasure of sharing their warmth and enthusiasm with another. There are exceptions of course—mean and anti-social Sulphurs, arrogant and even timid Sulphurs, but these are the exceptions that prove the rule.

Shakespeare's Falstaff is a classic example of a Sulphur who is larger than life in every way. Although he is both fictional and fantastic, he is also easy to relate to, since he fits the real essence of Sulphur so accurately. Falstaff is full of contradictions, most of which he is aware of, which make him all the more amusing. He is a knight—Sir John Falstaff—yet he has no money, and spends his time with common thieves in the tavern. He is an inveterate liar, yet he espouses and genuinely believes in honour, at least some of the time. He is intelligent, well-read and witty, yet he mixes with fools, and spends most of his time eating, drinking and chasing women. Despite his frivolous behaviour Falstaff retains a certain dignity. Like many Sulphurs, he is too irresponsible and too preoccupied with playing to live a socially acceptable, 'productive' life, and yet his wit, his outrageous tale-telling and his innocent self-acceptance make him not only tolerated but loved. Most of his lies are designed to entertain rather than to deceive, and in true Sulphur fashion they are as elaborate as they are unbelievable. Sulphur has a tendency to exaggerate, because he gets excited about things, and he loves to emphasise the more dramatic implications of a given subject, sometimes to the point of losing contact with reality.

Sulphur will also lie to get out of a tight corner, or to save face. Like Lycopodium and Phosphorus, he is an opportunist, and will bend or break the rules of accepted behaviour to avoid being found to be lacking in some way, or to gain a particular objective. In doing so he will often adopt rather grand motives to disguise the real ones, in keeping both with his pride and his tendency to 'enlarge' upon a given topic. Falstaff, when asked by Prince Hal why he ran away when the disguised Prince attacked him during a nocturnal caper, claimed that he recognised the Prince and hence could not attack him, "since a valiant lion would never attack a true Prince". In this way he turned his cowardice into valour. On a more prosaic level, Sulphur will often justify laziness and abdication of duty by saying that he is involved with more important matters, which usually means pursuing his pet interest.

Most Sulphurs love to talk. Some are highly intellectual, and will only talk to the few who they think will understand their theories and observations, but many will talk to anybody about anything. Sulphur generally has a far broader range of interests than other people, and usually knows enough to talk intelligently about a wide range of subjects. This is true even of the provincial Sulphur who has had no formal education. A great many of the latter disdain formal education, since they see the narrowness of outlook that it often produces, and also because they resent the fact that they are afforded less respect than those with a degree, even though the latter may have a more limited knowledge of life, and often far less 'personality' and spirit than Sulphur (Kent: 'He despises education and despises literary men and their accomplishments, and he wonders why it is that everyone cannot see that he is above education'.) I once treated a signmaker for eczema. It was apparent to me almost immediately that he was Sulphur constitutionally, from the way he loved to talk, not nervously, but with relish, humour and genuine friendliness. Somehow he got talking about borrowing money from the bank, and recounted how the bank-manager had asked him to fill out piles of forms, principally concerning guarantees for the loan. At first he was going to fill them in, and search for a guarantor, but suddenly he became angry, returned to the bank, demanded to see the manager, and said " I'm from the country, and where I come from, my name is my bond. If that's not good enough for you, you can stick your money." The manager was taken aback, but not wishing to lose a customer, he agreed the loan without the usual formalities. My patient recounted the story with pride, and ended by saying that he had once been afraid of standing up to authority figures like doctors and bank-managers, but no longer. He was trained to do his job, and they were trained to do theirs, and they were no better than he was. Sulphur, like Nux, is a natural leader, and cannot bear to be bossed about by beaurocrats with a degree but no spirit.

### The Modern Traditionalist

Sulphur's naturally expansive and optimistic spirit generally makes him rather liberal minded. Freedom is something he prizes highly; the freedom to do what he likes, to say what he likes, with whom he likes. He is an individualist, and is usually happier when he is in charge of his own destiny, preferring to be self-employed than to work for others. He will often defend the freedom of others when it is under attack, at least verbally, and he will always sympathise with those who are at odds with authority, especially with the government. One might expect such a buoyant and liberally minded type to be future-orientated and progressive, and this is generally true, but at the same time Sulphur individuals tend to have a great deal of respect for traditional values. There are several reasons for this. First of all, most Sulphur men have a love of wisdom, as opposed to mere learning, and hence they are attracted to the religious and philosophical teachings of the past, be they orthodox, mystical or radical. Secondly, for all his weaknesses, Sulphur is a proud type, and tends to have a natural dignity which he sees reflected in traditional values like Honour, Valour and Charity. The modern amoral materialistic way of life lacks soul for most Sulphurs, who tend to dream of a better future, which incorporates many of the old traditional values. Thirdly, for all his intellectual dexterity, there is something simplistic and rather childish about Sulphur's mentality. Rather than getting bogged down with subtle ethical distinctions, or agonising about the correct moral course of action, Sulphur prefers to adopt rather simple basic values, such as honesty and non-interference in the affairs of others, and then get on with his life without thinking too much about morality. He will often use the traditional values as a touchstone or easy reference in life, but unlike Arsenicum and some Natrums who stick rigidly to these values, Sulphur will bend them or even ignore them to suit his purposes at the time. Like Falstaff he will appeal to your sense of honour one minute, whilst lying the next to avoid some loss of face.

Although most Sulphurs admire much of the greatness of past civilisations, including their nobility and their wisdom, few are conservative in the sense of wanting to turn the clock back. They may read all of the classics, and may even dress in a rather traditional manner, but they are generally aware of the desirable progress that has been made both scientifically and socially over the past two hundred years or so, and look ahead to greater things to come.

### Earthiness

There are two poles within the Sulphur type, which one could call the Earthy and the Airy. By earthy I mean focussed principally upon the gratification of physical desires, and also this includes a certain crudeness or lack of refinement. Some Sulphurs are very earthy and not at all intellectual or idealistic. Generally they are the most selfish and stubborn of all Sulphurs, but this is not always the case. The earthy Sulphur is a simple soul who lives to eat, drink, have sex, and play, whether the games be sporting or simply social. He is physically robust, and either wiry or obese, depending upon the extent of his physical activities. He is not necessarily stupid, but his intellect takes second place to his senses, and also to his ego. The most earthy Sulphurs resemble some Baryta Carbonica individuals, in that they are simple in outlook, robust and usually rather uncouth (Kent: 'A state of refinement seems to have gone out of the Sulphur patient'.) The wife of such a Sulphur patient of mine once complained to me that her husband would embarrass her in public by picking his nose unselfconsciously, or by farting loudly at the theatre. He took no notice of her complaints, which is typical of the boorish stubbornness that one often encounters in the more earthy Sulphur individual. Unlike the more physical Baryta, the earthy Sulphur generally has a lot of self-confidence, and is quite given to boasting about his achievements. He is far more sociable than Baryta in most cases, and may be something of a leader within his own circle. He is also quite often bossy, and can easily lose his temper when frustrated or crossed. Even amongst the earthier Sulphurs there is quite a lot of variation of character. Some are very physical, but also easygoing and gentle, whilst others are selfish, domineering and aggressive. The former, like their more intellectual Sulphur brothers, generally have a buoyant, positive outlook on life, and a sparkle in their eye, whilst the latter can become narrow and embittered. These more negative earthy Sulphurs are difficult to differentiate from the more negative earthier types of Natrum and Tuberculinum. In common with other Sulphurs, they tend to have a large ego, to be indifferent to the opinions of others, and yet to expect respect from others. They are usually relatively fearless, especially when it comes to rough physical activities, and unlike the earthy Natrum they are not very prone to worrying. Some are wanderers, soldiers or sailors, who have a woman in every port, and a thousand tales to tell, and can often earn their supper with their tales. Others are burly labourers who spend their evenings drinking in the pub, chatting up women, and then going home to a wife who is already asleep in bed.

Even the most earthy Sulphur has a soft side, and will usually respond to tales of romance and tragedy with a tear in his eye. Falstaff is a good example of an earthy Sulphur, although like many, he also had a keen intellect, which he was too lazy to use all that much. He could easily be moved, both by his own tales, and by the misfortunes of others, and though he was a rogue, he was not without heart. Generally Sulphur is a warm and passionate type, and even the most selfish Sulphur tends to have his soft side, in contrast to the harder Arsenicums, Kalis and Nux', who can remain as cold as ice.

On the opposite pole to the earthy Sulphur is the airy or ethereal Sulphur, whose head is in the clouds, thinking about matters philosophical and spiritual. In between is the thinker, the scientist and inventor, the intellectual Sulphur. All these are distinct Sulphur types, but they are part of a continuum. Most Sulphur intellectuals and philosophers have their earthy side. Often this is merely a large appetite, or an irresistible attraction to women, but the further they move down the scale away from the philosopher, the more earthy they become. On a par with men like Falstaff is the Sulphur man of action, who is very handy and practical. Sulphur artisans are included here, as well as Sulphur adventurers, and Sulphur soldiers and sailors, many of whom rise to high rank. The Sulphur man of action is simple and direct, like the Nux man of action. He will usually perform his work with easy enthusiasm, working long hours without complaint when necessary, but enjoying his leisure when it comes. Most Sulphurs are gifted enough and enterprising enough to find work which they enjoy, and the Sulphur man of action is often equally enthusiastic about his work, his family and his hobbies. Such men inspire confidence in others, and are fun to be around. They are very resourceful, and are wonderful people to know when you are in need of practical help, which they generally are very willing to supply, providing you have not taken advantage of them. The Sulphur sign-writer I treated was an Australian, and like many Australians he answered both requests and thanks with the phrase 'No worries', which translates roughly as 'Certainly', 'No problem' and 'You're welcome'. Unlike most other Australians, he injected such enthusiasm into this phrase that I knew he meant it, and it made me smile to hear him say it.

As I write about the Sulphur man of action, I am reminded of the old pioneers of the Wild West. Many of them were not only resourceful craftsmen, who could build their own houses, wagons and ploughs, but were also fired with the positive mental attitude, and the self-confidence to get them across the new continent. Inside those weather-beaten crusty-looking faces were clear blue eyes which sparkled with a mixture of adventure and mischief. Their wide white moustaches only heightened their (ever so slightly comic) dignity, as did the proud poses they adopted for those early photographs. Without doubt many of those early pioneers were Sulphurs, whose courage and natural leadership inspired others to follow them, and whose allegiance to traditional values reassured their followers, and ensured a sense of identity and stability to the new communities.

### Ego, Selfishness and the Lovable Rogue
Sulphur is not the most egotistical of types (Platina probably wins that epi-

thet), but it is not far from it. It competes as a constitutional type with Lycopodium and Nux for the biggest ego, and is generally more egotistical than Tuberculinum and Phosphorus, and certainly more than Natrum Muriaticum. There are many facets of an expanded ego, and all can be found in the Sulphur individual. First of all, he believes in himself when all else have given up believing in him. On the one hand, this can be a great asset, since it allows him to persevere through difficult times without support, especially when he is engaged in an activity or project he feels strongly about. Inventors are very often Sulphur people, and they must often pursue their work without either recognition or financial investment. Similarly, a great many actors are Sulphurs, and they too must believe in themselves long before they gain the recognition of their public. Even in defeat, Sulphur tends to blame his failure on the short sightedness or the meanness of other people, rather than looking to his own deficiencies. It is here that Sulphur's faith in himself can sometimes be a liability rather than an asset. Some Sulphurs will pursue projects that are impractical, either because they will not appeal to a public whose support Sulphur depends upon, or because they are flawed or unrealistic in themselves. In these cases Sulphur may doggedly hang on to the bitter end, refusing to accept that his judgement was mistaken (Kent: 'Obstinate'). This is in part due to his undying faith in himself, and in part due to his obsessive passion for the project in question.

Another aspect of Sulphur's pride is his tendency to boast. This is generally a more subtle boasting than that of the Lycopodium strutter, who has a fragile ego and is seeking to boost it. Sulphur's ego is anything but fragile, and can take a great many knocks without appearing dented. A Sulphur father may show you a photograph of his daughter, and then beam with pride as he tells you that she is entering the local beauty contest. Like Nux and Ignatia, the Sulphur businessman and the Sulphur performer can be very forward in promoting themselves to the public. Generally they do so with flair, without resorting to outright boasting, which would put people off. Those Sulphurs who believe they have a monopoly of truth and wisdom (and here there are many) can be quite didactic about expressing their superior vision. Hahnemann is a classic case. Whilst it is true that he developed a wonderful new therapeutic tool, the arrogant way in which he went about proclaiming his new knowledge and attacking the 'old school' did nothing to enhance the popularity of homeopathy.

Modern day spiritual leaders and gurus are quite often Sulphurs, and it is especially the Sulphurs who make extravagant claims about their unique qualifications as spiritual guides of Mankind. They do so in earnest, believing what they say, but their 'spiritual arrogance' can be off-putting, especially when it involves denouncing all other spiritual leaders. Fire and Brimstone preachers are most likely Sulphurs in the main. They are totally committed to their vocation of saving souls, and use all their fiery passion to that end. Their sermons are enlivened by dramatic intonation and fantastic descriptions of the joys of Heaven and the torments of Hell, in a similar fashion to the speeches of Ronald Reagan, whose imaginative (if impractical?) vision of Star Wars technology was intended to protect the God-loving citizens of the United States from 'The Evil Empire'.

An amusing example of a particularly arrogant Sulphur from the works of William Shakespeare is that of the Welsh military commander Owen Glendower in Henry IV Part 1. When Glendower meets the equally fiery soldier Hotspur, who is supposed to be an ally, we are treated to a confrontation between the 'Welsh wind bag', who loves to claim supernatural powers, and the no-nonsense dry humour of his Nux guest. Repeatedly Glendower tries to explain to Hotspur that at his nativity the Earth trembled, and the heavens were ablaze with fiery portents, to which Hotspur replies, "Why so they would be if my cat had kittened". The powerful and self-important Sulphur Glendower comments that he would not take such impudence from anyone else, and in truth the stature of a Sulphur leader can only be matched by a Nux leader or another Sulphur. It is because Sulphur senses the greatness inside of him that he appears arrogant. Unfortunately, some Sulphurs sense more greatness than is really there (Kent: 'Foolish pride').

Chauvinism is an example of arrogance that is seen more in Sulphur and Lycopodium men than in any other types. Both have a tendency to take women for granted, and to assume that they are doing a woman a great service by granting her the favour of their company. Most Sulphur men consider that they are superior to other men (Kent: 'Haughty), and that men are superior to women, although few would say it so bluntly in this day and age. Sulphur, for all his arrogance, is generally a kind soul, and hence he adopts a paternalistic attitude to women, protecting them and complimenting them on their looks, whilst expecting them to wait on him, and assuming they have no brain. Sulphur husbands are often very lazy, thinking that their job is to be the bread-winner, and that all jobs at home are the woman's responsibility, including taking care of the kids, even on holidays. It is at home that Sulphur's selfishness most often comes to the fore. He may take his wife entirely for granted, thinking that he has more important things to do than pick up the children (like chat with his mate, or watch the football), and when his spouse finally loses her temper, he looks astonished, and calls her a foolish hysterical woman. I have seen this scenario a good many times between a Sulphur husband and his long-suffering wife, and have come almost to expect it (Kent: 'He will sit around and do nothing, and let his wife take in washing and work her fingernails off taking care of him; he thinks that is all she is good for'.) The Sulphur cook I mentioned earlier confided to me that his wife was a little simple, on account of her brain having been starved of oxygen during an emotional crisis. He emphasised that she was a wonderful woman and that he loved her dearly, but she was a little simple and could not understand a great many things. I eventually got to know his wife, and found her of above average intelligence, and a little tired of her husband's childish dreaming about world peace and mind-expansion.

As one might imagine, Sulphur's neglect of his wife (and children) is often in direct proportion to the amount of charm he expends upon pretty women. Like Lycopodium, a great many Sulphurs are womanisers, and because of their greater sense of self-importance, they tend to be less circumspect about their infidelity. The Sulphur cook told me that he believed married partners should allow each other the freedom to sleep with others from time to time, and said that he had discussed the matter with his wife, but strangely she was not very keen on the idea (Sulphur can be genuinely surprised by such 'women's logic'). The wife of another Sulphur patient told me that her husband flirted openly with her friends, and even attempted to take them to bed. In true Sulphur fashion, he justified his behaviour by claiming rather grand motives, namely that he had such a lot of love in his heart that it ought to be shared around. Such is the charm of the average Sulphur man, and such is the genuine warmth and generosity in his heart, that he is often forgiven a hundred times by his partner for his indiscretions. If she does walk out, however, he usually learns very quickly how hopelessly dependent upon her he was, both emotionally and practically. Sulphur is often very much a child emotionally, thinking he can have what he wants without having to take responsibility for it. When he suddenly loses his love or his job as a result of his negligence, he tends to be stunned and uncomprehending. I remember counselling a couple who were having marital difficulties. The wife complained that her Sulphur husband spent all of his time on his obsession, which was playing and coaching football, and none of his time with her and their children (unless they came to the football field). He sat impassively throughout the whole interview, and when I asked him what his reaction was to his wife's complaints, he said that she was mentally ill, and hence was grossly exaggerating. I said that I knew the kind of man he was, and that I knew that he meant well, but it was clear to me that his wife had genuine cause for complaint. At this he simply replied 'I am what I am, and I'm not going to change'. He was keen for his wife to have psychotherapy "to knock some sense into her", but when the therapy increased her self-esteem and she left him, he fell apart both physically and mentally. His attitude then alternated between pleading pathetically for her to come back, and blaming her for all the problems in his life. He even went on a weekend 'self-awareness' course, after which he told his wife that he was now free of his hang-ups, and could see how emotionally sick she still was. Such Sulphur men must learn the hard way that there is more to self-examination than a weekend course. When they fall they tend to react like children, crying and looking for sympathy, or for someone to blame. The degree of self-pity of a Sulphur man in distress is greater than I have see in any other type. At such times he may lose all motivation for living, and become the very opposite of the impassioned Sulphur. He will then neglect himself, eat rubbish, turn up late for work, or fail to turn up at all, and speak slowly as if in a mist (Kent: 'Too lazy to rouse himself up and too unhappy to live'). In such a state Sulphur will often depend upon a female friend to motivate him and pull him back into shape. (Occasionally all the King's horses and all the King's men can't put Sulphur together again, and he remains a confused, worn out reflection of his old self.)

As you might have gathered by now, many Sulphur men tend to consider themselves a law unto themselves. They may see the need for laws and regulations, but they don't worry too much about breaking the rules if and when it suits them. When this trait is combined with a love of adventure and alcohol, as it often is, we have the makings of a Sulphur rogue. Sulphur has a naturally exuberant nature, and a need to play, and since he is liable at times to get carried away with his enthusiasms, he may sometimes go wild and get up to antics which shock some, and amuse others. Two notable examples are both classical dramatic actors, are both Irish, and have both acquired a reputation in the past for drinking large amounts of alcohol. I am thinking of Peter O'Toole and Richard Harris. Both are larger than life characters off the stage as well as on, and are notorious for their wild and frequently drunken lifestyle. On the stage and screen they have usually played lovable rogues, which is not surprising, since that is what they are. As with Falstaff, these two firebrands are tolerated and loved by the public, since their charm is equal to their irresponsibility. This charm is not just a matter of cheek and self-confidence. In true Sulphur fashion their bearing is just as often noble and inspired as it is wild and debauched.

Most Sulphur rogues have a soft heart, and when their sprees have come to an end, they may find themselves genuinely remorseful for the damage they have done, both physically and especially emotionally. The wife of a Sulphur rogue would have to be a masochist, but just when she can take no more and has packed her bags, he is back imploring her to stay with tears pouring from his eyes, protestations of love, and promises to reform his ways. This show of feelings is liable to be genuine in the case of Sulphur, and it frequently succeeds, only to be followed by further broken promises, indiscretions and infidelities.

The Sulphur rogue is just as generous as any other Sulphur, and will frequently find 'partners in crime' to accompany him on his adventures. Some of these are less confident revellers, who are emboldened by Sulphur's example to let their hair down, whilst others are cynical users who take advantage of Sulphur's generosity and his gullibility. An excellent example of a Sulphur rogue being taken advantage of can be seen in the film 'Raising Arizona', a black comedy about a childless couple in the deep South of the United States, who kidnap one of five quintuplets born to a wealthy business-man. Herb, played by Nicholas Cage, (who usually plays Sulphur types, and is almost certainly a Sulphur himself) is a Sulphur petty criminal who falls a little more in love with police officer Edwina every time he goes back to jail and she takes his photograph for the files. Eventually he places a ring on her finger before being led off to the cells, and then claims her as his bride upon his release. Shortly after kidnapping Nathan Arizona Junior, the happy couple are called upon by two convicts who have just escaped from jail and turn up at the home of their old jail mate Herbert. In typical Sulphur fash-ion Herb is pleased to see his dubious friends, and shows them every hospi-tality, much to the alarm of Edwina, who knows they are a bad influence on Herb, and knows how easily he can be influenced. Herb is trying to go straight now that he is a family man, but the longer he spends drinking with his old mates, the more attractive his old life appears to him, and when they invite him to join them in a bank robbery, he can't resist, (since he has just lost his job, on account of punching his boss on the jaw for suggesting a round of wife swapping). Herb weeps copiously as he writes a farewell note to his wife before leaving in the night, saying that he will never be the man she deserves. He is an excellent example of the Sulphur rogue who has a warm heart, but is childishly irresponsible and cannot face or foresee the consequences of his hare-brained actions.

Sulphur people often have a peculiar block when it comes to learning from past experience, and will follow the line of least resistance again and again. Eventually they may shape up and become more responsible in later years, drinking less and moderating or ceasing their marital infidelities, and stick-ing to a regular job, and these mellowed Sulphur rogues are frequently very content with their lot, especially if they have a good wife and something to keep them occupied.

### Head in the Clouds

Irresponsibility is seen in all opportunistic types, including Lycopodium, Phosphorus and Mercurius, but in no other type is it so common as in Sul-phur. Sulphur is so bright, so warm and so inspired, that there has to be a catch, and the biggest catch is that he is so frequently an impractical dreamer, who does what inspires him, and neglects the physical and emotional reali-ties of his life. A common example is the Sulphur father who forgets his wife's birthday, because his mind is too occupied with its favourite obsession, whether it be his work or not. He makes regular promises to his children to take them fishing, or to the ball game, and regularly forgets and arranges to do something else instead. Each time he is genuinely sorry, and means it when he promises to get it right next time, but gradually his family learn to ignore his promises, and realise that in many ways he is just a child, who cannot be relied upon. Like a child Sulphur does what he wants to do, when he wants to do it, and can find it very hard to grow up and accept responsibility.

When I was a teenager my best friend was a Sulphur rebel, who was passionate about communism, and felt that it held the promise of uniting Humanity, and abolishing poverty and injustice. In typical Sulphur fashion he knew everything there was to know about communism, and his arch-enemy capitalism, and could talk for hours about the history of the Russian revolution, the French revolution, and cite detail after detail concerning the morally reproachable behaviour of past and present governments. He was an idealist who like many Sulphurs had a sense of mission, and this made him exciting to be around. His parents and my own parents were a little less enthusiastic than I was, since he was utterly devoid of manners, incredibly lazy (Kent: 'Indolence'), and quite unwilling to apply himself to those school subjects which didn't interest him. He eventually went to a radical university, where he studied political science, but was thrown out for doing no work whatsoever, and for spending most of his time organising political protests. He did gradually change his ways however, and applied himself to a teaching course with diligence and enthusiasm. Sulphurs make marvellous teachers, since they are more interested in conveying the wonder of their subject than in pushing facts.

The more intellectual Sulphurs are especially liable to neglect practical details. The stereotype of the absent-minded professor is based on the reality of Sulphur intellectuals, who have a brilliant understanding of their chosen field, but cannot remember where they left the car keys. Their neglect for practicalities and the immediate physical aspects of their lives (Kent: 'Indifference to external things') can in some cases result in the characteristic untidy appearance of the Sulphur intellectual (Hering's 'ragged philosopher'). It is rare these days for a Sulphur to be so eccentric as to wear rags. More commonly one sees Sulphur dressed reasonably cleanly, but with some aspect of his appearance out of place or neglected. For example, his shirt may be crumpled and unironed, or his tie may be askew, or his hair may be wild and dramatic, like that of Einstein, who according to all accounts relied upon his wife for every aspect of his material existence, from paying the bills to insisting that he eat regularly. Sulphur is famous for his untidiness, and there is good reason for this. He often pays little regard to material things, and that includes the state of his house, as well as the state of his body and of his bank balance. On the positive side, he is able to avoid the petty worries of other people, who have to have an immaculate house, or who con-

stantly count their pennies. Being relatively unfettered by material considerations, he can not only immerse his mind in intellectual explorations, but
also he can appreciate the sunset, the pleasure of a good meal, or congenial
company. Sulphur's detachment from material considerations is a two edged
sword, bringing with it as much freedom as it does trouble (such as when the
electricity is cut off for non-payment, or the car engine seizes for lack of oil).
Those Sulphurs who find down-to-earth wives tend to have the best of both
worlds; the freedom to be themselves, and the luxury of someone making
sure that the world doesn't tumble down around them whilst they play. For
the wife the rewards vary. At worst she is a slave who is neglected and taken
for granted, at best she has a loving and considerate mate who brightens up
her life with his enthusiasm and humour, for whom she is quite willing to take
care of much of the practicalities of their lives.

As I have mentioned previously, there is a scale of Sulphur from the most
earthy and physical, to the most ethereal and idealistic. It is the latter type
who is most liable to lose contact with reality, immersing himself in dreams.
The aforementioned Sulphur cook is a good example. He was so busy talking about philosophical matters in the kitchen that it cost him his job. There
is a thin line between rational or applicable idealism and foolish idealism,
and many times Sulphur idealists are simply ahead of their time, but if one
cannot judge the mood of one's own time, one cannot communicate with
the people, and one is left speaking to the wind. Some Sulphurs are so un-
worldly that they become objects of ridicule. The mild and innocent characters so often played by the actor Jimmy Stewart are frequently of this type.
They live in a world where people act from only the highest motives, and they
instantly forgive those who act selfishly and cruelly, excusing them on the
grounds of ignorance. Most Sulphurs are 'softies', in that they will give to
those in need, and forgive bad debts , to the point of being taken advantage
of in many cases, but some are so idealistic, and so indifferent to material
concerns, that they are their own worst enemies. Although such Sulphur
individuals may believe that they are acting from a superior, more spiritual
point of view, in reality they are often avoiding confrontation, and hiding in
a fantasy world where everything is lovely, and no tough decisions ever need
to be made.

There is such a subtle difference between true spirituality, and the kind
of dreaming indulged in by some Sulphurs. One good way to differentiate
between the two is that the truly spiritual person (whether Sulphur or otherwise) does not inconvenience others with his reliance upon them, and does
not harm himself through physical neglect. The Sulphur dreamer is very
relaxed and 'laid back', but he is not really all here; he is somewhere else,
in his mind of abstract thought and imagination. In contrast a truly healthy

Sulphur is 'reachable', and is happy to be here and now, rather than having to philosophise all the time.

The homeopath must be able to distinguish the Sulphur idealist from other idealists. Causticum is probably the most difficult to differentiate on the basis of the personality alone. The most helpful trait here is the righteous indignation that Causticum feels so often when he comes across injustice. Sulphur tends to be less obsessed with righting the wrongs of the world, and less angry about them, especially if they do not concern himself or his loved ones. Another useful difference is that Sulphur is generally more egotistical and proud than Causticum, and less willing to sacrifice his own leisure and pleasure for the cause. He is also more liable to be obsessed with intellectual matters for their own sakes.

The other common idealists that one comes across are Natrum and Phosphorus idealists. The Phosphorus idealist is more emotional, more sensitive, and less egotistical than Sulphur. Phosphorus is also less intellectual, placing more emphasis on relating to people than Sulphur, and is much more liable to be swayed by the opinions of others. In contrast, Sulphur idealists are usually dogmatic, and will not be swayed at all by differing opinions.

In medical school students are taught that syphilis is the great imitator, in that it can produce such a wide variety of clinical presentations that it can be mistaken for virtually every other disease. I tend to see Natrum Muriaticum in a similar light. There is such a wide spectrum of Natrum personalities that they may resemble superficially almost any other constitutional type. There are two types of Natrum man who may easily be mistaken for Sulphur types. Firstly there is the robust jovial type who is always laughing and joking. These Natrums are usually very fat. Their joviality is a disguise for the pain inside, and a careful probing by the homeopath will reveal not only a very sad past, but also a poor degree of self-esteem. In contrast, the jovial Sulphur tends to think highly of himself, even if he has had a painful past, and his joviality is not as easily punctured as that of Natrum.

The other Sulphur-like Natrum is the Natrum man who has adopted philosophy or religion as his main focus in life, and likes to talk about little else. Again, a careful probing will usually reveal typical Natrum characteristics, such as self-criticism (or a past history of such traits), a fear of intimacy, claustrophobia, and a fear of what other people think. The Sulphur idealist tends to be even more indifferent to what people think of him than are other, less idealistic Sulphurs, and is very self-tolerant.

### The Romantic
Closely allied to the idealist is the romantic, the principal difference being that the idealist is thinking, whereas the romantic is feeling. Very often the two go together. Most Sulphur individuals are romantic, even if they have a

tendency to be self-absorbed, and to forget their wedding anniversary. To many Sulphurs, life is one big romance, a journey of wonder and excitement, with love as its raison d'etre. Few Sulphur individuals are satisfied without a deep and enduring love in their life, and Sulphur's heart is generally open and capable of great love. One Sulphur patient of mine told me how he had wept for a deer he found dying in the road, and had killed it to put it out of its misery. This kind of empathy can be seen in many other types, but it is particularly characteristic of Sulphur, Phosphorus, Causticum and Natrum Muriaticum. Although Sulphur is often very intellectual, he is seldom a dry, unemotional person like Kali Carbonicum, Lycopodium and some Natrums. He is usually something of a poet, and he is liable to love rousing emotional songs of human tragedy and human triumph, as well as ballads about love. To be sure there are Sulphurs who are so wrapped up in their intellectual passion that they neglect their loved ones, but there are an equal number who cherish their personal relationships above all else.

The more sensitive Sulphur makes an indulgent and loving husband and father. He is liable to dote on his wife and children, and to be extremely proud of them. To such a man, his wife is truly his queen, which is only natural, since he is himself something of a king, having an inherent nobility and authority, irrespective of his background. The average Sulphur family man is very protective of his family, but that does not mean that he cuts himself off from others. On the contrary, he is liable to invite all and sundry home, because he enjoys meeting people, and he loves to bask in the human warmth of friends and family.

Kent lists Sulphur under the rubric 'sentimental', and this is true of some, particularly those who have fallen on hard times, and hence look to the past for comfort. More often though, Sulphur's romanticism is outward and forward-looking. Like a poet, his heart can be uplifted easily by beauty and by human love, and he may be prompted to speak in characteristically grand terms about the rapture he is feeling. A Sulphur man will tell his new amour that he loves her far sooner than most others, so soon that she probably does not believe him, yet he feels what he says, even though he may feel equally strongly about another woman in a month's time. I once treated an old Sulphur sailor who admitted proudly that he had a woman in every port. He had picked up a passable smattering of many different languages, but told me that he could only say two things in Russian—'Ice-cream' and 'I love you'.

The romanticism of Sulphur is somewhat impersonal compared with that of more sentimental types like Natrum and even Lycopodium. As with most other Sulphur traits, it is on a larger, more universal scale. By that I mean that beauty and love inspire Sulphur to feel a part of a greater whole, at home in the universe, with a sense that all is as it should be. For example, a Sulphur man, on hearing that his wife is pregnant, may be prompted to go out into the night and look up at the stars, feeling the wonder of existence, and giving thanks in his heart. Like Phosphorus, Sulphur feels himself to be a child of the universe, a citizen of the Earth, to a far greater extent than most other people. His horizons are broad, and his gaze is not only analytical, but also deeply romantic, not in the sense of a teenage Ignatia girl waiting for love, but rather like one who has tasted the mystery of life, and has an abiding faith in its meaning.

Not all Sulphurs are religious, but most that I have come across have had a sense of relationship with a greater power, to which they often give very little thought, but are silently nourished by. I once treated an elderly Sulphur man in hospital, who had broken his neck in a fall, and knew that he would not live to return to his home. I asked him about his religious beliefs, and he said peacefully, "Well, I haven't been in a church for donkey's years, but me and Jesus are mates", and I knew that he meant what he said, without any flippancy.

### Senility, Introversion and the Aged Sulphur

As Sulphur grows into his latter years, there is a tendency for him to become even more individualistic, to the point where he appears eccentric. He no longer cares at all how he appears to others, and he tends to do exactly what he wants, and says exactly what he means. (I am reminded of William Blake, a brilliant and flamboyant Sulphur, who once invited a group of respectable men of society to dinner, and then served them himself, entirely naked.). In the case of a reasonably well-balanced and contented Sulphur, this results in a quirky but kindly old gent, who knows a thing or two about life, but is not going to waste his wisdom on those who don't want to know. He is liable to be very good with children, since he is completely himself, and children can sense that he respects them, and speaks to them as intelligent beings. A genial old Sulphur makes a wonderful grandfather. He has a thousand tales to tell, loves good company (and by that he probably means people who are themselves, and call a spade a spade), and he still has that twinkle in his eye that is so characteristic of the happy Sulphur. His love for the dramatic may lead him to scare his grandchildren from time to time with all too realistic impersonations of bogeymen, but it also makes him tremendous fun to be around. He may like to be left alone a fair bit to just sit in peace, but then he will come out again with his sympathetic ear, and his brilliant wit.

Those Sulphurs who harboured a certain amount of discontent in their earlier years can become very crabby as they get older. They are liable to become increasingly antisocial (Kent: 'Averse to being spoken to', 'Wants to be left alone'), especially towards their wife and family. I once spent a few days with an elderly couple in a mountainous area of California. The old gent was tall and bony, and very active for his eighty or so years. He spent much of his time tinkering with old engine parts in the shed, having been an engineer and an inventor in his time. He proudly showed me a grandfather clock which he had designed and built, and explained its unique mechanism to me. He also brought out several beloved scrap-books in which his letters to local newspapers were neatly presented. He had a habit of writing to the press about virtually any subject under the sun, from the perils of chemical fertilisers, to the true interpretations of the gospels. It was clear that he was thrilled to have a captive audience to impress with his diverse achievements, and he was quite impervious to my increasingly blunt hints that I had had enough and had other things to do. His manner was quirky and quaint, if a little tiresome, except for the way he treated his wife, which was utterly disrespectful. He completely excluded her from his conversations, speaking to her only to demand more coffee, or to give other orders concerning the house, and she obliged in a miserable cowed fashion. She later confided to me that her husband had become increasingly selfish and dictatorial over the years, and took very little notice of her wishes. This kind of cruel and arrogant behaviour can be seen in some younger Sulphurs, but it generally gets worse in later years.

The elderly Sulphur who becomes increasingly irritable may be reacting to the disappointment of a life that has not been the wonderful adventure he expected. The more unrealistic were his dreams, the more likely he is to become disillusioned and resentful. He may then become quite unbearable to live with, expecting unreasonable obedience from others, arguing about petty matters, and sulking like a child when he doesn't get his own way. Many people become more childlike in their old age, and this is especially true of Sulphur, who was always more of a child than most. Any of Sulphur's more negative traits can become more extreme in his old age. Obsessiveness is a good example. Some Sulphur old men will talk about nothing but their pet interest, whether it be bee-keeping or Revelations, and with time they may lose all contact with their surroundings, as they drift into senility, increasingly indifferent to those around them, muttering to themselves about the same obsession they have nurtured for decades.

For some, the obsession they harbour is a grievance, which can be every bit as bitter and as persistent as the grievances of Natrum and Nux Vomica. One elderly and exceedingly eccentric gentleman came to see me to ask if I could help his wife, who had been hallucinating for years. His appearance was classically Sulphur - lean, bony and dishevelled, and he carried around an old tattered hold all, on the sides of which he had scribbled telephone numbers, addresses and other vital pieces of information (Sulphur people often scribble down things on bits of paper, which they have thought of on the spur of the moment, only to lose the paper in most cases.) During my interview with this old gent he began to weep pitifully as he described the state his wife was in. Then his tears suddenly turned to rage, as he told me between clenched teeth that his daughter in-law had put a spell on his wife, resulting in her hallucinations. He called the girl the Devil's daughter, and swore that if he had his way he would put a gun to her nether regions and blast her to Hell. This show of rage was in marked contrast to the gentle manner in which he spoke for the rest of the interview. Like many older Sulphurs, he was a religious man, and he cried when he expressed his fear that he too was damned, because he was the husband of a woman possessed (Kent: 'moaning with despair. He thinks he has sinned away his day of grace'.)

The elderly, eccentric Sulphur is often so rambling in his speech that inexperienced homeopaths will give Lachesis by mistake. Like the latter, the elderly Sulphur will jump from one subject to another (Kent: 'Speech wandering'), though his speech is generally slower than that of a loquacious Lachesis. Both types tend to spring from one subject to another which is related in some way, but the relation may be quite tenuous or irrelevant to the original topic in question. For example, the distressed Sulphur husband said to me "My father was a cold man—not a coal man. He didn't cry 'Coal!' or 'Fish!'" (He acted out little dramatic scenes like this, cupping his hands to his mouth, and shouting in the surgery as if he were really selling fish!)

Many elderly Sulphurs spend a great deal of time feeling sorry for themselves. If they get the chance, they will 'bend your ear' with a sorry tale of their multiple misfortunes, in a manner that is so self-indulgent that it appears childish. Like a child, many Sulphurs, particularly older ones, are unable to accept misfortune, and tend to blame others as a means of venting their frustration. Whether the loquacious Sulphur is resentful or not, he is liable to ramble on entirely oblivious to the lack of interest shown by his audience.

Naturally, the aged Sulphur tends to have more trouble with his memory than he used to. In particular, he forgets people's names. Even younger Sulphurs have difficulty remembering names. As soon as they have been introduced, the name has gone, and they have to awkwardly try and hide the fact, or ask again later on. Perhaps this is something to do with Sulphur's tendency to act as if he were the centre of the universe, and hence others are to some extent unimportant, like supporting cast for the main star.

Some intellectual Sulphurs become more and more cynical as they advance in years. I once worked with a Sulphur doctor who had been tremendously idealistic, and had written extensively about spiritual matters. I had been keen to meet him, having read one of his books, but when I did, I found that he had abandoned his spiritual interests entirely, and was both embarrassed and cynical about them. He had at one time practised homeopathy, but had also abandoned this, his old enthusiasm having turned to disbelief. He was still highly intellectual, and loved to discuss new scientific discoveries, but I was surprised to find how private and insular he appeared. There was none of the passion in his eyes that one normally sees in Sulphur individuals, and yet his appearance, his intellectual depth and breadth, and his somewhat aloof manner all confirmed to me that he was a Sulphur constitutionally. I have since come across Sulphur patients who have had difficult lives, or who have fallen upon hard times, who have lost much of their 'spark', and are quite guarded socially, and far less idealistic than the average Sulphur. They can easily be mistaken for Natrums or Causticums, being prone to melancholic periods, and to fears of all kinds, especially fear of people (Kent: 'Fear of men', 'Fear of people'). Their symptoms and their generals do not fit Natrum or Causticum, which makes me look a little closer, at which point I realise that the patient has a very curious and inventive mind, and a love of abstract and philosophical concepts. One such man was an inventor in his spare time. He appeared a serious man to look at, and he confessed that he had often suffered from both self-doubt and depression, which he related to sexual abuse in his childhood. He had consulted me for treatment of chronic headaches, which were associated with a chronic fatigue syndrome. I was unsure whether to give him Natrum or Sulphur, but I was swayed by the directness of his gaze, and the directness of his speech. Sulphur, like Nux, is generally very direct, and this helps to distinguish him from other types. My introverted Sulphur patient responded very quickly to Sulphur 1M, thus confirming that Sulphur is not always the confident extrovert. Like other introverts, the Sulphur introvert wants to be left alone much of the time (Kent: 'Averse to being spoken to') and may feel ill at ease in social gatherings. He is liable to either immerse himself in books and intellectual musing, or to seek solitude in the countryside, and in physical labour. He often still has the sharp Sulphur wit, but it is drier and more sardonic than that of his more spirited brothers. He may even show off occasionally in his more extrovert moments. Homeopaths must resist the tendency to stereotype constitutional types, which are born from heredity, but are moulded by life's experiences. It is the homeopath's art to see through the superficialities of a client's personality to the essence within. Only then can the majority of the type be identified.

### *Physical Appearance*

I have never seen a woman who appeared to be Sulphur constitutionally. This is not due to some presupposition upon my part, since in my early years of practice I was puzzled by the fact that I never saw Sulphur women, having never been taught that Sulphur was an exclusively male type. There are occasionally women who need Sulphur acutely or sub-acutely, or to remove a layer of pathology, but I advise homeopaths to be very cautious before assuming that a woman is Sulphur constitutionally. I have met several women who thought that they were Sulphurs, including one homeopath, but on taking their cases I found that they were all extrovert Natrums. (The homeopath took Natrum Muriaticum and was much surprised by the improvement she experienced.)

There are three types of physique which are characteristic of Sulphur, and they correspond reasonably well with three characteristic Sulphur personalities. First of all there is the ectomorph, who has a tall thin frame, and a large head, especially a high forehead. This type is usually highly intellectual, and often spiritually orientated.

Secondly there is the polymorph, who is fat, and may be either tall or short. He usually is more earthy and sensual, and eats a great deal, although he may also be practical and intellectual (e.g. Sir Winston Churchill). Thirdly there is the mesomorph, who has a firm muscular body, and is often but not always tall. He is the Sulphur man of action.

Sulphur people may have any complexion, but the most common are fair or red haired, with blue, green or grey eyes, and black-haired with blue or grey eyes. The eyes frequently appear to have a sparkling quality, and also often have a dreamy, far-away look. The eyebrows are frequently very bushy, and either curl up at both outer edges, or one end curls up and the other curls down, producing a somewhat comical appearance (like the bushy brows of the British politician Dennis Healy).

The face is generally angular, and usually broad, whilst the nose is prominent and is usually quite straight, or else hooked—what I call a "fire-nose," since it is associated with the element of Fire. Very often Sulphur will have a head that appears large in comparison with his body, which is in keeping both with his expanded ego, and his cerebral and spiritual interests. (The imposing visage of the Shakespearian actor Brian Blessed is a good example. The parts he plays are classic Sulphur 'larger than life' parts as well.)

Sulphur's chin is usually broad and firm, denoting self-confidence, except in the cases of some of the ectomorph intellectuals, where the chin is pointed in comparison with the broad forehead.

In keeping with their flamboyant personalities, Sulphur individuals will often wear flamboyant clothes. These may be chic and sophisticated, as in the case of the bow-tie and the cravat, both Sulphur favourites, or they may be simply eccentric. My Sulphur schoolfriend liked to wear a coat which resembled a yak-skin or a woolly mammoth, which turned his already large frame into something which looked quite spectacular.

# Syphilinum

*Keynote:* Morbidity

Syphilinum is a strange and hence fascinating constitutional type. It is uncommonly seen, and its mental features are very poorly dealt with in the older materia medicas.

We can analyse the three miasms simplistically in functional terms as follows:

Psora—Lack of function (e.g. constipation, apathy)
Sycosis—Excess function (e.g. diarrhoea, hurriedness)
Syphilis—Distorted function (e.g. ulcerated bowel, insanity)

Those remedies that correspond to mentally disturbed personality types, such as Stramonium, Hyocyamus and Anacardium, belong in the main to the syphilitic miasm. Small wonder then that Syphilinum itself has a strange and disturbed mental picture. I must point out at the start, however, that some Syphilinum individuals possess few or none of the more abnormal mental features of the remedy, and can be spotted almost exclusively on the basis of physical symptomatology, family history and general features.

## Death's Daughter

The strangest and most fascinating aspect of Syphilinum's personality profile is the tendency for the individual to be attracted to all things connected with death. One Syphilinum woman who appeared to all intents and purposes to be normal mentally told me during the interview that as a child she was so fascinated with death that she would keep the bodies of dead animals in a drawer, so that she could look at them from time to time. She buried her pet cat in the garden, but would repeatedly dig it up to examine the remains over several months, and felt no sadness, but only fascination with the process of decay. Her main complaint was crippling agarophobia, which she only experienced in unfamiliar surroundings, and which responded very well to Syphilinum 10M.

Syphilinum individuals may be attracted to anything that is associated with death. One patient of mine, a typically pale and emaciated-looking girl, said that her favourite animals were spiders and bats. She had a pet spider at home, which she fed occasionally with flies. She also had a love of cemeteries, and would often walk through them looking at the grave stones. It gave her a sense of peace. Like many Syphilinum people, she was relatively normal on the surface, and only revealed her unusual fascinations, and her distressing mental symptoms, upon closer examination. Some Syphilinums have something of a sadistic streak, in that they enjoy watching animals die, and will find themselves stepping on insects, or putting them in water and watching them drown. I have not come across cruelty towards humans amongst Syphilinums, but the potential is presumably there.

Syphilinum's fascination with death and the macabre is sometimes reflected in her dreams. (The majority I have seen have been female.) One patient told me that she often dreamt of skeletons or of skulls, or of being buried herself, and that these dreams were not distressing.

It is important for the homeopath to realise that this fascination with death is genuine and deep-seated, and not some fad that the person has embraced to appear interesting. Usually the Syphilinum person knows that her interests are 'weird', and for this reason she keeps them to herself.

I have not come across any patients with sexual fetishes related to deceased people, but the portraits of two people with such fetishes in the Australian film director Paul Cox' artistically delicate films 'Man of Flowers' and 'Golden Braid' are highly reminiscent of Syphilinum. Both characters not only have obsessions with death and deceased people, but are also obsessed with collecting objects of beauty. I have come across one Syphilinum patient whose main hobby was collecting beautiful vases, and most of the Syphilinum people I have treated have had a fine appreciation for beauty, and also a tendency to collect things.

### *Obsessive-Compulsive*

All 'syphilitic' remedy-types have an obsessional tendency. The most commonly seen is the fastidiousness of Arsenicum, and the most well-known mental feature of Syphilinum is usually the compulsion to wash. Not all Syphilinums have a compulsion to wash, but the majority that I have seen have had this compulsion to some degree at some point in their lives (Kent: 'Always washing her hands'). Most often, one finds a compulsion to wash the hands frequently. There is usually a sense of contamination and a fear of germs, and this drives the person to wash her hands tens or even hundreds of times a day. After shaking hands with you she may feel contaminated, and cannot relax until she has washed her hands. One Syphilinum patient, who reported all the classic fascinations with funerals and spiders and the like, washed in a different but equally compulsive manner. She spent about an hour in the bathroom every morning and every night, scrubbing every inch of her body clean. As a child this annoyed her family, who had to fit in around her cleansing 'ritual'. She said that she felt dirty and also anxious if she reduced the extent of her washing.

Sometimes the washing compulsion of Syphilinum is more subtle, or the patient attempts to rationalise it away. One woman who was very clearly Syphilinum said that she washed her hands frequently, but this was only because she worked as a cook. It occurred to me that she may have unconsciously chosen a profession which enabled her to keep up her obsessive washing.

Given the origin of the nosode, it seems somehow fitting that Syphilinum individuals often have a fear of contamination. One young woman came to see me for treatment of a bizarre syndrome which she claimed to have originated from exposure to a cyanide compound whilst she was working as a printer. Although the alleged exposure was said to have occurred about eighteen months previously, she said that she was still 'leeching' cyanide out of her skin, and that everything she touched became contaminated, so that if she touched it again a day later, she would experience symptoms of burning skin, headache and mental confusion. As a result of this belief of hers, she was unable to read books, to store any food in her refrigerator, or to wear clothes more than once without washing them. She was an intelligent woman, and she had gone to the trouble of obtaining laboratory reports which appeared to confirm that shortly after the time of the alleged exposure she did indeed have traces of isocyanates on her clothing. She could not, however, provide evidence that the toxin was still coming out of her skin a year and a half later, and I pointed out to her that even if it was, it would cause symptoms whether or not she touched something 'infected' by her previously. To this she had a rather sophisticated explanation, namely that the toxins coming out of her skin chemically changed when exposed to the air for a time, liberating free cyanide, which then caused her symptoms when she touched it. Her explanations seemed so thorough that I thought there was an outside chance that there was some truth to them, but in order to avoid a wild goose chase, I decided to treat her constitutionally in the first instance. There were few strong features to go on, but she had the ghostly pale complexion typical of Syphilinum, and the gaunt physique. In addition, she appeared to have a delusion of being contaminated, and so I gave Syphilinum 10M. After a few weeks she reported that the physical symptoms had subsided a little, but more importantly, they no longer dominated her life, since she took less notice of them. She eventually became open to the possibility that her symptoms were principally psychogenic in origin, and she told me an interesting piece of information. Shortly before the time when she was exposed to the chemical, she had been raped. It seemed to me that the rape had highlighted a tendency to feel contaminated that was constitutionally part of her make-up. Since the rape she had repeatedly thought that she had seen the face of the rapist in crowds whilst out shopping, even though the rape had occurred hundreds of miles away. After taking Syphilinum this disturbing phenomena also subsided.

The other common obsession of Syphilinums is a tendency to collect things, and then place them in an orderly arrangement. This is not so specific, since it can be seen in any of the syphilitic types. An example is the patient who collected vases, and then wrapped and stored them very neatly in her cupboards. It may manifest simply as a tendency to arrange the tin cans in the pantry in strict lines, or to collect stamps and display them in meticulously ordered arrangements. It is presumably a psychological defence mechanism, aimed at producing a sense of stability in a mind that is subconsciously (or consciously) afraid of disintegration.

## Self-Destructiveness and Despair

The syphilitic miasm is a destructive one. On the physical level it manifests as ulceration, wasting and congenital malformations. On the psychological level it can produce madness of various kinds. One of the characteristic features of Syphilinum is a tendency to be self-destructive - to harm oneself. Syphilinum is a more passive type than Hyoscyamus and Stramonium, and is generally more normal psychologically. Whereas these latter types may display overt self-destructive behaviour, such as self-mutilation, the self-destructiveness of Syphilinum is more often a kind of stoicism or neglect. For example, one patient reported that if she had a stone in her shoe, she would carry on walking without removing the stone until her foot bled, despite the fact that she was in considerable pain, She did not enjoy the pain. It was rather that it was not important to her. Another woman who was apparently normal psychologically, but had a fascination with death as a child, said that when she was learning to rock-climb she had an accident in which a large rock fell on her head, concussing her. Her party insisted that she abandon the climb and turn back, but she refused, although her head hurt a lot. There are all sorts of ways that one can be self-destructive. One Syphilinum woman endured an abusive relationship with a man for years, in which he did not allow her to go out of the house. She was ordered to stay and wait on him, and she did so. She even gave up a promising career as an artist to be with him. When I asked her why she did so, she could only reply that she loved him. This same woman had a tendency to get drunk when she was unhappy, and to dance to very loud music, having first covered her face in garish make-up. Her new boyfriend was present during the consultation, and told me that his partner seemed almost insane at these times, and would get violent if he tried to quieten her down.

None of my Syphilinum patients have been alcoholics, but many seemed to use alcohol to excess when they were depressed, and many had a family history of either alcoholism or suicide (which has been confirmed by many other homeopaths). Some Syphilinum people are subject to depressive episodes which are very stark and quite characteristic. They report a sense of emptiness, as if they were in a wasteland, and a sense that their life will never get better (Kent: 'Despair of recovery', 'Indifferent, no delight in anything'). One woman told me that at these times she would simply stare into space for hours, in a kind of limbo in which she felt little, and didn't think at all. If she were dragged out of this state by a friend she would feel suicidal. The same woman had a fear of going to bed, and would stand for hours at night on the same spot, staring into space until she fell down asleep on the floor. Her depression and her strange nocturnal behaviour both disappeared after a couple of doses of Syphilinum 10M, but were replaced by anger towards her husband which seemed unwarranted. She had been very suppressed as a child by an aggressive alcoholic father, and it seemed to me that this was the source of her depression and fear. In this light, the replacement of her depression by anger was a healthy sign, even though it was projected onto her husband. Prior to receiving Syphilinum this patient had a degree of passivity that was unhealthy. She would go along with anyone whose will was stronger than her own, and felt that she did not really matter. Only under the influence of alcohol and loud music was she able to feel her suppressed vitality, and also her anger. After taking the remedy she seemed a lot more in control of her life, and no longer depended upon her husband all the time to make decisions for her.

The empty, vacant feeling that some Syphilinum people report seems congruous with their deathly pale complexion, and their frequently emaciated looking physiques. It gives one the impression that they have a flimsy grip on life, which is further emphasised by their fascination with death. One Syphilinum patient told me that as a child she dare not go to sleep until she had seen her face in the mirror. It is as though she were afraid that she would simply cease to exist when she fell asleep, unless she first affirmed her existence by seeing her reflected image. The morbid fascination with death of the more classic Syphilinum personality, combined with the characteristic white complexion and pointed teeth, have led to comparisons with supernatural traditions of vampires and zombies. Syphilinum people may sometimes look as if they have one foot in the grave, but at least they still cast a reflection in the mirror!

### Fear and Psychic Sensitivity
Syphilinum, like Stramonium and Hyoscyamus, is often in touch with psychic contents that remain unconscious for most of us. With Stramonium these unconscious forces burst through dramatically into consciousness, and then recede. With Syphilinum the connection is more constant, and less dramatic. Those aspects of life (and especially death) that most people prefer to relegate to their subconscious mind are incorporated into the personality of Syphilinum, producing a relatively stable but highly unusual indi-

vidual. One aspect of Syphilinum's contact with normally subconscious material is her tendency to be quite psychic in many cases. Many Syphilinums are prone to psychic experiences, such as precognition and out of body experiences, and also to hallucinations. One Syphilinum woman I treated could not drive a car, because after a while she would start to hallucinate, seeing imaginary people by the side of the road, or even in the road. Another found that street lamps would go out as she passed them by. I accompanied her one evening and confirmed that this actually happened. She eventually discovered, to her delight, that she could turn them back on again by concentrating on them. This was significant to her, because she had always felt that she was 'jinxed', since bad events seemed to follow her. When she found that she could turn lights on as well as off, she began to think that she had constructive as well as destructive capabilities.

Psychic and hallucinatory tendencies tend to make the mind less stable, and this results in some Syphilinum people fearing for their sanity (Kent: 'Fears loss of reason'). It also can produce a general fearfulness that appears as free-floating anxiety, or as agarophobia. One Syphilinum patient used to feel panicky if she were in town for too long. As a girl she had dreamed of being invisible, and when she went out she dressed in a huge coat and hat which covered up her identity and made her feel safer. Many Syphilinum people appear meek and rather passive in company, yet they have a wild side which comes out when they drink alcohol, and also sometimes during sex.

I am sure that Syphilinum as a remedy will cover some states of dementia and of madness (Kent: 'Imbecility', 'Laughing and weeping without cause'), but I have not seen them. As homeopaths we seldom see the more florid examples of mental instability, as our counterparts in the last century must have.

### A Complex Male Syphilinum Case

The majority of the Syphilinum patients I have seen have been female, and in these cases rage was either absent from the picture, or it arose only under the influence of alcohol. Ihave treated one male Syphilinum patient who expressed a great deal of rage, as well as other very classic Syphilinum traits such as self-destructiveness and fear of dirt. His case is quite differeent from that of my female Syphilinum patients, and it resembles more closely the popular image amongst homeopaths of Syphilinum being an aggressive self-destructive type. This leads me to suspect that the gender of the patient has a big influence upon how the syphilitic miasm will be expressed. As with Stramonium, it appears that male members of the Syphilinum constitution are more liable to express the more active and aggressive aspects of the type, whilst female Syphilinum tend to express the more passive aspects of the type. My male Syphilinum patient, who I shall call Dave, was a gifted musician, who was able to tap into an almost mystical stream of musical inspiration, enabling him to write songs very spontaneously. (This reminds me of the gifted Mercurius poet who was similarly inspired. There is a lot in common between these two types.) When I first saw him I thought immediately of Syphilinum, because his irises were of two completely different colours. He attributed this to his mother having been exposed to nuclear radiation in the outback of Australia. Whether this was true, or another example of Syphilinum's fear of contamination, was not clear to me. In his first consultation with me, Dave was in a very active state indeed. His mind was racing and his speech was fast and somewhat scattered. In other words, he was manic. He said he had a chemical disorder which gave him dramatic mood changes. It appeared these moods were an alternation of suicidal despair, rage and inspired elation. In between these states he might feel normal for a while, but when he ate, the 'attacks' would return. He said he would often fast in order to avoid attacks. During an attack he would feel that his mind was disintegrating, and that his limbs were scattered and unconnected (like Baptisia and Phosphorus during a fever). During his attacks he would let out his anger upon inanimate objects, bashing metal gargage cans flat on one occasion, and cutting his hands in the process. His rage was especially aggravated by any sexual contact, so much so that he could not make love with his wife. When he did so, he wanted hard violent sex, which made him feel ashamed afterwards. He was clearly a very tormented man, who was not insane, but was not far off from insanity.

Dave had been a hyperactive child. Curiously, he had not talked till he was six. This kind of markedly unusual development is often found in the histories of Syphilinum patients, although the exact manifestation varies a great deal. He said that he had not stopped talking since! Dave's birth was a very difficult one. He had got stuck and had 'split open' his mother, who nearly dies. He says he was thrown away as dead, but later noticed to be breathing. This image is for me quite symbolic of Syphilinum. These people are usually born into a difficult environment, or they have a violent, alcoholic or suicidal family background. They are often physically or mentally disturbed, and will often lead quite tortured lives. In Dave's case sexual abuse had contributed to his life-long rage, and this also is more common in the kind of severely abnormal soil from which the Syphilinum seed sprouts forth.

Dave had said that he felt suicidal every day, except when he drank alcohol. He had none of the morbid attraction to death that I have seen in Syphilinum women, in the form of love of cemetaries, etc., but instead he had frank suicidal despair. (I suspect that the morbid fascination of some female Syphilinum is a sublimated form of suicidal impulse, a kind of vicarious exploration of death.) Curiously, he only needed to drink one beer a day to keep the mental disintegration at bay. Thus he was not alcoholic in the usual sense, but he was dependent upon alcohol, and said that his cravings for alcohol were intense. Another way Dave would defuse his mental tension was to hurt himself. Here we have an explanation for the self-destructiveness of Syphilinum. He said that at times he had to inflict pain upon himself to suppress the energy flowing through him. He had done this previously by putting his hands into hot coals and also by sleeping on a bed of nails! He said that the pain would bring him a sense of calmness.

Dave had the typical Syphilinum fear of contamination, in several forms. At times he could not bear to get dirty, and would vomit if dirt got on him. At other times he would enjoy getting dirty, when he was feeling more re-laxed. He was very hygienic, and had a great fear of catching viruses. In this case his fear appeared justified, since he said he would become deathly sick whenever he caught a virus, losing weight and even stopping breathing at times. Perhaps this is the origin of the Syphilinum's fear of contamination, a (normally subconcious) knowledge that infection will be too devastating for their system, which is presumably related to the inheritance of the Syphilis miasm itself, a devastating disease in pre-antibiotic times. Dave's food sensi-tivities were legion, so much so that any food could send him off the deep end. This is really another version of Syphilinum's fear of contamination, whether it was based upon a physical sensitivity or not. Dave also had a para-noid fear of radiation of all kinds, including X-rays, and also microwave machines. In addition, he was very psychic, and said he was too sensitive to the radiation given off by other people, and could tell telepathically what they were thinking on occasions. He gave an example of a patient he met whilst visiting a relative in a psychiatric hospital. This lady had not spoken for years, and just made 'meaningless' gestures with her hands. Dave instantly knew what these gestures meant, and he replied to her. Dave said that this break-through in the woman's communication led her to recovery and discharge from the hospital. (If this story sounds fantastic, it is almost exactly the same as the story recorded in Dr. Carl Jung's early psychiatric notes. Dr. Jung also intuitively understood the peculiar behaviour (in this case 'nonsensical rav-ings') of a 'mad' patient, and by replying to her he apparently cured her.)

Dave's psychic sensitivities led him to dread going to bed at night. At night he would travel to other realms in his dreams, and talk to spirits there. Some-times these were wonderful conversations with spiritual beings, but at other times they were frightful encounters with demons. He also had precognitive dreams, and he had a habit of intuiting the future of other people. On one occasion he felt he suddenly could not breathe, and shortly afterwards the baby of a friend was found dead.

One aspect of Dave's symptoms was clearly syphilitic, but I had not seen it before in Syphilinum cases. He said that he was very analytical, so much so that sometimes he could not comprehend a whole sentence, because he was so absorbed in analysing each individual word a person spoke. As a result, at school he would have difficulty, since he would get confused and reply to questions which had not been asked. Hyper-analytycal thinking is seen in other syphilitic types, notably Arsenicum and Kali Carbonicum, but I have never seen it taken to such an extreme degree as in Dave's case. Dave's excessive analyzing is related to Syphilinum's well known obsessive-compulsive tendency, which involves an excessive focus upon detail. Once again Syphilinum takes on the appearance of an extreme version of Arsenicum.

Although Dave was a sensitive person, he created a dominating, aggressive persona to protect himself. He was very clear about this. He called this persona 'The Dictator'. As the Dictator he could cope with sex, albeit in a dominating way, but he said that the Dictator suppressed both his vulnerability and his creativity as a musician. Thus he was torn between the safety of the Dictator, and the creativity of his undefended self. This protective mechanism of Dave's sheds light on the dictatorial tendencies of other syphilitic types, including Veratrum and Mercurius. The latter two types are also prone to feelings of great vulnerability, and this is presumably the origin of their dictatorial tendencies.

Upon taking Syphilinum 10M Dave felt 'speedy' for a few hours and then felt very calm. He lost the need for alcohol almost immediately, and had ceased to 'spin out' mentally when I saw him a week later. He was much calmer, and spoke clearly and normally. Dave required weekly doses of the remedy for a while to keep him in balance, but gradually he was able to stay centered taking it less and less frequently. He still takes the remedy occasionally when he feels his mind is beginning to go out of control. Dave's case illustrates quite dramatically how violent is the disturbance of the mind in some Syphilinum people, who teeter at the edge of insanity, but do not become mad. It amplifies the impression of self-destructiveness that we have seen in cases of female Syphilinums, as well as the psychic tendency of Syphilinum, and the manifold ways of expressing fear of contamination. Dave's case suggests that the suicidal impulse is a strong feature of Syphilinum, and it confirms the classic rubric of a strong craving for alcohol (Kent: 'Longing for strong drink').

### Physical Appearance

Physically, there are several characteristic features that are often seen in Syphilinum people. First of all, the physique is generally very thin, and the complexion is usually very pale. There is usually some abnormality of the teeth, most commonly taking the form of pointed teeth, or 'saw toothed' as it is called. These three features can all be seen in the striking appearance of the famous rock musician and singer David Bowie. In addition, Bowie has irises of markedly different colour and size. Such developmental abnormalities are far more common in Syphilinum people than in other types. I have seen Syphilinum children who grew only their canine teeth, and others who had a layer of skin missing, producing an almost transparent effect.

The face is generally thin and angular, and the features may be either sharp or blunted. Some Syphilinum people have relatively normal, well-balanced personalities, but markedly abnormal physical appearances, and others are abnormal mentally but relatively normal physically. Still others are relatively normal both physically and psychologically. In these latter cases one must rely on the physicals, and upon isolated mental features, to spot the remedy type.

# *Thuja*

*Keynote:* Sexual guilt

There tends to be a rather extreme picture in most Thuja people, with a combination of unusually positive and unusually negative characteristics in the same person, particularly in women. The men tend to be far more ordinary. What follows applies principally to Thuja women, unless otherwise specified.

### *Beauty and the Beast*

The central polarity for understanding Thuja is that of beauty and ugliness. Most Thuja women have a very fine sensitivity to beauty, comparable only with China, Phosphorus and Medorrhinum. Thuja's sensitivity to beauty is mystical rather than merely aesthetic. She becomes one with the beauty perceived. Such experiences give Thuja a mystical philosophy of life which sets her apart from most people, and which is based more on experience than on intellectualisation or belief. In order to experience the immediacy of beauty in a mystical way, an innocence of heart is required, and this is usually present in Thuja. There is something childlike about the wonder which Thuja experiences when she looks at a beautiful scene, or recognises the beauty in a person's eyes. There is also a childlike enthusiasm and playfulness when she is happy. At such times she has an impish quality which is similar to that seen in Phosphorus and Mercurius. She loves to have a good time, and tends to do so with a little wildness, even recklessness.

Closely allied to Thuja's sensitivity to beauty is her sensitivity to love and emotional pain. Although she can fall intensely in love if she lets herself, she soon learns how painful this is, and thereafter tends to guard her heart from such vulnerability. Her defence is only partial however, since she is much more sensitive than other defensive types like Natrum Muriaticum and Ignatia, who tend to succeed more completely in walling off their heart once hurt. The result is an uneasy hovering between emotional openness and avoidance of intimacy. Often Thuja will appear nonchalant and detached, but one word of perceived criticism or rejection from somebody she cares about and Thuja will collapse in tears or strike out.

It is when Thuja has been hurt that she begins to feel ugly, either physically or emotionally. She has an in-built tendency to reject herself once she has felt rejected by another. If she was hurt or rejected by her parents to any degree, then she carries with her a lifelong tendency to feel bad about herself; that she is ugly, or stupid, or a bad person. The degree of hurt determines the degree to which this self-hate overshadows her natural love of life in all its beauty. Those Thuja women who were very unhappy as children tend to feel that they do not deserve happiness, since there is something intrinsically wrong with them. This happens to some extent to anyone who was hurt as a small child, but the result is much more pervasive in Thuja. Natrum Muriaticum and Carcinosinum develop low self-esteem when they do not experience unconditional love as a child. Thuja develops self-loathing.

Thuja's self-loathing can show itself in a thousand and one ways. Frequently Thuja women will speak excessively negatively about themselves (Kent: 'Reproaches self'). They will overreact to misdemeanors on their part. If they were slightly less warm than usual toward an acquaintance they will consider that they have behaved really awfully, and fear they will lose the latter's respect or friendship (Kent: 'Delusions—that he is a criminal').

It is common for Thuja to expect rejection, since she feels she is bad. One Thuja woman whom I saw for psychotherapy would come in every other session expecting and dreading that I had decided I would not see her anymore because she said something 'wrong' in the last session. Thuja will often restrict her activities and interaction with people in order to avoid the rejection she anticipates. This is particularly true when it comes to asking for help. She will not ask a good friend for a small favour, for fear that she is imposing and will be rejected as a friend. Actual rejection is extremely painful for many Thujas. It confirms their worst fears that they are horrible people. And it ensures that they will not ask for help again. Similarly, Thuja may avoid attempting new activities because she is afraid of failure. There are many ways in which Thuja may think that she is an awful person. Usually they are not true, and when Thuja is in a more positive frame of mind she may be able to see this, but it doesn't stop that deep-seated self-loathing from haunting her.

One Thuja woman I treated for smoking addiction appeared entirely healthy emotionally. She was relaxed, confident and fulfilled in her work. She was an artist, and she was highly intuitive, with a sense of quiet wisdom and attunement to life's inner harmony. She showed no signs at all of low self-esteem until she mentioned a fungal infection on her toenail. She became agitated when I asked to see it, initially saying 'No'. When asked why, she replied, 'Because it is so ugly'. I did get a look at the toenail, which was just a minor case of fungal infection, and she blushed with shame and embarrassment that I had seen her imperfection.

### Dark Secrets
A great many Thuja women appear secretive once their initial friendliness

has been seen through. They will deflect a question which approaches too close to the guilt and loathing that they feel inside. A typical Thuja characteristic is the trailing off of sentences, which are left unfinished. She initially begins to say something, then her internal antennae pick up a danger of revealing something shameful, and she aborts the sentence automatically. If she is pressed to finish the sentence, she may become tearful and reveal something she is ashamed of, such as the fact that she smokes. She will then look at you for signs that you have discovered what a wretch she is.

Thuja's internal psychodynamics tend to be very complicated, at least in the average or more unhealthy individual. There is such a tangle of half-truth hiding in Thuja's own self-image that she trips herself up all the time. The whole structure is unstable and prone to crisis, since at any time a secret may slip past the veil and threaten to reveal other secrets. One reason Thuja may react so catastrophically to the revelation of a minor fault is that there really are major secrets hidden inside, and the failure of the veil may lead to far greater shameful revelations, like a thread unravelling. By far the most common awful secrets in Thuja's subconscious are her sexual ones.

Thuja is a passionate type, with a high sexual drive. When she is healthy emotionally, her sexual life is enjoyed as part of her love life and begets no shame. However, once Thuja has been really hurt, she will close off her heart. This tends to be an all or nothing event, rather than a gradual closing. Once closed, she will still enter into relationships, but her heart will not be fully available. This scenario can give rise to promiscuity, since emotional intimacy has become threatening, and the libido is still high. A history of promiscuity is quite common among Thuja women. They may speak without shame about their sexual life, because they have adopted a strong belief that there is nothing wrong with it. Thuja has a remarkable ability to cut off from unwanted feelings and beliefs, and this can make her vulnerable to a kind of self-destructive hardening. When such women gradually open up during psychotherapy, they do feel shame about their promiscuity, but even more they feel the emotional pain that made their hearts close in the first place.

The picture is often complicated in Thuja women by a past history of sexual abuse. For some reason, Thuja appears to be more prone to childhood sexual abuse than other types. Because of Thuja's natural tendency to feel guilt easily, sexual abuse has an even greater inpact upon Thuja women than upon other types. The sense of self-loathing becomes enormous and gives rise to self-destructive behaviour. The unconscious has its own simple logic. In this case it thinks, 'Something terrible happened to me. Nobody protected me. I must have deserved it. I must be really bad. I must be punished. I don't deserve to live'. Or, 'I am in Hell. Death would be preferable to this'. Either way, the abused Thuja child grows up feeling she is very very bad, and when she falls into depression, she is tempted to kill herself, or just to stab herself till she bleeds. Such feelings of self-hate are often temporarily relieved by Thuja inflicting injury upon herself.

Abused Thujas are prone to very deep depression. One Thuja patient of mine would go to bed for days when she was depressed. She had no will to do anything, because she had no will to live. If she became suicidal, a dose of Thuja 10M would quickly bring her out of it. Thuja's self-destructive behaviour can take many forms. Substance abuse and sexual promiscuity are two of the most common. A damaged Thuja individual will often turn to psychotropic drugs, cigarettes or alcohol to dull her sense of unease. Quite often such addictions bring Thuja in for homeopathic treatment. In these cases the trauma and self-loathing that lie behind the addiction are often unknown to the patient. She knows that she is moody and prone to anxiety, but she has forgotten why. Since past trauma must usually be brought to consciousness before it can be healed, the Thuja patient who presents with a cigarette addiction may be in for more than she bargained for. The remedy will bring up suppressed memories, and this may be extremely traumatic in itself. However, with skilled psychotherapy and continued Thuja medication, the pain from the past can be gradually dispelled, and with it the self-destructive tendencies. It is when Beauty kisses her Beast that his spell is broken and his ugliness disappears. Similarly, when Thuja faces and forgives her dark side, it too disappears, or rather, it is transformed into strength.

One common form of self-destruction in Thuja women that is driven by sexual guilt is gynecological pathology. Thuja is very prone to gynecological problems, including infections, endometriosis, severe period pain and premenstrual tension. When the remedy is given these symptoms gradually abate as the underlying shame and trauma are healed.

### Wildness
Thuja is a passionate type, sharing with her sister type Medorrhinum a wild streak. In the healthy Thuja this shows itself as adventurousness. Thuja can be a tomboy who is oblivious to danger and gets thrills from wild physical adventure. She is more mischievous than Medorrhinum, playing pranks and laughing with abandon when they are discovered. The healthy Thuja woman may be adventurous sexually as well, but not to a self-destructive extent.

Thuja's wildness makes her more independent than other women. She needs to be free to express herself, and this will often be translated into non-committed relationships or committed relationships where each partner allows the other plenty of space. Her wildness has a distinctly physical quality. She needs to use her body to feel free, whether making love, dancing, or engaging in vigorous sports. It is a more intense need than that of Sepia, who needs to be physically active, but not in such a passionate way as Thuja.

In the unhealthy Thuja woman, there is a driven and self-destructive flavour to her wildness. She will impulsively get drunk, and then jump into bed with a loathsome man, only to hate herself for it the next day. Or she will fly into a rage with anyone who 'presses her buttons', screaming uncontrollably. Thuja is very prone to rage but will normally control it unless she is drunk, or in a therapy session. The more she has been hurt before, the more dangerous will her wildness be, especially to herself. She may find herself attracted to the dark side of life, watching dark and violent films, indulging in sadomasochistic sex, and wearing black clothes. Such activities are Thuja's attempt to face the darkness within, albeit vicariously. They do not dispel the darkness, but they discharge some of the tension associated with it. When one gets to know such a wild Thuja woman (usually a young woman), one finds a sensitive, gentle soul who is terrified of life, hates herself, and is prone to bouts of rage. One also sees the beauty that lies just below the surface, the delicate refinement and the innocence that is natural to Thuja and never completely obscured.

Thuja is very prone to fear. She is one of the most sensitive types, and this sensitivity includes sensitivity to emotional pain, and also to danger. When she has been abused in her childhood, Thuja is even more prone to terror. She may develop a free-floating anxiety that is especially strong when she is with people (Kent: 'Fear of strangers'). Thuja develops a tendency to run away to cope with this fear. She will bolt from a party when she cannot bear the fear, and she will be evasive when invited out. Her defence mechanisms are not as robust as those of more stable types like Natrum or Sepia, who will go through with social activities despite fear and not show their fear. Thuja is more brittle, and when she snaps she will break down or run away.

Thuja's fear tends to show very clearly in her eyes, which tend to resemble that of a frightened animal when she is scared.

Fleeing is not Thuja's only defence against anxiety. She may also adopt a tough, masculine appearance, dress in men's clothes, learn karate, and engage in the kind of tough adolescent banter that teenage boys use to assert themselves. Use of sexual swear words is very common in such Thuja women, who toughen themselves to protect their vulnerability. Commonly such women avoid touch, unless it is rough touch like wrestling, because it is harder to steel against than words, being so intimate (Kent: 'Aversion to being touched'). Despite this masculine exterior, their sensitivity still shows through, both in their appearance (especially in their beautiful eyes) and their words. One young Thuja woman came to see me for treatment of extreme mood swings. She had medium-length straight dark hair, an angular, impish face dotted with freckles, and beautiful clear green eyes. She was very aggressive in her behaviour towards men, including her rather sweet boyfriend, and adopted a tough, invulnerable stance in the consulting room, which included a playfully aggressive side. Whenever I steered her towards uncomfortable self-truths, she would laugh nervously and say 'Oh fuck!' Despite her tough exterior, she was gentle with her friends to the point that she would help whenever they were suffering. In fact she felt their suffering acutely. Her sensitive heart was quite visible beneath her macho posturing, and this is usually the case with Thuja women, who are far too sensitive to hide it, unlike many Natrum and Ignatia women.

### On the Verge of Madness

I have not seen a Thuja case that deteriorated into madness, but it seems as if the potential is there. The materia medicas are full of references to the strange perceptions that Thuja is prone to, especially the delusion that her legs are made of glass, or that there is a fetus in her stomach. I did not take these references very seriously for years, having never come across them in my Thuja patients, but when I came to have Thuja patients for psychotherapy, I began to encounter these strange perceptions. In particular, when one patient was beginning to get in touch with distressing emotions which had been suppressed, she would feel it first as strange physical sensations. There were many of these, but the most frequent were movements in her abdomen, sometimes like a whirlpool inside her stomach, and sometimes like a feeling of a moving lump. At other times she would have a vision that her pelvis was filled with blood, or that something was rotting inside her. These experiences would no doubt be alarming to a great many Thuja people if they had them, but in the context of psychotherapy we were able to make sense of their symbolism, and this made them far less threatening.

My Thuja patients were certainly far less stable psychologically than most of my psychotherapy patients. At times they would 'flip out', entering dreamy, almost comatose states when they could not face the emotions that were surfacing (Kent: 'Stupefaction'). Thuja will often leave her body rather than face painful emotions. Those Thuja women who have been sexually abused will often experience terrible physical pain when the memories emerge, not to mention the accompanying emotional pain. At such times they will either cut off and be back in the present, or they will leave their body for some dream-like space. At other times they will rage, and their anger is again more dramatic than I am used to seeing in other patients. Like Lachesis, Thuja can be thought of as something of a taut string, but whereas Lachesis either becomes nervous as a result of suppressing this tension, or loses her temper, Thuja tends to be more self-destructive.

Occasionally Thuja becomes unstable when, as a result of past trauma surfacing, she loses her ego-defences and becomes too open to the psychic world. At these time she may be more frightened of spirits than of people (Kent: 'Delusions—see images, phantoms'), and she may interpret ordinary events as symbolic, a milder version of the schizophrenic's ideas of reference.

### Right Brain

Thuja has many similarities with Medorrhinum, both physically and emotionally. One difference is the degree of objectivity. Medorrhinum usually has a good balance between left- and right-brain functioning, making her both analytical and artistic. Thuja is far more biased towards right-brain functioning. She is not an analytical type. She tends to experience the world in a childlike, innocent manner, which includes a lot of intuitive perception. Unfortunately, as Thuja becomes unhealthy emotionally, she begins to doubt her intuition, and eventually to dismiss it altogether.

Thuja's combination of right brain 'thinking' and her intense and often tortured emotionality can result in confusion. It is common for Thuja to have difficulty thinking clearly, particularly when she is feeling emotional. This is one reason why she may hesitate before answering questions. Sometimes Thuja will be quite unsophisticated, and yet intelligent. She may grapple with unfamiliar words in an attempt to appear more intelligent, and this only makes her more confused. Her sensitivity, her intuition, her vulnerability and her artistic sensibility may cause the homeopath to confuse Thuja with China. Both can claim to be the most sensitive of constitutional types, in the positive and the negative meaning of the word. The principal difference is that China is analytical as well intuitive, and far less earthy. Also China tends to be more introverted than Thuja. Thuja will have a rollicking good time at a party, whereas China is more shy and needs to be coaxed out. Despite her analytical ability, China appears more feminine because she is more delicate, lacking the robust earthiness of Thuja. This combination of earthiness and delicate sensitivity is uniquely characteristic of the Thuja woman.

### The Thuja Man

Thuja men are uncommon, and difficult to spot. They can be divided into two kinds, the ordinary type and the secretive type.

## The Ordinary Type

This type is something like a cross between a Natrum and a Graphites man. He is introverted, stable and moderately emotional. He is moderately expressive of his feelings and prone to moderate anxiety. He tends to be rather conventional, and often enjoys family life. He is somewhat materialistic and tends to be unimaginative, and not oversensitive. He is conscientious and reliable. He may have some difficulty asserting himself, since he does not like confrontations, but he is capable of being irritable when stressed. Such a normal man is hard to identify constitutionally from the mentals. The physicals are usually what lead to a diagnosis of Thuja constitution. In particular, a history of prostatitis is highly characteristic, though asthma and sinusitis are common, as is seborrheic dermatitis. Dreams of falling are not commonly reported, and the sexuality is normal. The physical appearance may help, being dark and swarthy. In the presence of typical physical features, the very ordinariness of the personality helps to confirm Thuja!

### The Secretive Type

This type is rare. It shares many features with the unhealthy female Thuja, but is tougher and more manipulative. The secretive Thuja man is vulnerable emotionally, and he generally develops a manipulative and aggressive persona to protect himself. One such man took part in a psychotherapy group I was running. He tended to accuse other people of whatever traits he was trying to hide from in himself. In particular, he would get up, walk over to some small vulnerable woman, tower his bulky frame over her, and accuse her of trying to dominate him. He had very large sexual and gastronomic appetites, and his sexuality was distinctly sadistic. Here we see the twistedness that often gets incorporated into Thuja's sexuality as a result of past trauma.

The secretive type gives little away in the interview until he trusts you, when he reveals the aggressive impulses he is prone to. These may include a desire to dominate others, a tendency towards rage, sadomasochistic sexual practices, and other self-destructive tendencies such as those seen in Thuja women. The secretive Thuja male is thus something of a tortured type, with a hard exterior. He is prone to being judgmental and vengeful, but is also easily hurt emotionally, and he may be aware of self-loathing and thus prone to suicidal depression. Like the unhealthy Thuja woman, he tends to become suspicious, even paranoid, and is unable to keep friends. He can be very evasive in the consulting room, weaving around questions or becoming vague rather than revealing his inner truths. Also like Thuja women, he has an attraction for the mystical and can be quite intuitive and artistic.

### Physical Appearance

Thuja generally has a dark complexion and may have sallow skin or fair skin with dark hair. The hair is usually straight. Freckles and moles on the skin, as well as warts, are common. Thuja women are more sensitive than the men, and this is reflected in their faces, which tend to have more refined, delicate features. The face is more angular than rounded, and the Thuja women I have treated had a light sprinkling of freckles on their faces, whereas the men did not. The men had 'average' physiques, whereas the women all had light builds, reflecting their quick, lively minds. Thuja's eyes are often beautiful in that they express the innocence and childlike wonder to which Thuja is open. The eyes are often blue or green.

# *Tuberculinum*

*Keynote:* Restlessness

Some homeopaths treat Tuberculinum simply as a nosode, to be given when there is a family history of tuberculosis. Kent warns against this superficial approach in his Lecture Notes, pointing out that Tuberculinum is a distinct constitutional type, to be given only when the whole picture fits. The mentals of Tuberculinum constitute a personality profile as distinct and specific as any other type, but unfortunately it is poorly understood by the majority of homeopaths, and this is one reason the remedy is used more as a nosode than as a constitutional remedy.

The remedy is made from tuberculous lymph nodes, and as usual there is some correspondence between the origin of the remedy and the characteristics of the patient who needs it, including their personality. The image of the consumptive writer racing against time to complete his work of intellectual romanticism, living off bread, wine and tobacco, poignantly embodies the spirit of Tuberculinum. Tuberculinum individuals have a kind of hunger to experience a great many things in a short period, as if time were really running out for them. They cannot bear a steady routine, unless it is packed with excitement. More than any other type they are subject to that awful feeling that they are missing out, whenever the hectic pace of their life slows down, and they are left without stimulation.

In previous times the tubercular patient lived with his disease for many years, gradually losing strength and drawing closer to a premature death. This long lingering pattern of disease seems to have produced a 'miasm'. In other words, it affected every aspect of the health of the infected person, changing them at a cellular level, producing new characteristics which were then passed on to their children. It is the slow nature of the disease which allows it to create a characteristic and inheritable mental picture. The Tuberculinum individual has inherited from his consumptive ancestors a restless hunger to experience more of life before he expires. I remember one very fit man in his fifties who came to see me for treatment of his allergic asthma. He was a carpenter, and he found that certain woods made him wheeze. I was surprised when he told me his age, since he looked much younger. His body was very slim and firm, and he wore casual and very stylish clothes, which added to the appearance of youth. He was something of a health fanatic, working out at the gym several times a week, cycling regularly up mountains, and eating nothing but the best health foods. It turned out that he had a profound fear of dying early, at fifty six years old to be precise. His father had died suddenly at this age from a coronary thrombosis, and he was determined to do everything he could to avoid the same fate. Any constitutional type could have reacted in this way to his father's 'premature' death, but on further questioning I realised why my patient's tubercular inheritance had contributed to his fear. He told me that his father had worked all of his life in a factory, had hated his work, and had died before he had a chance to enjoy life. It was this that appalled my patient so much, the prospect of being trapped in an unstimulating existence and then dying, having left his greatest desires unfulfilled. Like his father, he did not enjoy his work, and he was trying desperately hard to find easier ways to make enough money to be free to enjoy himself. He studied creative tax accountancy, and made some money doing people's tax returns. He also planned to give seminars on how to achieve one's goals in life, and how to be financially independent (presumably he thought he would learn these skills himself in the process). Finally, he was attempting to break into the world of multi-million dollar loan broking, and on the three times I saw him he was always on the verge of making the big deal that would set him up for life. All this because, like most other Tuberculinums, he could not bear the tedium of regular nine to five work, especially work which was not all that exciting, and he craved the freedom to go where he wanted and do what he wanted, without sacrificing his comfortable standard of living. He sensed even more keenly than most Tuberculinums that time was running out, and there was so much he had not yet experienced. He was married to a woman who wanted nothing but stability and to be loved by her husband, but he was restless and dissatisfied with her also, and he craved the stimulation of younger, more adventurous women. He told me that his primary need in life was to play, and that he was directing all of his energies toward that goal. Tuberculinum 1M greatly reduced his bronchospasm, but I did not see him again to discover whether a 10M would reduce his dissatisfaction with life.

· Many Tuberculinums find an outlet for their restlessness through an aggressive pursuit of sports. Tuberculinum's restlessness is not aimless. It is accompanied by a drive for stimulation, which prompts Tuberculinum individuals to aggressively enter into new experiences. Their sporting activities satisfy several needs; the need to remain fit so that they can maintain the hectic pace of their lives, the need for a challenge to stimulate them, and the ever present need of Tuberculinum to play.

Probably the most widely known aspect of Tuberculinum's restlessness is his desire to travel (Kent: 'Desire to travel, always wanting to go somewhere'). Many Tuberculinums do spend years travelling around the world, working as they go. The constant variety of such a shifting lifestyle helps to satisfy their restlessness, and enables them to avoid the boredom that they are otherwise prone to experience when life is too predictable.

Tuberculinum individuals are well suited to a nomadic way of life, since they do not form strong attachments to either places or to people. Their detachment reminds one of Sulphur and Lycopodium, but it is generally greater than that seen in either of these types. Lycopodium is very often highly dependent upon his spouse, both emotionally and practically, and the same can be said for many Sulphur individuals. Tuberculinum is more independent, and very often gives the impression that he needs nobody, at least not emotionally or practically. What he does need is stimulation, and hence he likes to surround himself with interesting people. On his travels he meets many interesting people, and he does not miss them when he moves on, since he does not look back, and there are always more people to get to know. Tuberculinum is not closed like Natrum. He is more like Nux, in that he is open about what he feels, but he tends not to feel much personal attachment. He lives for today, and loves for today, and the devil take the morrow.

The lucky few Tuberculinums find work which allows then to travel and still earn a living doing something interesting. I have come across many Tuberculinum travel guides, and also ski and diving instructors. They have the light airy appearance of somebody who floats effortlessly through life, playing instead of working. Unlike Natrum guides and instructors (the other commonly encountered type), the Tuberculinums don't try all that hard to please their clients. They simply play and demonstrate their knowledge and their skills, and they don't concern themselves overmuch with what the client thinks. The only time they may lose their cool is when their clients are late, or don't turn up, or are too slow. Tuberculinum is not a particularly tolerant type, and is more impatient than most.

Another occupation that is ideal for many Tuberculinums is that of newspaper foreign correspondent. It not only involves a lot of travel, but also exercises Tuberculinum's detached and discriminating intellect. Even home-based journalism attracts quite a few Tuberculinums, since it involves a lot of travel, variety, and intellectual stimulation.

Most Tuberculinums are not so lucky that they can earn a good living seeing the globe, and many will eventually cease their wanderings when they tire of living close to the bread line, and performing unstimulating casual labour. They will then settle for a while and find a steady well paid job, and a regular partner, but all too often it isn't long before they are restless again, and dreaming of new distractions. Their restlessness can turn to irritability, and a sense of dissatisfaction with everything, until they can bear the stability of their life no longer, and they are on the move again. This restless, nomadic way of life is also seen in most Wild Staphysagrias, and in most Subdued Staphysagrias. There is an important difference between the wandering of Tuberculinum and that of the Staphysagrias. Tuberculinum wanders in search of stimulation, and becomes bored when he is in one place doing the same thing for too long. (Many Tuberculinums can settle, providing their work and their partners are interesting enough.) Staphysagria moves on to distract himself from the emotional turmoil within his breast, and in the case of the Subdued Staphysagria to avoid the relationships which he fears. There is something vague or nebulous about most Staphysagrias, and the Subdued Staphysagria in particular is a fugitive, always on the run. In contrast, the personality of Tuberculinum is far clearer and less complicated. If he is running away, it is from boredom rather than fear. He is a relatively unemotional type, and is usually very clear-headed, and also confident. Like Nux he goes after what he wants, but unlike Nux he is liable to tire of it quickly when he achieves it.

### Intellectual Curiosity and Detachment

Tuberculinum is predominantly a mental or intellectual type, like Lycopodium, Kali and Sulphur. Like these other types, Tuberculinums are more often male than female, by a factor of about five to one. As with all mental types, the intellectual interests and attitudes of Tuberculinum are highly characteristic. A Tuberculinum intellectual is quite different in his thinking from a Sulphur or a Kali intellectual. In keeping with his restlessness and hunger for new experiences, the Tuberculinum individual is curious intellectually, but lacks depth when compared with intellectual heavyweights like Sulphur and Kali Carbonicum. (Depth is perhaps the wrong term for Kali; thoroughness is more appropriate.) Tuberculinum is attracted by novel information which captures his imagination. He is often something of a dilettante intellectually, flitting from one theory or school of thought to another, moving on when something more interesting comes along. When he does explore a subject in more detail, it is either for some practical purpose, such as his work, or it is a means of pursuing and justifying his constant search for freedom. Very often he tries to combine the two. The carpenter who longed to be free from the restraints of his work not only studied and presented workshops on how to become financially independent. He also worked as a rebirther (a 'New Age' therapist who uses breathwork to induce emotional release in his clients). There are several schools of rebirthing, with different approaches and different aims. One school stresses the need for emotional release, and encourages its clients to explore their past, whilst another encourages the experience of bliss during the therapy. My Tuberculinum patient was very firmly in the latter's camp. He was not interested in messy things like emotional release. It didn't appeal to his sense of fun. Instead he embraced the theory that one can let go of all previous emotional blocks painlessly by dissolving them in bliss. As part of his theoretical background to the rebirthing he studied the works of a teacher who maintained that one can attain physical immortality through the practice of breathwork and the denial of negative thought patterns. This idea was very attractive to him, since he had a terrible fear of dying early, before he had had enough fun. Like many Tuberculinums, he embraced those theories and attitudes which gave him the most sense of freedom, and which helped to liberate him from the prison of the past, and the mundane ordinariness of the present.

Most Tuberculinums are very much future-orientated. The future holds the promise of fantastic discoveries which will liberate Mankind from the drudge of routine existence, giving him the time and the means to play and to explore the inner and the outer universe (Kent: 'Hopeful'). Tuberculinums are often attracted by progressive scientific and psychological ideas, such as parallel universes, and virtual reality, which expand the possibilities of mental and physical stimulation ad infinitum. Others tackle 'deeper' subjects like the meaning of existence, and the phenomenon of consciousness, but even here they have a peculiarly superficial or detached approach, which seeks to avoid restriction and justify their constant search for an elusive freedom. The best example I can think of in this regard is Existentialism, and its principal exponent, Jean Paul Sartre, who I presume to have been a Tuberculinum, judging from his writings. The Existentialist vision promotes all the qualities that Tuberculinum already possesses, or at least aspires to; intellectual clarity, freedom from the restraints of morality, and freedom from attachment to existing conditions. What it lacks is heart. To the Existentialist there is no inherent meaning to life. Underneath the constant activity of the mind is the Void, an altogether empty and inhuman vacuum which threatens to swallow up Tuberculinum when he is still for more than a moment. Whereas Staphysagria and Natrum keep running from the seething mass of unruly feelings below the surface of consciousness, Tuberculinum runs from the Void, the emptiness within. Underneath the Void that Tuberculinum experiences when he stops thinking or indulging his senses is a world of feeling. Tuberculinum is familiar with transient ecstasy, which comes from an immersion in physical pleasure, or from flights of the imagination. It is his estrangement from deeper feelings of personal love that results in the silence within feeling so empty. Those Tuberculinums who overcome their fear of stillness long enough to explore their emotional side more fully tend to become less restless and less cynical. They discover that there may be something worth 'sticking around' for after all.

### The Sophisticated Bohemian
Tuberculinum individuals are very often hedonistic as well as intellectual, and they crave freedom. This combination often results in a Bohemian quality.

Tuberculinum seldom conforms to accepted social traditions, and yet he is seldom a revolutionary either—he is too self-orientated for that. He is attracted to the avant garde because it is novel and exciting, and many of its leading lights will resonate to the restless tubercular miasm. D.H.Lawrence, the English romantic novelist whose passionate romanticism combined a rejection of old social values, and a celebration of personal freedom, was probably Tuberculinum constitutionally. Another famous writer who was almost certainly a Tuberculinum is Henry Miller. His autobiographical trilogy 'Tropic of Capricorn' illustrates the wild restlessness of the type, its amorality, its romanticism, and its mental agility. Miller found a second home in Paris, where the Bohemian artist has always been amongst his own. The whole essence of the artistic avant garde in Paris at the turn of the century was in tune with the essence of the tubercular personality. It was sophisticated, hedonistic, stylish, modern and emotionally superficial. The Bohemian is romantic (in the sense that a poet is romantic, that is; inspired by beauty and by the imagination), but he makes no commitments. He looks toward a brave new world where technology has liberated Mankind from work and suffering, and also from outmoded moral restrictions, leaving him free to play, both physically and intellectually. Like Sulphur he may become more cynical as he gets older, and his vision of Paradise seems to be no closer. Then he will use his intellectual resources to attack the status quo, rather than concentrating on building something better.

Style is very important to most Tuberculinums. The national characteristics of the French people suggest a great deal of tubercular influence. After all, it is the French who are famous for enjoying themselves with style. They are very often chic, sophisticated, and rather detached. French films in particular display the tubercular qualities of the nation. The style is usually artistic and amoral, and very often concentrates on the search for individual freedom, as well as highlighting the 'existential dilemma' or sense of futility and meaningless that so often lies beneath the restlessness of Tuberculinum. The French also tend to be individualistic. They do their own thing to a greater extent than most other people, and allow others to do theirs. It is thanks to this highly individualistic tendency that France remained outside of NATO during the Cold War, even though it had nuclear weapons and was a part of Western Europe. Tuberculinum individuals are very much their own person. Like Sulphur and Nux they chart their own course in life, and pay little heed to social expectations. Unlike Sulphur and Nux, they are not born leaders, since they like their freedom too much to take on the responsibility of leadership, and they tend to lack the discipline it requires.

An English writer whose work expresses Tuberculinum's sophisticated modern style very well is Aldous Huxley. The characters of his earlier novels are often very clever, but lack depth. They float amongst a highly intellectual elite, playing games with one another, competing with each other's sophistication, and achieving only very transient satisfaction. In his later novels Huxley was far more spiritual, having embraced the philosophy of mystical traditions. His novel 'Brave New World' can be read as a Tuberculinum's realisation of the emptiness of physical progress when it is divorced from emotional and spiritual satisfaction. The denizens of his future world have all the physical stimulation they could dream of, including drug-induced psychic 'holidays' which last for weeks at a time, but they have lost their soul. Huxley himself sought freedom through the experimental use of hallucinogenic drugs, and his book 'The Gates of Perception' was a kind of manual for seekers of drug-induced mind-expansion. Even in his later years of spiritual quest he sought the short-cut of chemical hallucinogens to broaden his vision, like those Tuberculinum individuals who are too impatient to seek the satisfactions of stillness naturally.

### The Pussycat

The Bohemian has a feline quality, which I have seen very often in Tuberculinum individuals. Like a cat, Tuberculinum is sensual but detached. (The only famous personality I can think of to illustrate this quality who is probably a Tuberculinum is the actor David Niven.) He will abandon himself to sensual ecstasy very easily, having none of the inhibitions of a Natrum or a Kali, but whereas other 'ecstatic types' like Phosphorus and Medorrhinum will lose themselves entirely in the experience, Tuberculinum maintains a certain detachment even in the thralls of ecstasy. Like Nux he is alert and can be on his feet in a moment, rather like a cat who purrs as he is being tickled, and then is off in a flash when he sees a mouse in the corner of his eye. Tuberculinum has a sharp quality that is very similar to that of Nux Vomica. Both are lean, hungry types, who are principally self-serving and have fast reactions, both physically and mentally. The differences are numerous, but the two can be easily mistaken on superficial acquaintance. Nux is focussed, and will stick one-pointedly to his focus until he has achieved his aims, which usually involve the acquisition of power in some way. Tuberculinum is far less constant in his focus, needs to play more, and is far more romantic than Nux. There are many Tuberculinum poets, but few Nux poets. Nevertheless, the two share a mental sharpness and a tendency to physical agility, as well as a detached and relatively self-orientated approach to life.

Like many cats, Tuberculinum people tend to be friendly and yet aloof at the same time. If they find you interesting, (either intellectually or sexually), they will be bright and animated, with a self-assurance that is not easily dented. It can be disconcerting, however, to find how quickly a Tuberculinum's interest can wane, and how suddenly they become indifferent, or at best politely cool. It is easy to get the impression that a Tuberculinum person has taken a dislike to you, when actually he is treating you with the same indifference that he displays towards most other people.

Another feline characteristic of Tuberculinum people is their adaptability. Drop them into almost any situation or surroundings, and they will not only survive, but thrive. Tuberculinum individuals are generally quick-witted, wily and resourceful. This is partly because they have travelled a lot, and been in many different situations, but it is also an innate quality which Tuberculinum shares with the feral cat. Mercurius is also highly adaptable as well as being detached and intellectual. However, Tuberculinum is far more 'grounded'. Whereas Mercurius tends to be 'in his head' a lot, Tuberculinum is more physical, hence his liking for sports, and his good practical ability. He is also less scattered in his focus that Mercurius, and is a little less agile intellectually.

Whilst we are on the theme of 'felinity', it is appropriate to mention Tuberculinum's nonchalance—an appropriately French word. (Many French words are more useful in describing Tuberculinum's character than their English counterparts; words such as 'chic', 'savoir faire', and 'ennui'.) It is seldom that one sees a Tuberculinum person looking ruffled. In the main Tuberculinum does what he wants, and if things don't work out he moves on to something else, without fretting too much. This 'laid back' approach is similar to that seen in Sulphur individuals, and in some Phosphorus and Lycopodiums. Sulphur is often laid back in part because he is oblivious to what is going on around him. This is not the case with Tuberculinum, whose sharp and subtle mind is usually very well connected to his surroundings. His nonchalance is more a result of his intellectual detachment, and also his adaptability. He needn't worry, because he knows that whatever happens he can get by, and in any case, worrying isn't any fun, and is therefore not worth doing. This relaxed attitude appears very attractive to a great many people, and when it is combined with Tuberculinum's wit, and his fun-loving nature, it tends to make Tuberculinum a popular person. Tuberculinum individuals can generally be themselves with strangers, and have none of the nervousness that many people experience at a party where they know few of the other guests. Like Sulphur they can strike up a conversation with anybody, and generally they will enjoy it, as long as it doesn't last too long. Their cosmopolitan outlook makes them interesting to talk to, and if they are talking to the opposite sex, they are likely to ooze a lot of natural charm.

Another constitutional type with a distinctly feline quality is Phosphorus. Tuberculinum and Phosphorus are very closely related, as can be seen by the similarity of their physiques, as well as their physical symptomatology. I have come across many instances where a Tuberculinum individual was mistaken for a Phosphorus, either by homeopaths, or by the individual himself, if he has some knowledge of homeopathy. I remember one such person who worked as a psychotherapist. He led a workshop that I was taking for a week, so I came to know him quite well. The most distinct quality about him was his dynamism. In the workshop he was fired with energy, which he directed towards the group as a whole, and towards any participant whom he was addressing. The workshop was concerned with personal growth, and our leader saw to it that nobody was allowed to sit and hide behind his own personal limitations and fears. He was as gentle with those in pain as he was confronting with those who refused to face their issues directly, and many a time he would shout with frustration and anger at someone who was wasting his time by avoiding being true to themself. I wondered what constitutional type this man was, and I considered Phosphorus, because he had a boyish quality, as well as a great deal of charisma, but it gradually dawned on me that he was too aggressive and too 'hungry' to be a Phosphorus. By hungry I mean restless to experience more, and impatient when he was made to wait. Furthermore, this man did not seek intimacy with people in the way that Phosphorus does. For example, he preferred the dynamic excitement of a group situation to working individually with people. Eventually we got talking about homeopathy, and he said that he thought he was a Phosphorus. I said that I thought otherwise, and he let me take his case, which confirmed that he was a restless, hungry Tuberculinum, with a tendency towards asthma, not a dreamy, innocent Phosphorus. I tend to see Tuberculinum as something of a cross between Phosphorus and Nux Vomica, having something of the lightness and romantic sensitivity of the former, and the sharp, driven quality of the latter.

I once knew another Tuberculinum psychotherapist, who was quite different from the latter. He was much older, being about fifty or so, but he also had that boyish spritely quality that is so common amongst Tuberculinums. He was much more relaxed and sanguine than his younger colleague, having mellowed over the years. He had made for himself a very idyllic existence, in which virtually everything he did was a pleasure. He lived in a beautiful house on a hill overlooking the ocean, close to the town where he worked and ran workshops. He was single, and seemed to have one attractive lady after another staying with him and sharing his bed. At work he was far more patient than his younger colleague, and more interested in working one to one with people. His particular style was the most passive of all the therapists that I have seen. One of his principal techniques was to reflect back to the client whatever they were saying, including their intonation and physical posture. He maintained that all the therapist has to do is be a reflection for the client, and the client will work out the rest. This puts me in mind of the Tuberculinum rebirther who felt that all his clients had to do to overcome their emotional problems was to dissolve them in bliss. Both therapists took a light, 'laid back' approach to their work, which enabled them to avoid much of the pain and 'ugliness' that arises when clients are confronted, and forced to face deeper feelings of sadness and despair. In true Tuberculinum style, this older therapist took a more detached approach, which enabled him to interact with and help a great many people, without 'getting his hands too dirty'. One evening he was talking to a group of participants, and he commented that he had everything he could want in life, and he was still dissatisfied. He said that he was frustrated because he could not find enough time to do all the things he wanted to do. Such is the lot of even the most mature and contented of Tuberculinums.

The above example illustrates Tuberculinum's tendency to use his innate intelligence to enable him to enjoy the sweet life. Naturally there are a great many people of all types who seek an easier, more stimulating lifestyle, but in my experience Tuberculinum succeeds more often than most, since he is so dedicated to the task, is not held back by consideration of family and duty to any great degree, and is generally very enterprising.

### The Tuberculinum Woman

I have said nothing specifically thus far about the Tuberculinum woman, although all that I have said applies. Tuberculinum women are not very common, and are not often seen by homeopaths, partly, I suspect, because Tuberculinum, like Sulphur, tends to be fairly robust physically. Those few Tuberculinum women that I have treated were relatively assertive and masculine. One was a medical doctor, who was far more interested in windsurfing than in medicine, and for this reason had emigrated from England to Australia. She told me that she couldn't wait to finish work most days, so that she could be off windsurfing, or going to one of a constant stream of parties which occupied most of her evenings. She drank heavily, and swore copiously, and had a reputation for being rather curt and unsympathetic with her patients. Despite this, she was of a fairly feminine and attractive appearance, and was very popular with the men. I found her a fun-loving but rather cold person, ironically colder than most of the Tuberculinum men that I have treated, but perhaps had I known her more personally I would have found a warmer side.

Another Tuberculinum woman I treated was also relatively masculine, but appeared much warmer and more personable than the latter case. She was a lesbian, and dressed in a very masculine style, and because of her sporting enthusiasms she had a very muscular body for a woman. Nevertheless, she appeared both friendly and approachable, and during the interview she was somewhat sad when talking of her emotional life, which was rather turbulent at the time. Unlike many homosexuals and also many Tuberculinums, she had a steady partner, who was more feminine than herself, and also more insecure. Like many Tuberculinums she had travelled a great deal, and was still very restless when she stayed for long in one place. She said she had a tremendous amount of physical energy, which 'drove her crazy' if it were not released, hence she did a great deal of sport, including canoeing and mountaineering. Her principal physical complaint was asthma, which was mild and related to hayfever. It settled quite rapidly after a few doses of Tuberculinum 200c, but once again I did not see her for long enough to see what effect a high potency would have on her restlessness.

I have seldom treated a Tuberculinum mother or housewife. They do exist, but they are as rare as hens' teeth. I can imagine nothing more terrifying to the average Tuberculinum woman than being tied down by a brood of children, or more boring than having to stay at home and look after the house and her husband.

### Dissatisfaction, Destructiveness and Hyperactivity

Tuberculinum does not always keep cool and calm. When things are not going his way, he can become not only restless, but also irritable. He will generally keep his cool for a while, and then become more and more tetchy, adopting a cold authoritative manner to voice his complaints. The more annoyed he becomes, the more he will curse. Being a relatively uninhibited type, Tuberculinum swears easily (Kent: 'Cursing'), and I have seen Tuberculinum individuals using 'obscene' language for the pleasure of the 'punch' in it, even when they are not angry.

Tuberculinum has something of a reputation for destructiveness, but I have not seen this born out to any great degree, except in Tuberculinum children. I have never seen a Tuberculinum person really lose his or her temper, but some Tuberculinums do seem to have a lot of aggressive energy, and admit in the case-taking to having a rare but violent temper.

It is in children that the Tuberculinum temper seems to be most common and most destructive. Tuberculinum children are very often hyperactive. Some of these children are allergic to one or two foods or additives in food, and will settle when these are withdrawn, but many are hyperactive irrespective of their diet. I have the impression that the hyperactivity of Tuberculinum children is more focussed than that of Natrum and especially Stramonium hyperactive children. By that I mean that the child is always on the go, but knows what he is doing. He may run around all day playing and pestering his parents, and in the consulting room his excessive physical energy may cause him to fidget and tap his feet, but at least his activity is purposeful, in contrast to the apparently aimless activities of some hyperactive children.

Not all Tuberculinum children are hyperactive, but whether they are or not, they are frequently wilful children, who test their parents' patience to the limit by insisting upon their own way, and by throwing a tantrum if their will is denied. A Tuberculinum child's tantrum can be very violent, and may include smashing of toys or later of crockery, but it is seldom as violent as that of the Stramonium child, who will deliberately harm any nearby person with his teeth, his nails or an implement. I have come across Tuberculinum children who went through a stage of swearing obscenities at their parents, but I have not seen this as a lasting feature of the personality. Since Tuberculinum is so intent upon being free to do as he wishes, it is not surprising to find that aggression is quite common in Tuberculinum children, who are subject to restrictions like any other child.

The Tuberculinum child is generally bright intellectually, but he is easily bored at school, and he may make a nuisance of himself by distracting other children in the classroom. He is likely to love playing vigourous games, unless he is one of the highly intellectual Tuberculinums, and he will tend to do what he wants much of the time, and resist pressure do what he finds boring, much like the Sulphur child.

### *Physical Appearance*

Tuberculinum tends to resemble Phosphorus physically, but is more wiry and muscular, and not so graceful or ethereal in appearance. The physique is generally thin and compact, and the complexion is usually, but not always, fair. Freckles are very commonly seen on the face and body. The Tuberculinum face is generally narrower than that of Phosphorus, and the eyes are not so large, though the lashes tend to be long like those of Phosphorus. The face is usually angular, and often has a 'lean' look to it. The hair is generally straight and quite fine, and the lips are usually thin, but not absent.

The condition of Pectus Excavatum or sunken breast-bone is quite common.

# Veratrum Album

*Keynote:* Dogmatism

Veratrum is a rare constitutional type, one of the handful of remedies which correspond to people who live their lives on the verge of insanity. It is closely related to Stramonium and Syphilinum, but has its own very unique characteristics.

Most homeopathic consultations with Veratrum individuals involve those who are relatively stable mentally. Nevertheless, even during stable periods the Veratrum individual appears somewhat odd from the outset, as do many stable Anacardium patients. The most obvious abnormality initially is often the speech itself. Veratrum is a very rigid type psychologically, and this is reflected in his voice. One Veratrum patient spoke inappropriately loudly throughout the interview, whilst another spoke in a tense staccato fashion, as if he were a robot. Kali Carbonicum often speaks a little stiffly, but he is not nearly as stiff in either thinking or in speech as Veratrum, who is probably the most rigid of all types mentally. The next unusual feature that becomes apparent is the pushy, overconfident manner in which the patient speaks. This is of an order altogether more inappropriate than that seen in other confident types such as Nux and Sulphur, since the Veratrum personality is mentally off-balance, and does not interpret reality in a normal fashion.

Those Veratrum patients who seek help for physical complaints may appear only a little stiff and loud, until one investigates the mental picture. The social etiquette that we take for granted is often poorly mastered by Veratrum, who is liable to laugh a little too loud, or to launch into a description of his symptoms immediately upon sitting down, without waiting for the homeopath to address him (Kent: 'Rudeness'). When one arrives at a consideration of the mental picture, the most striking characteristic that is revealed is usually the arrogant way in which Veratrum insists upon his own way, and the dogmatism with which he expresses his opinions. Two Veratrum patients have said to me that other people have called them 'a little Hitler', and have admitted that they are very bossy people. One was always arguing with his flatmates (Kent: 'Quarrelsome'), because he thought their music was too loud, they were too untidy, or he didn't like the friends that they brought home. He knew that he was somewhat dictatorial, but he said so with a smile, and not the slightest sign of regret. Another Veratrum patient told me how he had been sacked from his job as an accountant as a result of his 'attitude'.

He showed me a pile of correspondence between himself, his old boss, and their respective solicitors, which was highly instructive of his character. His old boss, a bank manager, had written that my patient was 'didactic, intolerant and quite unable to maintain reasonable relations with his colleagues'. This was not the only reason he had lost his job. He had also suffered episodes of mania, during which times he would not care what figures he put on the ledger sheet. Although there were clearly ample grounds for his dismissal, he kept up a relentless legal battle to be reinstated, which must have cost him a fortune in legal fees, and which was ultimately unsuccessful. All this because he was sure that he was in the right, irrespective of the evidence. As he told me about this affair, he became more and more incensed and I had to drag him away from the subject to calm him down (Kent: 'Offended easily'). His principal complaint was headaches, and these cleared rapidly after a dose of Veratrum 10M, but he was not interested in coming back for follow-ups, so I cannot say to what extent the remedy affected his overall personality.

Veratrum's know-all attitude naturally makes him rather difficult to live with or be around. One of my Veratrum patients was married, and he told me that his wife wished he was less bossy. I asked him in what way he was bossy, and he told me that he had to have his own way in almost every matter. For example, he had to choose the colour to paint his living-room, and he would not listen to his wife's opinion. He also told me that he reported neighbours quite regularly who parked illegally in the street (even though they were not obstructing his drive), and he often complained to the authorities if he found people smoking in non-smoking public areas.

The way in which the Veratrum patient interacts with the homeopath is often a good example of his arrogance. One patient asked me a great many questions about the remedies and how they worked, and then responded with a cynicism that bordered on frank disbelief (Kent: 'Haughty'). I found that the only way that I could avoid this cross-examination and get on with the interview was to be very firm in the way I expressed myself. This seemed to surprise him and make him more cooperative.

### Manic Depressive Psychosis and Religiosity

Veratrum people are often prone to manic-depressive psychosis, but the manic phase is generally more prominent than the depression. The accountant who lost his job described all the typical features of mania when describing his behaviour during a manic episode. At these times he was extremely restless (Kent: 'Propensity to be aimlessly busy'), spent too much money, propositioned strangers sexually (Kent: 'mania-erotic'), and would not eat for days (Kent: 'Refuses to eat'). Veratrum is a very restless type at the best of times. Even outside of manic episodes he is liable to have some difficulty sitting still for long. One patient told me that he often paced up and down at home in the evening, and when this pacing became more frantic his wife knew he was heading for another manic attack (Kent: 'Restlessness-anxious').

Following manic phases Veratrum may enter into a depressive phase, which is characterised by brooding despair. The depressed Veratrum will sit silently for hours thinking about how wretched he feels, and imagining that he will never feel any better (Kent: 'Despair of his recovery'). At these times he is liable to be more anxious than usual, especially when alone, and he may contemplate suicide as a way out of his misery.

One very characteristic feature of the Veratrum personality is a tendency towards religious fanaticism. Of the three Veratrum patients that I have treated in recent years, one was not religious, one said that he used to be obsessed by religion, and the third was fanatical about his religion. Usually such religious fanaticism involves the threat of damnation and the possibility of redemption. Veratrum may be obsessed with the thought that he is damned (Kent: 'Anxiety about salvation'), and try hard to be pious and make amends for his sins, (Kent: 'Praying'—black type), or he may adopt an evangelist's role and try to convince others that they must repent and turn to the Lord (Kent: 'Exhorts to repent, preaches'). In a manic phase this religiosity may be fuelled, and Veratrum may stand on street corners and preach excitedly at passers by. He may at these times believe that he has been chosen by Christ to save the multitudes, or even that he is himself Christ (Kent: 'Exalted state of religious frenzy'). This is similar to the religiosity of Platina women, but here the delusions of grandeur are more prominent than the preaching.

The materia medicas are full of references to Veratrum's potential for violence (Kent: 'Abusive', 'Biting', 'Delirium—raging'). Some of my Veratrum patients have admitted to a violent temper, but it was seldom a prominent feature of the history they gave of themselves. I suspect that one would have to be there at the time, or talk to witnesses, to assess the extent of the Veratrum temper. Certainly Veratrum is dogmatic, aggressive and out of his mind at times, and it is easy to see how these attributes could lead to violence, especially during manic episodes. I believe that Adolf Hitler was probably a Veratrum. (The alternative is Stramonium.) Not only was he dogmatic, and had to have his own way in all things, he was also close to insanity, and felt that he had an almost divine mission to produce and lead a super-race. He was deeply involved with occult traditions, which he felt substantiated his claim to power over the earth, and he used a great deal of religious imagery in his speeches.

### Fear and Obsession

Like other syphilitic types, Veratrum can be prone to obsessive/compulsive disorders. The more unhealthy the syphilitic type mentally, the more likely these are to occur. Thus Arsenicum and Kali Carbonicum often exhibit a mild degree of obsession, whilst Syphilinum, Veratrum and Hyocyamus are often markedly obsessive. One of my Veratrum patients was obsessive about punctuality. He was not only punctual himself, and extremely indignant when others were late, but also lived his life to a highly regimented regime, closing the curtains at exactly the same time each evening, and reading the paper for exactly half an hour after supper. Other Veratrums are generally pedantic about every little detail, whether it be the number of raisins in their bowl of cereal, or the way their wife arranges her hair. Whereas other obsessive types feel anxiety when their rigid routines are broken, Veratrum is more likely to feel irritable, or to lose his temper.

The fears that I have seen in my Veratrum patients were not prominent parts of the history from their point of view. Nevertheless, I have come across an irrational fear of death in Veratrums, and also a degree of paranoia, as illustrated by the Veratrum accountant who felt he had been unfairly dismissed.

I have not seen a female Veratrum patient, although Kent describes its usefulness in hysterical or insane women with rather intense premenstrual symptoms ('Veratrum is a remedy that would keep many women out of the insane asylum, especially those with uterine troubles').

### *Physical Appearance*
Veratrum tends to have a very angular face, in keeping with his rigid mentality. The nose is usually strong and straight, a reflection of determination, and the eyes tend to look intense or manic. The body is usually taut and wiry. A good example of a Veratrum appearance is that of David Koresh, the late fanatical preacher who died along with many of his followers in Waco, Texas when he ordered them to set fire to the compound.

# *Appendix*

An Elemental Analysis of Constitutional Types

The four elements—Earth, Air, Fire and Water, have for thousands of years been used by mankind to represent the different qualities that make up his constitution, and that constitute the material world. They correspond to the four humours known to the physician in the Middle Ages—Phlegmatic, Sanguine, Choleric and Melancholic.

Several systems of psychological analysis have used this fourfold division to help describe the differences between different personality types. Carl Jung was the first to my knowledge to use the four elements in this way, and his work on the four resulting character types has been developed further in the Minnesota Multiple Personality Inventory, which is in popular use today.

Jung made his analysis sound more scientific by using functional terms to describe the four types. Thus the Earth type is described as the Sensation-Oriented type, the Air type as the Intellectual, the Fire type as the Intuitive or Inspirational type and the Water type as the Emotional type. His descriptions of these four types correspond quite closely to the medieval understanding of the four humours, and also to psychological astrology.

Jung further refined his analysis by saying that each person has a dominant function and an inferior function. Thus for predominantly emotional people the Water element is dominant, but one of the other three elements is least developed. I have used my knowledge of Jung's system to analyse the personalities of the constitutional types. I believe that this rather novel approach has value in helping to illustrate the basic nature of each remedy type, and how it differs from other types. For example, when we compare Phophorus and Pulsatilla, two remedy types that are often confused by inexperienced homeopaths, we see that both have Water or emotion as the dominant way of relating to the world, but in Phosphorus the least developed element is Earth, leading to 'unboundedness' and lack of grounding, whereas in Pulsatilla the least developed element is Air or intellect, resulting in a lack of objectivity and intellectual clarity.

The following analysis is in no sense definitive, but I believe that it is accurate at least with regard to the most and least developed elements for the majority of constitutional types.

Let us first consider the qualities of each elemental function in more depth, before considering the remedies in turn.

## *Earth*

This element relates to the physical senses. Earthy people are primarily sensation orientated. Their view of the world is based on sense perceptions, and this makes them practical and matter of fact. If they cannot see or touch something, it does not exist for them. Earthy people are the most practical people, and also have the most 'common sense'. Their focus is on the physical reality in front of them, not in their emotions, or off somewhere in the imagination. They are practical and reliable, cautious, stubborn and often inflexible. They are also often hedonistic, since they live so much through their senses. Physically, the Earth element is associated with the skeleton, with connective (structural) tissues, and with the digestive tract, which assimilates the 'building bricks' of the physical body from the food it eats. As we shall see, constitutional types which are predominantly Earthy tend to have problems with these physical elements.

| Positive | Negative | Lack of Earth |
|---|---|---|
| realistic | materialistic | unrealistic |
| practical | narrow-minded | impractical |
| reliable | inflexible | impulsive |
| intuitive connection | | |
| with the earth | | |

## *Air*

Air represents the mental or intellectual faculty. Airy people live in their heads, thinking about everything, rather than feeling with their emotions and their senses. They have a tendency to rationalise, and to discriminate and analyse. Airy people can stand back and see the broader picture, and are good at working with abstract concepts. The Air element tends to produce a detached, 'laid-back' approach to life, and a youthful physical appearance. Physically it is associated with the lungs and respiratory tract, the nervous system (especially with vision), and also the stomach and intestines (which are hollow and filled with air to some extent).

| Positive | Negative | Lack of Air |
|---|---|---|
| intellectual | over-analytical | fuzzy thinking |
| objective | insensitive | subjective |
| detached | aloof | attachment |
| broadminded | | |

## *Fire*

This is the element of personal magnetism, faith, courage and inspiration. It is also the element of egotism, desire and anger. Fiery people are optimistic, proud, and often egotistic and selfish. Like Air, Fire has an intellectual aspect, but whereas the Airy intellect is primarily analytical, the Fiery intellect is inspired and intuitive as well. Fire provides the creative insight, which then requires Air to analyse the details, and Earth to put them into practice. Physically, Fire corresponds with the heart and circulatory system, to muscle and metabolism, to the liver and gall-bladder, and to the nervous system (along with air).

| Positive | Negative | Lack of Fire |
|----------|----------|--------------|
| confidence | arrogance | timidity |
| independence | selfishness | lack of self-worth |
| inspiration | delusions of grandeur | apathy |
| assertive | angry | passive |

## Water

This is the emotional element. Watery people have strong emotions. They are generally sensitive and nurturing, and also intuitive.

| Positive | Negative | Lack of Water |
|----------|----------|---------------|
| sensitive | oversensitive | insensitive |
| intuitive | subjective | superficial |
| nurturing | dependent | cold |

Let us now consider the constitutional types elementally, grouping them according to their dominant function.

## The Earthy Types

| Remedy | BARYTA | CALC | GRAPH | SILICA | NUX | ARS-ALB | KALI-CARB |
|--------|--------|------|-------|--------|-----|---------|-----------|
| dominant | Earth | Earth | Earth | Earth | Earth | Earth | Earth |
| second | Water | Water | Water | Air | Fire | Fire | Air |
| third | Air | Air | Air | Water | Air | Air | Fire |
| inferior | Fire | Fire | Fire | Fire | Water | Water | Water |

According to the above classification, the Earthy types divide into three groups when the second most developed element is considered. (Most people are relatively strong in at least two functions.)

Calcarea, Baryta and Graphites all have Water or emotion as the second function. Each of these is a down to earth type, without pretensions, and each has a certain simplicity about them. This simplicity is due to a combination of the straightforwardness of the Earth element, combined with the innocence of the Water element. Furthermore, each of these types tends to be rather emotional and sensitive when compared to the other Earthy types. Graphites is the most emotional of the three, and can be said to be equally emotional and 'physical'.

The chart shows that these three types also share the same inferior function—Fire. Consequently, each of these types tends to be rather fearful. In the cases of Baryta and Graphites this fear is expressed as timidity, whilst in the case of Calcarea it is seen as a reluctance to reach one's full capacity in life.

The second group, comprising Arsenicum Album and Nux Vomica, have Fire as the second strongest element. Thse are very different types from the first group. Since they are Earthy types, they are both practical kinds of people, and tend to call a spade a spade. Furthermore, they both tend to focus on material realities. Nux does this by building up a power-base in the world, whilst Arsenicum does this by attending to physical security and physical comforts, as well as by teaching others practical knowledge.

It is the Fire element that marks these two types apart from the other Earthy types. It gives them a determined, one-pointed will which enables them to achieve a great deal in the world. It also gives them an ambitious streak (especially Nux), and a tendency to become angry when their will is obstructed. Nobody is better at getting things done than these two types. They can enter into an organisation and streamline it from top to bottom before anyone knows what is happening, and Nux in particular is liable to have plenty of creative ideas for further projects.

The combination of sensual Earth and hungry Fire also tends to produce hedonistic appetites, and this is especially true of Nux Vomica.

Both of these fiery Earthy types have water as the least developed element. The result is that they can both be insensitive, rude, or downright cruel. They have little time for emotional interaction, finding it either boring or perplexing.

The third group of Earthy types comprises Silica and Kali Carbonicum. (Kali Bichromium probably belongs with the first group of watery Earth types.) Both of these are relatively intellectual types, having Air as the second element. In fact both could be said to be equally Airy and Earthy, since the intellect and the down to earth aspect are both very strong. Silica is earthy in the sense that a sculptor or a painter is earthy—having a natural aesthetic feel for physical form. She also has the stubborness that is seen in many earthy types. Her intellect is subtle and discriminating, in comparison to that of Kali Carbonicum, which is analytical but prosaic. Kali is earthy in the sense that he is sceptical, and can only recognise what is there in physical terms in front of him. His intellect is highly analytical, but it is imprisoned in an earthly straight-jacket, which prevents him from appreciating anything poetical or abstract.

Silica's least developed element is Fire, resulting in timidity and hesitancy. Kali's least developed element is Water. He is the driest of all constitutional types, the least emotional of them all.

## The Airy Types

| Remedy | ARG NIT | MEDOR | MERC | LYCOPOD | TUB. BOV. | PHOS-AC |
|---|---|---|---|---|---|---|
| dominant | Air | Air | Air | Air | Air | Air |
| second | Fire | Fire | Fire | Earth | Earth | Water |
| third | Water | Water | Water | Water | Fire | Earth |
| inferior | Earth | Earth | Earth | Fire | Water | Fire |

When we consider the Airy types, we can again separate them into three groups according to the second strongest element. Argentum, Medorrhinum and Mercurius are relatively fiery types. Argentum is very warm-blooded, and generally buoyant and optimistic unless adverse circumstances generate fear. The combination of Air and Fire is an unstable (combustable) one, and all these types have a tendency towards mental instability. Argentum's mind is very quick, as these are the quickest of the elements, and his mental agility can easily be upset, resulting in erratic thinking. This is compounded by the weakness of the fourth element Earth, which is needed to 'ground' or stabilise an individual. Lacking the common-sense of the Earth element, Argentum is prone to 'foolish' impulses, as well as unrealistic fears. Exactly the same can be said of Mercurius.

Medorrhinum is interesting because all four elements are usually well developed. Medorrhinum generally has a sound intellect, is assertive and relatively optimistic, as well as being intuitive and imaginative. Furthermore, Medorrhinum is generally relatively 'deep' emotionally.

The second group comprises Lycopodium and Tuberculinum, who have Earth as the second element. These are the most stable of the Airy types. They are seldom particularly innovative like Sulphur or Argentum, but they can use their sharp and steady intellect to analyse and dissect information in a detached way, being relatively free from the influence of both emotions and passion.

The Earth element also results in a tendency towards materialistic thinking in Lycopodium, and a hedonistic streak in Tuberculinum. Unlike the former, Tuberculinum has a relatively strong dose of Fire as well, resulting in both self-confidence and a strong desire-nature. Tuberculinum is far more 'hungry' for experience than Lycopodium, who shares Kali Carbonicum's 'dryness' to some extent (since both types have Air and Earth as the dominant elements, and Water as the least developed).

Lycopodium lacks fire, leading to the lack of faith in himself that is so characteristic of the type. Tuberculinum lacks water, and hence is generally emotionally detached, and often emotionally insensitive. (Lycopodium's emotional sensitivity is also often rather poorly developed as well, a case of a weak third element). The reactive pride that we see in some Lycopodium individuals is an example of the principle described by Carl Jung, that the undeveloped element is often expressed in a negative or immature fashion.

Phosphoric Acid is rather difficult to analyse from an elemental point of view. I have put Air as the dominant element, since Phosphoric Acid individuals are so detached. Indeed they feel as if they are living in a vacuum, devoid of all feeling. The placing of the second and third elements is especially difficult. It can be argued that as Phosphoric Acid is so devoid of feeling, Water should be the least developed element, yet these individuals do feel a lot of fear at times, and I believe this is due to a lack of Fire or self-confidence. Furthermore, they feel as if they have no personality and no motivation, a case of deficient (fiery) ego.

## *The Fiery Types*

| Remedy | SULPHUR | VERAT | CAUST | LACHES | HYOS | PLATINA | BELLA |
|---|---|---|---|---|---|---|---|
| dominant | Fire | Fire | Fire | Fire | Fire | Fire | Fire |
| second | Air/Earth | Earth | Air | Water | Water | Air | Earth |
| third | Earth/Air | Air | Water | Air | Air | Water | Water |
| inferior | Fire | Water | Earth | Earth | Earth | Earth | Air |

All the fiery types are prone to inspiration of one kind or another. Sulphur is the most fiery of all types, exibiting every aspect of the fiery element. He is intellectually inspired in most cases, passionate, generous, courageous, determined, and also often selfish, obsessed with self-gratification, and prone to rage. Sulphur's tend to divide into Airy Sulphurs and Earthy Sulphurs, the former being the most spiritual and intellectual, the latter the most coarse, and also the most practical. The combination of Air and Fire is inspired but often 'ungrounded' and impractical, hence the dreaminess of the Airy Sulphur. Sulphur's least developed element is water, a reflection of the emotional insensitivity and immaturity that we often see in the type.

Veratrum is often inspired in a manic fashion with a saviour complex. He feels chosen to save the world, usually in a religious sense, and may stand in the street and preach to the wind. He is extremely willful (Fire and Earth), and very prone to anger. He is also often very selfish. Veratrum can be surprisingly practical for one close to insanity (I have known a Veratrum farmer who managed a large farm successfully with very little help, although he was both paranoid and a drug addict at the time), a reflection of the strong Earth element. This combination of Earth and Fire is also seen in Arsenicum, a very closely related type. Both are obsessive, especially about material things, and both are emotionally insensitive, having Water as the inferior element.

Causticum is one of the most inspired of the Fiery types, at least in the extovert cases. His inspiration is usually one of passionate championing of individual rights, and service to the needy. It may take an overtly political turn, in the form of revolutionary zeal. Most Causticums are intellectuals, and hence can back their idealism with cogent reasoning. They are also often intuitive, a function of the Fire element. Most Causticum individuals are well rounded, in that they have at least three well developed functions, and often all four. Thus they are often emotionally sensitive (and weep in the presence of another's suffering), and can be very practical too. The more introverted Causticum is generally very analytical, and less inspired, hence we could say that the Fire and Air are reversed, with the latter dominating.

Lachesis is often inspired artistically. He is also fiery in his sexual and other sensual appetites, hence his attraction to alcohol and other stimulants (like Sulphur and Medorrhinum). Unlike most Fiery types, Lachesis tends to be sensitive emotionally, and the combination of Water and Fire is responsible for Lachesis' highly intuitive nature. It is an unstable combination, which results in moodiness and powerful emotions, as can be seen in Ignatia and Hyoscyamus individuals as well. Lachesis is usually sharp intellectually, and even the Earth element is often well developed. Some Lachesis individuals are quite eccentric, and their minds are flighty and inreliable. This is an example of a weak Earth element.

Hyoscyamus is like Lachesis exaggerated. The temper and the sexual obsession are greater, as are the religiosity and the jealousy. The emotions are more volatile, and the intellect is less stable. We could say that only the first two elements are developed, and the lack of Air and Earth results in a far more unstable individual than Lachesis.

Platina is the most proud of all the constitutional types, and is prone to extreme delusions of grandeur, a case of extreme Fire. The sexual desire is also extreme in most cases, and anger is experienced in the absence of emotional sensitivity, leading to cruelty and even murder. The intellect is usually quite strong in most cases, and this adds to the aloof impression that Platina gives. The lack of Earth results in a highly unstable individual who is prone to hallucinations and delusions.

Belladonna is as fiery as Sulphur, but less stable. The strong Earth element gives physical strength (like Nux, also Fire and Earth), as well as stubborness. The lack of Air results in passion being untempered by objective reason, hence the rashness and obsessiveness of Belladonna.

## The Watery Types

| Remedy | NAT.M | AURUM | THUJ | CHINA | PHOS | NAT.C | PULS | SEPIA | IGNAT |
|--------|-------|-------|------|-------|------|-------|------|-------|-------|
| dominant | Water | Water | Water | Water | Water | Water | Water | Water | Water |
| second | Air | Air | Earth | Fire | Air | Earth | Earth | Earth | Fire |
| third | Earth | Earth | Air | Air | Fire | Air | Fire | Fire | Air |
| inferior | Fire | Fire | Fire | Earth | Earth | Fire | Air | Air | Earth |

All of these types are predominantly emotional people. The emotions are strong, and relatively deep, except in the case of Phosphorus, where they are strong but superficial in most cases.

Natrum Muriaticum is a very emotional type, but in many cases the emotion is suppressed, and a detached front is presented to the world. In other words, the Air element is developed to mask the emotion. Natrums are often highly analytical, but they are always sensitive underneath. The degree of Fire and Earth is variable in Natrum. Often all four elements are quite developed, prodicing an individual who is both practical and relatively confident. Fire is most likely to be underdeveloped, as can be seen by the lack of self-esteem that is so common in Natrum individuals. As with Lycopodium, this sometimes gives rise to compensatory pride.

Aurum is very similar to Natrum, but more suppressed emotionally. The elemental configuration is the same. Because the emotions are more suppressed, they erupt with more force when they surface, giving rise to extremes of rage and despair. These two types share almost all of their typical psychodynamics, with differences in degree rather than kind.

Thuja is another sensitive, emotional type who usually has a strong intellect. The men tend to be repressed emotionally, but the women are not. The elemental make-up is similar to the preceding types, with lack of Fire expressed as timidity and lack of self-esteem, in particular a sense of being 'dirty' in some way. Thuja's psychic tendencies can be seen as an example of unrestrained Water. The strong Earth element is expressed as sensuality and an intuitive connection with nature.

Phosphorus has a unique elemental make-up. The emotional sensitivity of Water is very evident, though the order of the next two elements, Fire and Air is not so obvious. Phosphorus is a light, 'Airy' type, not because he is analytical, but because he is 'laid back' and playful. He is also often inspired and visionary, hence Fire is also strong. Only Earth is clearly deficient, which is why Phosphorus is so flighty and often 'flaky'.

China is similar to Phosphorus, having a mystical, inspirational nature. However, China is more of a visionary than Phosphorus, hence the Fire element is stronger. She is also even more 'ungrounded' than Phosphorus.

Natrum Carbonicum and Pulsatilla both have a lot of Earth element, but it is expressed very differently. Natrum Carbonicum is down to Earth, sensible and cautious, but also somewhat emotional and fearful. Pulsatilla is very emotional, and the Earth element is expressed and sensuality and also in the practical arts. Natrum Carbonicum lacks Fire, being rather timid and unadventurous, whereas Pulsatilla lacks Air, and hence has very little objectivity.

Sepia is also predominantly Water and Earth. She is an emotional person, who is generally sensible and grounded in her body, which she has an intuitive connection with, hence her love of dancing and yoga. She also has an intuitive connection with the earth. Some Sepias are also quite Fiery.

Ignatia is highly emotional and often volatile, a combination of Water and Fire. The Fire element is seen as a sharp intuitive intellect, as well as in a passionate nature. Ignatia tends to have a highly analytical mind (Air element also strong) which is often inspired by spiritual or artistic impulses coming from the realms of Fire and Water.

I have not included Staphysagria in the main tables, because it seems to have a more complicated elemental configuration. This is partly because there are four different sub-types of Staphysagria, and partly because the anger of Staphysagria is often powerful but very suppressed, and hence the Fire element can be judged as either strong or weak. The following table is only an attempt at analysing the Staphysagria sub-types.

| Staphysagia | SWEET | WILD | SUBDUED | SMOOTH | HIPPY |
|---|---|---|---|---|---|
| dominant | Air | Fire | Air | Air | Air |
| second | Water | Water | Earth | Water | Water |
| third | Earth | Earth | Fire | Fire | Fire |
| inferior | Fire | Air | Water | Earth | Earth |

The Sweet Staphysagria is a very mild person, who is easily confused with Lycopodium. The passions are not strong, but she is sensitive, and usually has a fine intellect, hence Water and Air predominate. Her anger or Fire is so suppressed that she is very passive and unnassertive.

The Wild Staphysagria is passionate and out of control much of the time, since the suppressed anger is close to the surface. He is usually an adventurer, and can be a very practical person, hence the Earth element seems to be well developed. His greatest weakness is a lack of objectivity, which results in him getting into all kinds of trouble, and interpreting events from a very personal point of view.

The Subdued Staphysagria is a dry withdrawn person, who is hiding from his anger. He usually has a keen intellect, and sound practical skills, and is emotionally guarded.

The Smooth Staphysagria has a light Airy social persona, and comes across usually as light and intelligent (like Lycopodium). However, he is more emotionally sensitive than Lycopodium.

The fifth Staphysagria type is the Hippy drop-out who is usually addicted to drugs. He appears weak and passive, and has very little individuality. He is generally very out of touch with his emotions, and is quite impractical. Even his intellect is clouded much of the time. He is thus an Airy type with all four elements relatively underdeveloped, and he generally has a difficult passage through life.

I have also omitted from the main tables some of the rarer psychologically unstable types, again for the sake of clarity. They are difficult to analyse elementally, but I shall make an attempt below:

| Remedy | ALUMINA | ANACARDIUM | STRAMONIUM | SYPHILINUM |
|---|---|---|---|---|
| dominant | Water | Fire | Fire | Earth |
| second | Air | Air | Air | Air |
| third | Earth | Water | Water | Water |
| inferior | Fire | Earth | Earth | Fire |

Alumina is prone to extremes of emotion, hence can be said to be a Watery type. The intellect is strong until pathology intervenes, and Alumina is prone to feelings of separation and detachment from other people, a reflection of the Air element. Fire is lacking, resulting in fearfulness and Alumina's characteristic lack of a sense of self.

Anacardium and Stramonium are similar types. Both are volatile, with a propensity for violent eruptions of rage, reflecting a strong Fire element. During calm periods, these types can have an unnaturally detached attitude that is characteristic of many of the more abnormal constitutional types, reflecting the strength of the Air element and the releative weakness of Water. The lack of Earth is seen in the tendency towards delusions and hallucinations.

Syphilinum is not easy to classify elementally. Most Syphilinum people are quiet and down to Earth, and often obsessively orderly, reflecting the dominant Earth element. They also have a relatively strong intellect, hence Air is strong, and a lack of self-confidence, suggesting that Fire is weak. The fascination with death can be understood to be a combination of cold detached Air (death is the ultimate in detachment) and a lack of vibrant Fire.

# Index

# Index of Remedies

417

# About the Author

Philip Bailey trained as a medical doctor at Westminster Hospital Medical School. He studied homeopathy at The Royal London Homeopathic Hospital, and with Greek homeopath George Vithoulkas. He spent three months at Esalen Intitute studying gestalt therapy, and has had personal experience of Jungian, Primal and breathwork therapies. Dr. Bailey works in Perth, Australia as a medical doctor and homeopath, and lectures frequently on homeopathy.